Mentalizing

in Clinical Practice

Mentalizing

in Clinical Practice

Jon G. Allen, Ph.D.

Helen Malsin Palley Chair in Mental Health Research and Professor of Psychiatry, Menninger Department of Psychiatry and Behavioral Sciences, Baylor College of Medicine, Houston, Texas

Peter Fonagy, Ph.D., FBA

Freud Memorial Professor of Psychoanalysis and Director of the Sub-Department of Clinical Health Psychology, University College London; Chief Executive of the Anna Freud Centre, London, England

Anthony W. Bateman, M.A., FRCPsych

Consultant Psychiatrist in Psychotherapy, Halliwick Unit, St. Ann's Hospital, Barnet, Enfield, England, and Haringey Mental Health Trust

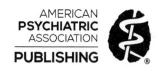

AMERICAN
PSYCHIATRIC
ASSOCIATION
PUBLISHING

Note: The authors have worked to ensure that all information in this book is accurate at the time of publication and consistent with general psychiatric and medical standards. As medical research and practice continue to advance, however, therapeutic standards may change. Moreover, specific situations may require a specific therapeutic response not included in this book. For these reasons and because human and mechanical errors sometimes occur, we recommend that readers follow the advice of physicians directly involved in their care or the care of a member of their family.

Books published by American Psychiatric Association Publishing represent the findings, conclusions, and views of the individual authors and do not necessarily represent the policies and opinions of American Psychiatric Association Publishing or the American Psychiatric Association.

If you wish to buy 50 or more copies of the same title, please go to www.appi.org/specialdiscounts for more information.

Copyright © 2008 American Psychiatric Publishing, Inc.
ALL RIGHTS RESERVED

Manufactured in the United States of America on acid-free paper
25 24 23 22   8 7 6 5
First Edition

Typeset in Adobe's Palatino and Kabel

American Psychiatric Association Publishing
800 Maine Avenue SW
Suite 900
Washington, DC 20024-2812
www.appi.org

Library of Congress Cataloging-in-Publication Data
Allen, Jon G.
  Mentalizing in clinical practice / Jon G. Allen, Peter Fonagy, Anthony W. Bateman. — 1st ed.
      p. ; cm.
  Includes bibliographical references and index.
  ISBN 978-1-58562-306-8 (alk. paper)
  1. Psychotherapy. 2. Mental healing. 3. Self-perception. I. Fonagy, Peter, 1952- II. Bateman, Anthony. III. Title.
  [DNLM: 1. Awareness. 2. Psychotherapy—methods. 3. Psychoanalytic Theory. 4. Social Behavior. 5. Social Perception. WM 420 A427m 2008]

  RC480.5.A454 2008
  616.89'14—dc22

                                                    2007044458

British Library Cataloguing in Publication Data
A CIP record is available from the British Library.

Contents

PART I
Understanding Mentalizing

PART II
Practicing Mentalizing

About the Authors

Jon G. Allen, Ph.D., holds the positions of Helen Malsin Palley Chair in Mental Health Research and Professor of Psychiatry in the Menninger Department of Psychiatry and Behavioral Sciences at the Baylor College of Medicine, and Senior Staff Psychologist in The Menninger Clinic, Houston, Texas. He conducts psychotherapy, diagnostic consultations, psychoeducational programs, and research, specializing in trauma-related disorders and depression. He is past editor of the *Bulletin of the Menninger Clinic*, associate editor of the *Journal of Trauma and Dissociation*, and a member of the editorial board of *Psychiatry*; he also serves as a reviewer for several professional journals and book publishers. He has authored and co-authored numerous professional articles and book chapters on trauma-related problems, depression, psychotherapy, hospital treatment, the therapeutic alliance, psychological testing, neuropsychology, and emotion. Previous books he has authored, co-authored, or co-edited include *Traumatic Relationships and Serious Mental Disorders; Coping With Trauma: Hope Through Understanding; Coping With Depression: From Catch-22 to Hope; Diagnosis and Treatment of Dissociative Disorders* (with William Smith); *Borderline Personality Disorder: Tailoring the Treatment to the Patient* (with Leonard Horwitz, Glen Gabbard, and colleagues); *Restoring Hope and Trust: An Illustrated Guide to Trauma* (with Lisa Lewis and Kay Kelly); and the *Handbook of Mentalization-Based Treatment* (with Peter Fonagy).

Peter Fonagy, Ph.D., FBA, is Freud Memorial Professor of Psychoanalysis and Director of the Sub-Department of Clinical Health Psychology at University College London; Chief Executive of the Anna Freud Centre,

London; and Consultant to the Child and Family Program at the Menninger Department of Psychiatry and Behavioral Sciences at the Baylor College of Medicine. He is Chair of the Postgraduate Education Committee of the International Psychoanalytic Association and a Fellow of the British Academy. He is a clinical psychologist and a training and supervising analyst in the British Psycho-Analytical Society in child and adult analysis. His work integrates empirical research with psychoanalytic theory, and his clinical interests center around borderline psychopathology, violence, and early attachment relationships. He has published over 300 chapters and articles and has authored or edited several books. His most recent books include *Psychoanalytic Theories: Perspectives From Developmental Psychopathology* (with Mary Target); *What Works for Whom? A Critical Review of Psychotherapy Research* (with Anthony Roth); *Psychotherapy for Borderline Personality Disorder: Mentalization-Based Treatment* (with Anthony Bateman); *Mentalization-Based Treatment for Borderline Personality Disorder: A Practical Guide* (also with Anthony Bateman); *Reaching the Hard to Reach: Evidence-Based Funding Priorities for Intervention and Research* (with Geoffrey Baruch and David Robins); and *Handbook of Mentalization-Based Treatment* (with Jon Allen).

Anthony W. Bateman, M.A., FRCPsych, is Consultant Psychiatrist in Psychotherapy, Halliwick Unit, St. Ann's Hospital, Barnet, Enfield, and Haringey Mental Health Trust; Visiting Professor, University College London; and Visiting Consultant, The Menninger Clinic and the Menninger Department of Psychiatry and Behavioral Sciences at the Baylor College of Medicine. In collaboration with Peter Fonagy, he has developed mentalization-based treatment for personality disorder and is conducting clinical research trials on its effectiveness. He is an expert member of the National Institute for Clinical Excellence (NICE) development group for treatment guidelines for borderline personality disorder in the United Kingdom. He has authored numerous research articles and book chapters on personality disorder and the use of psychotherapy in psychiatric practice. His several books include *Psychotherapy for Borderline Personality Disorder: Mentalization-Based Treatment* and *Mentalization-Based Treatment for Borderline Personality Disorder: A Practical Guide*, both co-authored with Peter Fonagy.

Disclosure of Interests: The authors of this volume have no competing interests to declare.

Foreword

The Ox Cart

An ancient philosophical riddle asks the following question: *"What is the most important part of an ox cart?"* Most people answer, "The wheel." "The ox." "The cart." "The driver." "The axles." "The apparati connecting the ox to the cart," etc. One seasoned psychoanalyst even quipped, partially in jest, "The whip." The answer to this riddle that I prefer is, "The *concept* of an ox cart." I believe that this is, by far, the best answer to the riddle, because the answer demonstrates how important and how powerful concepts *can be*—even if concepts are unable to be seen, palpated, or imaged with MRI.

A related question is, "What, among the vast universe of concepts, makes a particular concept potent or valuable?" I propose that there are four elements that measure the merit of a concept: 1) the clarity of its definition; 2) its utility; 3) its longevity; and 4) its elaboration into future concepts. Applying these four elements to the ox cart: the concept of joining a pair of wheels to a pair of axles, fastening these to a wooden box, and then attaching the wheeled box to an ox is clearly defined (element #1); of obvious use for transportation of people and goods (element #2); and after 3,000 years since its initial conceptualization, remains in use to this very day in many parts of the world (element #3). Further, the ox cart has evolved into more potent concepts (element #4)—such as the automobile and truck, which, like the ox cart, are four-wheeled vehicles for transportation of humans and material goods, with the power source in the front and a seated human responsible for the guidance. Note that I do not propose that "originality" and "novelty" are requisite measures of the potency or value of a concept. Rather, as implied above, great concepts are evolved from preexisting ones—such as wheels, boxes, yokes, and using animals for transportation and labor. I believe, in fact, that the most valuable concepts are so derivative of preexisting concepts that when they are initially elaborated, they do not seem to be at all original or novel.

What's New?

Since I began my residency training in psychiatry more than three decades ago, I would estimate that I have attended about 1,500 departmental grand rounds. Among the presentations that stand out most prominently in my memory was a talk given by Aaron T. Beck, M.D., during my residency at Columbia University's New York State Psychiatric Institute; this took place several years before the 1979 publication of his landmark book *Cognitive Therapy of Depression*. At this grand rounds, Dr. Beck described cognitive-behavioral therapy and posited that it was a new psychotherapeutic approach that had many advantages, among which was the fact that its effectiveness could be tested. In essence, Dr. Beck had the temerity to claim that he had devised a new and better ox cart. My recollection of this event is framed less by the originality and far-reaching relevance of the subject matter of Dr. Beck's brilliant presentation than by the heated reactions of the many attendees who contended just the opposite: "This is really nothing new. We all have been doing that 'stuff' forever in our clinical practices." "All Aaron has done is to put old wine in new bottles." "Cognitive treatment is basic to all types of psychotherapy." "I think he is making something very complicated out of something that is fundamentally quite simple."

Curiously, when I first heard Jon Allen, Peter Fonagy, and Anthony Bateman present on "mentalization" at a symposium in Houston several years ago, the emotional reactions of and remarks by many of the seasoned clinicians in the audience were eerily identical to those evoked by Dr. Beck so long ago. Given the transformational effects that Dr. Beck's work has had on the mental health profession and for the people whom we serve, these reactions alerted me to the possibility that Drs. Allen, Fonagy, Bateman, and others working on the concept of "mentalizing" might be on to something very important. Manifestly, Dr. Beck's new concept has met all four of my criteria for a potent new "ox cart." Let us now apply these criteria to mentalizing, as illuminated in Allen, Bateman, and Fonagy's new book.

Criterion #1: Clarity of Definition

My first criterion for the potency and value of a new concept is the clarity of its definition. Early on in their book, the authors of *Mentalizing in Clinical Practice* advance a terse and lucid definition of mentalizing and, in the same sentence, throw down the gauntlet by making the following extravagant proposition: "We propose boldly that mentalizing—attending to mental states in oneself and others—is *the most fundamental common factor* among all psychotherapeutic treatments and, accordingly, that all mental health professionals will benefit from a thorough understanding of mentalizing and from familiarity with some of its practical applications." The authors also maintain: "our view [is] that understanding the nature and significance of mentalizing will help clinicians and patients make the best use of *all* forms of mental health treatment; this entire book strives to buttress that claim." In other words, the authors audaciously state that they have invented a new and better ox cart.

As we have seen, when anyone makes such a claim, the reflexive response of others is incredulity, challenge, and, often, pique. I suspect that the readers of this book might join me in asking: "Are the authors implying that understanding and applying the concept of mentalizing are more fundamental and important to psychotherapy than the therapeutic alliance, or than a patient's capacity to form attachments, to abstract, to think rationally, or to be objective? Are the authors implying that mentalizing is so basic as to be a seminal component of therapeutic alliance, attachment, and vital cognitive capacities?" Anticipating such challenges, the authors directly counter the readers' resistances by restating, with minor embellishment, their definition of mentalizing:

> The gist of mentalizing is holding mind in mind.... We are mentalizing when we are aware of mental states in ourselves or others—when we are thinking about feelings, for example.... More elaborately, we define mentalizing as imaginatively perceiving or interpreting behavior as conjoined with intentional mental states.

Manifestly, this definition requires in-depth contemplation by the reader and skillful further explication by the authors—the latter of which is admirably and successfully achieved in Part I of this text, "Understanding Mentalizing." In arriving at such an understanding, the reader is taken on a lush tour through a fascinating terrain of the integral *facets* of mentalizing, wherein such related, enlightening, and otherwise elusive vistas as imagination, mindfulness, mindblindness, mindreading, metacognition, emotional intelligence, insight, agency, mental representation, attachment, and intergenerational transmission are brought into sharp relief and explored. A strength of their book is the authors' skillfulness in linking vital components of mentalization-based therapy to illustrative clinical examples that immediately refine and enlarge the reader's therapeutic armamentarium.

As a devoted, card-carrying (American Neuropsychiatric Association) neuropsychiatrist, I was, not surprisingly, delighted with Chapter 4, "Neurobiology." From my perspective, this consideration, which relies heavily on the most current progress in developmental and neuroscience research, is a critically important component of their theses about and definitions of mentalizing. The authors do not shy away from examining and critiquing their concept of mentalizing through the lenses of modern evolution theory, structural neurobiology, neurophysiology, and neurochemistry. Readers not entirely familiar with this landscape will be treated to a gem-like, enticing review of one of the most exciting and promising areas of biological science. Additionally, neuropathology classically sheds important light on normative brain functioning (for example, stroke has proved to be an important probe in enhancing our understanding of regional brain function), and their examination of emotional dysfunctions, impaired socialization, attachment, and interpersonal relationships—with special focus on such "mentalizing disorders" as autism and sociopathy—opens new frontiers of understanding. The net result is that the authors, in Part I of their book, have succeeded famously in satisfying my Criterion #1, clarity of definition, for establishing a potent and valuable new concept.

Criterion #2: Utility

My second criterion for assaying the potency and value of a new concept is its demonstrated utility. Part II, "Practicing Mentalizing"—comprising approximately 40% of *Mentalizing in Clinical Practice*—is allocated constructively for this purpose. Fortunately, Drs. Allen, Fonagy, and Bateman are active and master clinicians, and they are thus able to draw from a treasure trove of recent and relevant clinical experience that features mentalization-based treatments. Their goal in this section is to help the reader "find out how to translate theory into practice...", and they succeed admirably in this aspiration. They begin with a confession: "*doing it* at any given moment is an art, not a science." We all understand that even though "science" is challenging to teach, however, instruction in the transformation of a skill into "art" is even more difficult. Accordingly, the first chapter devoted to this consideration, Chapter 5, is entitled "The Art of Mentalizing." They characterize their distinction between science and art in the practice of psychotherapy as follows:

> we have no doubt that systemizing plays a role in conducting psychotherapy; without knowledge, principles, and strategies, the process would founder for lack of direction—nor could we improve our effectiveness through research. But the moment-to-moment interactive process requires empathizing.

I agree fully that the optimal practice of the latter in the psychotherapeutic setting approaches "art." What follows is an extraordinarily adept exegesis of the art of mentalizing, embellished constructively by the writings of Daniel Stern, by whom I had the privilege of being supervised during my residency—an experience that provided the opportunity of a glimpse of a therapist who truly is an artist. All art occurs within boundaries, whether a frame for the canvas of an oil painting or the out-of-bounds markers for most sports involving spheres. The authors add such structure to their explication of mentalizing by strongly recommending that therapists conduct formal "mentalizing case formulations," by reviewing a profusion of technical aspects of mentalization-based treatments, and by providing practical tips about how to apply concepts of mentalizing in "everyday" therapeutic practice.

One unique, moving, and compelling inclusion in this book is the firsthand account of the therapeutic experience of mentalization-based treatment by a patient with borderline personality disorder who received such care. Together with the careful outcome data of the authors published in this and other books and in their plethora of papers in peer-reviewed scientific journals, this patient's account of her personal experience of receiving mentalization-based therapy, fully affirms my Criterion #2 (does this new concept have utility?). Further corroboration of the usefulness of mentalization-based therapies is readily gleaned from the chapters on treating attachment trauma; on parenting and family therapy; on treatment of people with borderline personality disorder; and on psychoeducation, which integrates therapy and education in working with family members of people with psychiatric disorders. For the reader who desires further consideration of the "two cultures," science and art, I heartily recommend these two books: *The Two Cultures and the Scientific Revolution,* by C. P. Snow, and *Consilience,* by Edward O. Wilson.

Criteria #3 and #4: The Future

Without question, the psychoanalytic concepts proposed by Freud have both persisted in application and acceptance for more than 100 years (Criterion #3) and have spawned many other robust, derivative, conceptual applications (Criterion #4). Included among these derivations, as discussed, is Beck's cognitive-behavioral therapy as well as the mentalization-based therapies advanced in this book. Given the freshness of the latter, the jury is still out regarding its longevity and derivational impact. Nonetheless, there are preliminary indications that mentalization-based therapies are destined to demonstrate both potency and value over time.

One among many examples that I could detail derives from the Brown Human Neuroimaging Laboratory (HNL) of Baylor College of Medicine, where Drs. Fonagy and I are collaborating faculty members. Utilizing powerful magnetic resonance imaging devices and novel computer programs, the HNL is a research laboratory that specializes in highly advanced functional brain imaging applications. A technique called "hyperscanning" enables scientists to image the brains of two or more individuals while they are interacting in specific research tasks. These technologies have enabled our scientists, for example, to image regions of the brain involved in decision making related to an interactive task. The scientists in the HNL—primarily neuroscientists, mathematicians, behavioral scientists of many disciplines, and radiologists—were captivated by the concept of mentalizing and mentalization-based therapies, as these helped encapsulate quite specific and important functions in so-called "normal subjects" as well as models for the primary brain-based dysfunction in people with relatedness-based disorders ranging from autism to personality disorders. There is broad and shared interest in localizing the brain regions and brain systems involved in mentalization, as well as in determining if there are brain-based changes wherein patients with dysfunctions of relatedness improve with mentalization-based therapies. Such potential discoveries could lead to enhanced understanding of the genetic, cellular, molecular, and neurophysiological concomitants of these conditions.

The availability of a well-defined, useful, and tested concept like mentalizing thus might advance significantly our understanding and evidence-based treatments of people who have suffered from disorders of relatedness and relationships, heretofore thought of as inevitable and inalterable scourges of the human condition. This is but one of multifarious examples of how the concept of mentalizing and the applications of mentalization-based treatments are likely to be utilized, applied, and, most likely, adapted over the years to come. Now that's an ox cart worth riding.

Stuart C. Yudofsky, M.D.
Baylor College of Medicine

Preface

M *entalizing* refers to the activity of understanding behavior in relation to mental states such as thoughts and feelings. We envision the evolution of interest in mentalizing as having expanded in three waves. The first wave occurred when Uta Frith, John Morton, and their colleagues construed mentalizing impairments as the core psychological problem in autism. Shortly thereafter, Peter Fonagy, Mary Target, and their colleagues created a second wave in extending mentalizing to trauma-related developmental psychopathology as it is manifested in borderline personality disorder; in this clinical context, Anthony Bateman and Peter Fonagy developed residential and intensive outpatient treatment programs expressly designed to enhance mentalizing. More recently, a third wave has been building in relation to the wider clinical applications of mentalizing to a broader range of disorders, treatment modalities, and theoretical approaches. As well as in numerous conferences, this third wave of interest is represented in our *Handbook of Mentalization-Based Treatment*, published in 2006. The present book aspires to bring this third wave to a crest in inviting clinicians to consider mentalizing as the foundation of all psychotherapeutic treatments. Over the course of this book we hope to make it plain that this ostensibly audacious proposal merely rests on a truism: perforce, clinicians mentalize in conducting psychotherapies and also engage their patients in doing so. This book aspires to strengthen this foundation of psychotherapeutic practice by acquainting clinicians with the broad base of rapidly accruing knowledge about mentalizing.

We have been surprised by the sheer enthusiasm of participants in conferences and workshops on mentalizing as well as the broad international scope of this interest—from the Americas, the United Kingdom, Europe, and Asia to Australia and New Zealand. Of course, we are not surprised that therapists are eager to learn about anything that promises to be of help with the challenges inherent in treating patients with borderline personality disorder, where mentalization-based treatment has become solidly established. But the enthusiasm seems to go beyond this challenge as mental health professionals of diverse orientations begin to grasp the broader significance of mentalizing. Yet, alongside enthusiasm, we have become accustomed to meeting with some resistance as we advocate that our colleagues join us in embracing the concept of mentalizing. Mary Target boiled down this resistance to two forms. First, many clinicians find "mentalizing" to be foreign and alien—our colleague Jeremy Holmes rightly characterizes it as an "ungainly" word. We, too, have reservations about using such a technical word to characterize what we regard as our quintessentially human capacity. Incorporating the word into one's natural vocabulary takes some time, but many clinicians and some patients are doing it, an effort justified by what we will articulate as the unique boundaries of the concept. Hence, fully understanding the concept and coming to apply it in clinical practice—as we hope to inspire you to do—will overcome the initial alien sense.

Second, having overcome the first resistance and gaining some superficial understanding of the concept, clinicians are liable to believe that there is nothing new here and that they already know it all. A brisk flip through the pages of references at the end of this book might begin to dispel that conclusion. We authors would hardly claim to know everything there is to know about mentalizing, much less to be consistently successful in mentalizing in our clinical practices—or our daily lives, for that matter. Indeed, our own excitement is sustained by the fact that this is a relatively new field and we have so much yet to learn. We have strived to make that point amply clear throughout this book.

After we completed the *Handbook*, Stuart Yudofsky, chairman of the Menninger Department of Psychiatry and Behavioral Sciences at the Baylor College of Medicine, suggested that an accessible guide to help clinicians of diverse backgrounds understand the concept of mentalizing and its various applications would be a useful contribution to the field and that American Psychiatric Publishing would be the best publisher for it; we agreed. As an edited volume, the *Handbook* has the advantage of representing many voices, but we also believed that it would be helpful to take stock of current knowledge and present it in one voice (or three morphed into one). The pertinent scholarly literature is diverse and burgeoning, and we have endeavored to pull it together and present it clearly to our fellow clinicians who are unacquainted with the technical literature. The practice of mentalizing is generally common-sensical, such that we have maintained a conversational style throughout much of this book. Yet just as mentalizing itself often entails hard mental work, so does understanding the subtleties of the concept and its extensive scientific footing. Accordingly, giving the sheer richness of mentalizing its due, we have not stinted on technical material that demands some intellectual effort. Yet we can reassure readers that after a few hard climbs in the early stages, the trek is generally easy. Also, readers will encounter innumerable long quotations from the writings of other authors whose fine work we showcase—notwithstanding that many of these authors never heard of "mentalizing."

The overall organization of the book is simple: following an Introduction that presents our view of mentalizing as the most basic common factor in effective psychosocial treatments, Part I explains mentalizing in depth and Part II covers clinical applications. Of course, clinicians might get by with a general definition of mentalizing and then endeavor to apply it in practice, bypassing Part I and going straight to Part II. Yet we believe that a thorough understanding of the concept of mentalizing and firm knowledge of its scientific foundations greatly enhances its applications. The significance of this project cannot be overstated: we are striving to fathom how the human mind comes into being. Moreover, the developmental conditions that promote and undermine mentalizing translate directly into psychotherapeutic practice. Thus we have written Part I as a kind of book within a book to provide a comprehensive review of the scholarly literature pertinent to mentalizing, covering its many facets and relations to similar concepts, its developmental origins in attachment relationships, and its neurobiological underpinnings. Part II begins with a chapter proposing that although there is plenty of science behind it, the activity of mentalizing in psychotherapy is an art; this spirit sets the stage for the next chapter on mentalizing interventions in psychotherapy. Subsequent chapters illustrate the applicability of these interventions to trauma treatment, parent-child therapy, borderline personality disorder, psychoeducation, and violence prevention in social systems.

Acknowledgments

Although this book speaks with one voice, it reflects the thinking of a large international team of devoted clinicians and researchers as well as a consortium of supportive institutions comprising the Anna Freud Centre, University College London, Yale Child Study Center, The Menninger Clinic, the Menninger Department of Psychiatry and Behavioral Sciences at the Baylor College of Medicine, and the Human Neuroimaging Laboratory at Baylor. Thus we have evolved the clinical thinking represented in this book in collaboration with many like-minded colleagues, including Efrain Bleiberg, Pasco Fearon, Elliot Jurist, George Gergely, Jeremy Holmes, Linda Mayes, Richard Munich, Lois Sadler, John Sargent, Carla Sharp, Arietta Slade, Howard and Miriam Steele, Helen Stein, Mary Target, Stuart Twemlow, and Laurel Williams.

In addition, we have expanded the mentalizing team at The Menninger Clinic by including patients; as we discovered many years ago, one of the best ways to understand clinical problems is to try to explain them to patients in psychoeducational groups—and to learn in the process. Thus we have benefited from discussing mentalizing with a large number of inquisitive and insightful patients, and a number of our colleagues, including Efrain Bleiberg, Toby Haslam-Hopwood, Noelle McDonald, and April Stein, have made significant contributions to this educational project.

In addition, we are grateful to several colleagues for their critical reading of various parts of the manuscript: Susan and Yvonne Allen, Melvin Berg, Throstur Björgvinsson, Norma Clarke, John Hart, Toby Haslam-Hopwood, Leonard Horwitz, Lisa Lewis, James Lomax, Noelle McDonald, Richard Moran, Richard Munich, Carla Sharp, and Roger Verdon. We also thank Cassandra Shorter for help with literature searches and acquiring reference materials, and we are grateful to Katherine Connor Martin for tracking down the etymology of *mentalizing* in the *Oxford English Dictionary*. Finally, we are grateful to Robert Hales, Editor-in-Chief, and John McDuffie, Editorial Director, of the Books Department at American Psychiatric Publishing, Inc., for helping to shape this book at its inception as well as for continuing to do so as we brought it to fruition, and to Roxanne Rhodes, Senior Project Editor, for her skillful editorial direction in the final production.

J.G.A., P.F., A.W.B.

Chapter 1

Introduction

W hat Jerome Frank (1961) wrote decades ago in his classic *Persuasion and Healing* remains true: "much, if not all, of the effectiveness of different forms of psychotherapy may be due to those features that all have in common rather than to those that distinguish them from each other" (p. 232). Establishing a therapeutic alliance, for example, is critical to the success of any treatment, regardless of the clinician's theoretical orientation (Bordin 1979; Roth and Fonagy 2005). We propose boldly that mentalizing—attending to mental states in oneself and others—is *the most fundamental common factor* among psychotherapeutic treatments and, accordingly, that all mental health professionals will benefit from a thorough understanding of mentalizing and from familiarity with some of its practical applications. In advancing this thesis we acknowledge that we are more invested in what's important than what's new.

To be effective—in establishing a therapeutic alliance, for example—we clinicians must mentalize skillfully; concomitantly, we must engage our patients in mentalizing. Clinicians who work with patients who are reasonably skillful mentalizers can get by with taking mentalizing for granted—although we believe that attention to mentalizing is always in order. Clinicians working with patients who are distinctly impaired in mentalizing capacity, such as those with borderline personality disorder, must be more single-minded in promoting mentalizing.

The fact that we are employing an unfamiliar concept, mentalizing, for a familiar process—understanding ourselves and each other—calls for some orientation. We begin by introducing the concept of mentalizing and our view of its role in treatment. Next we launch our book-length project of elucidating the richness of the concept of mentalizing by describing its origins in psychoanalysis and attachment theory. Then we illustrate our thesis that mentalizing is the core common factor among psychotherapies by considering a few well-established treatments (cognitive therapy, interpersonal psychotherapy, and client-centered therapy) from the perspective of mentalizing. We conclude this orientation by reiterating our view that understanding the nature and significance of mentalizing will help clinicians and patients make the best use of *all* forms of mental health treatment; this entire book strives to buttress that claim.

Basic Questions

We start by giving sufficient definition to mentalizing to provide an orientation to this book. Although mentalizing lies at the core of our humanity, the conceptual territory is daunting: with the dominance of logical positivism and behaviorism, many philosophers and psychologists gave up on understanding the mind for some decades in the middle of the twentieth century. And when we are concerned with mentalizing, we not only must understand the mind but also must *understand our understanding* of the mind. We proceed undaunted.

Chapter 2 ("Mentalizing") explicates the various facets of mentalizing, and the entire book further elucidates the concept and its myriad applications. This Introduction first clears some ground: once we have an orienting definition in hand in this section, we will convey the general spirit of focusing on mentalizing in treatment, then return to a question that is bound to follow: what, if anything, is new here?

What is Mentalizing?

We are mentalizing when we are aware of mental states in ourselves or others—when we are thinking about feelings, for example. To get discussions of mentalizing off the ground, we and our colleagues employ a number of handy phrases, listed in Table 1–1.

TABLE 1–1.   HANDY DEFINITIONS OF "MENTALIZING"

- Holding mind in mind
- Attending to mental states in self and others
- Understanding misunderstandings
- Seeing yourself from the outside and others from the inside
- Giving a mental quality to or cultivating mentally

The gist of mentalizing is *holding mind in mind*. To most ears, "mentalize" has an unfamiliar ring—as it should, because it is not listed in many contemporary dictionaries. As we noted in the Preface, the sheer foreignness of the word is an obstacle to clinicians adopting the concept. Yet this sense of foreignness is inherent in all new words, as Mikhail Bakhtin articulated:

> The word in language is half someone else's. It becomes "one's own" only when the speaker populates it with his own intention, his own accent, when he appropriates the word, adapting it to his own semantic and expressive intention…. many words stubbornly resist, others remain alien, sound foreign in the mouth of the one who appropriated them and who now speaks them…. Language is not a neutral medium that passes freely and easily into the private property of the speaker's intentions; it is populated—overpopulated—with the intentions of others. Expropriating it, forcing it to submit to one's own intentions and accents, is a difficult and complicated process. (quoted in Wertsch 1998, p. 54)

Well said; we have found expropriating "mentalizing" to be an exceptionally difficult and complicated process, especially when we aspire to engage patients in doing so. A quick look at the history of "mentalize" might begin to surmount aversion to its alien ring. Although it does not yet appear in many dictionaries, "mentalize" is not a new word. "Mentalize" first appeared in the *Oxford English Dictionary* a century ago, in 1906. The *OED*'s etymology indicates that the first recorded use of the word was two centuries ago, in 1807. The *OED* quoted G. Stanley Hall, a founder of American psychology, as having written in 1885, "The only thing that can ever undermine our school system in popular support is a suspicion that it does not moralize as well as mentalize children." So began the first professional use of the word. Currently, the *OED* gives two senses for mentalize: first, to construct or picture in the mind, to imagine, or to give a mental quality to; second, to develop or cultivate mentally, or to stimulate the mind of.

Our use of "mentalizing" is consistent with the *OED* definitions, although we delimit the content of mentalizing to mental states: not all mental activity is mentalizing; rather, mentalizing is concerned with mental states. We generally use the word "mentalize" in the first sense of "giving a mental quality to" (e.g., interpreting a scowl as indicating condemnation) while endeavoring in our clinical work to mentalize in the second sense of "cultivating mentally" (e.g., fostering self-awareness as we aspire to do in conducting psychotherapy). More elaborately, we define mentalizing as *imaginatively perceiving or interpreting behavior as conjoined with intentional mental states*. We often say that mentalizing entails interpreting behavior as *based on* mental states or involves inferring the mental states that *lie behind* overt behavior, as if "behavior" and "mental states" are always separable. This way of thinking about mentalizing applies to a situation like the following: a patient is sitting quietly and reflectively, and then tears start running down his cheeks and he begins clenching his fists. The therapist is bound to inquire about what came to mind; in effect, what mental state prompted the tears and clenched fists. Often, however, mental states and behavior are inseparably *conjoined;* that is, so thoroughly intertwined that one cannot be disentangled from the other—as in giving out a cry of pain or leaning forward when paying keen attention and engaging in rapid-fire conversation.

Mental states are intrinsically *intentional;* that is, they are representational or *about* something: a feeling is about some state of affairs, whereas a material object like stone is not about anything—it just *is*. We will emphasize this critical point about the representational nature of mental states throughout. To underscore it here, Bogdan (2005, p. 190) rightly construes "the core of understanding minds" as entailing "ascriptions of representational states or attitudes, such as desires or beliefs, whose relation (or directedness) to what they represent is registered in some fashion." He dubbed this relation "representingness." Bogdan makes a subtle and important point: optimally, we have a sense of representingness regarding mental states, an implicit awareness that a mental state is always a particular *take* on a situation. The capacity to reflect on the various meanings of mental states, as we routinely invite our patients to do, depends on the sense of representingness. As we will describe, acquiring this sense of mental states as such is a major developmental achievement, and much of psychopathology entails losing this capacity.

More concretely, clinical practice requires continual mentalizing on the part of both the patient and the clinician. Table 1–2 illustrates various ways in which patients and clinicians might mentalize in the treat-

---

TABLE 1–2. COMMONPLACE EXAMPLES OF MENTALIZING

For the patient

- Explaining why he or she is seeking treatment and providing a history of symptoms
- Describing his or her spouse's view of the presenting problems and considering the impact of the presenting problems on their children's well-being
- Considering the impact of relationships in the family of origin on current relationships
- Articulating the basis of his or her distress and apprehension in the clinical interview
- Evaluating the accuracy of the clinician's observations and correcting the clinician's misunderstandings
- Reporting on the effects of medication

For the clinician

- Enabling the patient to feel safe in the session
- Understanding the meaning of stressful life events in relation to a history of trauma
- Formulating a diagnostic understanding and explicating it to the patient
- Explaining to the patient how a particular treatment approach might help
- Helping the patient to appreciate signs of progress or regression in treatment
- Managing the patient's distress stemming from the patient's own experience or behavior

Nonclinical interactions

- Reassuring a frightened child
- Ascertaining what gets in the way of holding to a diet
- Understanding the reasons for one's unreasonably angry response to a request
- Asking a harried supervisor for time off
- Mediating conflicts between children, friends, or family members

---

ment process as well as ways in which mentalizing is inherent in everyday situations. These commonplace examples make two points immediately evident: first, effective treatment depends on the mentalizing skill of the clinician; second, effective treatment depends on the mentalizing skill of the patient. We do not take the clinician's mentalizing skill for granted; research on the psychotherapy process indicates that clinicians' mentalizing capacities vary, for example, from patient to patient (Diamond et al. 2003). Thus, a focus on mentalizing potentially can make a significant contribution to clinical training (see Chapter 6, "Mentalizing Interventions"). Yet while by no means ignoring the clinician, treatment primarily addresses mentalizing deficits in the patient, for the purpose of enhancing mentalizing in everyday life.

We devote much of this book to diverse ways of focusing on mentalizing in treatment (see Part II, "Practicing Mentalizing"); while the contexts are varied, these methods have been developed with one primary goal in mind: *enhancing the mentalizing capacities of the participants.* Plainly, the point of enhancing mentalizing capacity is not to foster skill in being a psychiatric patient; rather, we aim to enhance the quality of life. As this book will explicate, impaired mentalizing capacity plays a major role in problems in living as well as in psychiatric disorders. Conversely, enhanced mentalizing plays a central role in resilience, that is, the capacity to cope with adversity—including psychiatric illness (Stein 2006).

Focusing on mentalizing in treatment faces a "catch-22": to participate in treatment and to benefit from it, the patient must mentalize; yet many patients who seek treatment have substantial impairments in mentalizing capacity. Clinicians' mentalizing skills come into play largely in navigating around this catch-22; the knack of treating patients with impaired mentalizing capacity involves establishing the therapeutic conditions that promote mentalizing in a bootstrapping process that enables patients to build on whatever mentalizing skills they have already developed so as to learn how to mentalize more consistently and effectively, especially in emotion-laden attachment relationships.

As this book shows, mentalizing can become a relatively singleminded focus of treatment in various different modalities. Yet, as we explain next, given the cardinal role of mentalizing in all forms of psychotherapeutic treatment, attention to mentalizing can be of general benefit to clinicians and patients.

What's New?

To head off confusion at the outset, clinicians must grasp one point: mentalizing-focused treatment is the *least novel* therapeutic approach imaginable, simply because it revolves around a fundamental human capacity—indeed, the capacity that makes us human (Allen and Fonagy 2006b). Given the generic role of mentalizing in treatment as we have construed it, we are not inclined to "sell" mentalizing interventions as yet another new brand or type of therapy in an already overcrowded field; rather, we advocate keen attention to enhancing mentalizing in extant therapies. Yet when impaired mentalizing is a primary clinical problem, mentalizing-enhancing interventions might become the main therapeutic agenda. We would add that despite the challenges of conducting it, the goals of mentalizing-focused treatment are modest: skillful mentalizing alone does not solve problems or resolve disorders but rather enhances participants' abilities to do so (Williams et al. 2006).

Much of what we do in mentalizing-focused treatment—including using the word "mentalizing"—aims merely to *draw attention* to mentalizing. We agree with Meins and colleagues' (2006) distinction between *acquiring* a capacity and *using* the capacity. They considered that their measure of *mind-mindedness* (see Chapter 3, "Development"), might turn out to be "as much a measure of motivational and personality differences as it is an index of an underlying cognitive capacity" (p. 194). Taking some mentalizing capacity for granted and working on the motivation to use it, we explicitly promote a *mentalizing stance* with patients and therapists, that is, an inquisitive, curious, open-minded—and even playful—interest in mental states in self and others (Allen 2006b; Haslam-Hopwood et al. 2006). By modeling this mentalizing stance, clinicians engage their patients in mentalizing. Notably, this attitude toward mentalizing requires a high *tolerance for ambiguity*—itself a marker of psychological health—namely, "a capacity for coping with unstructured or open-ended stimulus situations" (Foxman 1976, p. 67)—as the situations calling for mentalizing invariably are.

In sum, we consider our focus on mentalizing to be *a refinement rather than an innovation*: we are merely sharpening attention to a common factor inherent in psychotherapeutic treatments. Helpfully, we now have considerable scientific resources to sharpen our understanding of this core factor—namely, a substantial research literature in attachment theory and developmental psychopathology (see Chapter 3, "Development") buttressed by burgeoning research in social cognitive neuroscience (see Chapter 4, "Neurobiology"). A thorough understanding of the developmental and neurocognitive conditions that facilitate and impede mentalizing capacity is no small refinement; this is the agenda of the first part of this book.

Origins in Psychoanalysis and Attachment Theory

To actualize means to make something actual; to mentalize means to make something mental—or more *elaborately* mental. We are indebted to Freud for this bedrock sense of mentalizing. Thus, as we sketch next, the concept of mentalizing remains rooted in psychoanalysis, although it has flourished in the framework of attachment theory (Fonagy 2001a; Fonagy et al. 2002a; Holmes 2006).

Psychoanalysis

It is little wonder that mentalizing has deep roots in psychoanalysis; as Loewald (1970) wrote, "The psychoanalytic process is the arena *par excellence* for studying the underlying psychic activities which enter into the organization, maintenance, and growth of the individual mind" (p. 61). Although Freud did not use the term "mentalizing," he originated the fundamental idea in construing mental processes as arising from the *binding* of somatic drive energies into thought, that is, transforming something that is non-mental into something mental (Freud 1895; Pribram and Gill 1976). Thinking before acting on impulse is therefore paradigmatic of mentalizing. In effect, thinking is a holding action that provides a realistic pathway from feeling impelled by a drive to finding the object of satisfaction. In educating traumatized patients about coping with strong emotions, we often use the metaphor of "pushing the pause button" by mentalizing (Allen 2005); in so doing, we are merely epitomizing Freud's early theory.

In this Freudian view, the mind develops out of frustration inherent in the need to wait. Holmes (2006) pithily summarized Freud's conception that thinking arises in response to an absence of the need-gratifying object: "no breast, therefore imagine [mentalize] a breast" (p. 36). Freud recognized, of course, that other persons are the primary source of satisfaction and, foreshadowing our understanding of the development of mentalizing, he wrote, "it is in relation to a fellow human-being that a human-being learns to cognize" (quoted in Pribram and Gill 1976, p. 116).

Akin to Freud's view of binding energy with thought is Bion's (1962a, 1962b) useful conception of the *containment* function of thinking, whereby pressing internal impulses are transformed into tolerable and thinkable experiences. Insightfully, Bion (1962b) proposed that "a capacity for tolerating frustration thus enables the psyche to develop thought as a means by which the frustration that is tolerated is itself made more tolerable" (p. 307). Thus, Bion's fundamental insight about frustration tolerance is crucial to our understanding of the adaptive function of mentalizing: mentalizing *per se* helps to modulate strong needs and emotions and thus to make them more bearable. Moreover, as Freud also articulated, the process of containing strong impulses and feelings while thinking of realistic pathways to satisfaction is the essence of adaptation. This containment process requires mentalizing as we construe it.

Also proceeding in the spirit of Freud, French psychoanalysts were the first to introduce the term *mentalisation* into the psychiatric literature in the late 1960s. Lecours and Bouchard (1997) have traced the development of this line of thought and also refined it. As we also will do, they construe mentalizing as a process of *mental elaboration*: "we propose to explain mentalisation as referring to a general class of mental operations, including representation and symbolisation, which specifically lead to a *transformation* and elaboration of drive-affect experiences into increasingly organised mental phenomena and structures" (p. 858, emphasis in original). Highlighting its cardinal role in affect tolerance and modulation, they characterize mentalizing as "the 'immune system' of the psyche" (p. 857). Lecours and Bouchard also emphasize the crucial point that mentalizing is not an all-or-none phenomenon but rather "a continual, never-ending transformation of psychic contents through the multiplication and organisation of representations" (p. 857)—indeed, a "slow and progressive process, perhaps the venture of a lifetime" (p. 865). Accordingly, they delineate five levels of drive-affect containment and mental elaboration associated with increasing mentalizing, as displayed in Table 1–3.

Reflecting its Freudian origins, the psychoanalytic thinking we have just sketched highlights the transformation of fundamentally bodily processes (somatic and motoric) into psychic experience; to repeat, strictly speaking, mental-*izing* entails making something non-mental into something mental. Thus the *OED* definition of mentalizing as *giving a mental quality* to something or *cultivating mentally* is a fundamentally Freudian concept that we will employ throughout this book.

Yet mentalizing is not something that takes place solely inside the head of the individual. Although Bion (1962b) as well as Lecours and Bouchard (1997) and their psychoanalytic predecessors made this point, Winnicott (1971) most plainly articulated the role of maternal mirroring in the development of a mentalized sense of self. As Fonagy and colleagues (2002a) summarized, "the psychological self develops through the perception of oneself in another person's mind as thinking and feeling" (p. 28). To foreshadow a way of thinking to be elaborated in Chapter 3 ("Development"), the mind does not develop solely from within but rather largely *from the outside in:* infants, in effect, find their mind in the mind of the caregiver; thus mentalizing depends on being mentalized, that is, on the caregiver's mentalizing. The same applies to psychotherapy, and this point brings us to attachment.

TABLE 1–3.   INCREASING LEVELS OF MENTAL ELABORATION

Level	Examples
Disruptive impulsion refers to relatively uncontained, unmentalized experiences, often characterized by an unstoppable urge to do something.	Violent behavior; self-mutilation; sudden attacks of headache or nausea
Modulated impulsion refers to somewhat better contained and adaptive expressions of affect.	A spell of inexplicable crying or a fantasy of hitting someone
Externalization entails mentally representing a wish or affective state but disowning it somewhat by projection or by attributing it to an external situation.	Ascribing anger to another person's provocation; or, more generally, simply claiming that anyone would feel the same way in a certain kind of situation
Appropriation entails fully owning desires and affects as subjective— and subjectively tolerable— experiences.	Attributing physiological arousal to anxiety and, more generally, identifying and labeling specific emotional states
Meaning associations refers to an abstracting and reflective stage requiring complex verbal representation through which mental experience gains depth.	Insight—not intellectualization, but rather instances of reflection associated with genuine emotion in which the patient gains a fresh perspective

Attachment Theory

Winnicott's (1971) pinpointing the central role of the caregiver's mirroring in the development of the self foreshadowed the contribution of attachment theory to understanding the development of mentalizing. Specifically, mentalizing develops optimally in the context of *secure attachment* relationships. Bowlby (1973, 1982) characterized secure attachment as providing not only a *safe haven* (i.e., emotional comforting and a feeling of security) but also a *secure base* for exploration, the archetypal manifestation of which is the toddler who makes confident forays into the playground while periodically checking back to make sure that mother or father remains nearby. Accordingly, Bowlby (1988) construed the psychotherapist's role as being "analogous to that of a mother who provides her child with a secure base from which to explore the world" (p. 140). But Bowlby recognized that the secure base of attachment provides the platform not only for exploring the outer world but also the inner world, the world of the mind: the therapist's job is to provide the patient with a secure base from which he can explore the various unhappy and painful aspects of his life, past and present, many of which he finds it difficult or perhaps impossible to think about and reconsider without a trusted companion to provide support, encouragement, sympathy, and, on occasion, guidance. (p. 138)

A patient in a psychoeducational group on trauma brilliantly crystallized Bowlby's point: when the leader proposed that "the mind can be a scary place," she exclaimed, "Yes—and you wouldn't want to go in there alone!"

As advocates of mentalizing, we agree with Bowlby's (1988) contention that "No concept within the attachment framework is more central to developmental psychiatry than that of the secure base" (pp. 163–164). Grossman and colleagues (1999) captured the significance of what they dubbed the *security of exploration* (though we would give primacy to *mental* exploration):

Secure attachment provides the best-known psychological precondition for tension-free, playful exploration. Thus, when their adaptation is challenged, secure children can flexibly explore possible solutions or perspectives while retaining a secure feeling during exploration, and if their competence is depleted, they can rely on and summon social resources. We have called this a "wider view of attachment," in which the freedom to explore in the face of adversity and the freedom to call for and accept help are both necessary and important aspects of security. (p. 781)

Taking Bowlby's lead, Fonagy and his colleagues used the concept of mentalizing as a fulcrum for synthesizing psychoanalysis and attachment theory while anchoring the treatment in developmental psychopathology (Fonagy 2001a, 2006; Fonagy et al. 2002a). Fonagy's work was one of the two lines of thought that introduced the word "mentalizing" into the English clinical lexicon in the early 1990s. In advocating that research from developmental psychology be incorporated into the psychoanalytic theory of mental representation, Fonagy (1991) proposed "For the sake of brevity,…to label the capacity to conceive of conscious and unconscious mental states in oneself and others as the capacity to *mentalize*" (p. 641, emphasis in original). In a parallel line of thought pertaining to the most profound failure of attachment, Frith and colleagues (1991) proposed that "the whole symptom complex of autism arises from a single cognitive deficit" (p. 437)—namely, a lack of mentalizing capacity owing to stable neurobiological impairment. In the context of autism, Morton (1989) defined mentalizing more narrowly as a set of skills that enables "the ability to predict relationships between external states of affairs and other people's internal states of mind" (p. 46).

Although we will consider the relatively stable impairments of mentalizing capacity associated with autism later in this book (Chapter 4, "Neurobiology"), we concentrate on mentalizing as Fonagy and his colleague have elaborated it, namely, as a more variable dynamic skill (Fonagy and Target 1997a). In this line of thought, impairments in mentalizing are *context dependent* and mentalizing is most often compromised in the context of attachment relationships—not incidentally, the context in which mentalizing develops more or less adequately.

Owing to this synthesis of psychoanalytic theory and clinical practice with attachment theory and developmental psychopathology, the seemingly mundane attention to mental states in psychotherapeutic treatments now rests on a more secure base of theory and research, and we believe that this recently acquired knowledge has the potential to sharpen our daily practice. Moreover, when established treatments are viewed from the perspective of mentalizing, they too can be seen to rest on this new foundation. We are not inclined to tamper with brand loyalty when it comes to the practice of psychotherapy; as we illustrate next, mentalizing cuts across all "brands," and more knowledgeable attention to mentalizing can be employed to the benefit of all.

Mentalizing in Established Treatments

We have noted how the concept of mentalizing first emerged in psychoanalysis: Freud implicitly employed the concept of mentalizing in his initial neurobiological theory of the development of the mind, and a group of French psychoanalysts was the first to employ the concept explicitly and to refine it as such. Given the attachment context that gradually came to be appreciated as providing the developmental crucible for mentalizing, it is no accident that within psychoanalysis, object relations theory has been especially compatible with focusing on mentalizing in treatment (Fonagy 2001a). Plainly, the therapeutic relationship assumes paramount importance in mentalizing-focused treatment.

Psychoanalysis, potentially the most thoroughgoing exploration of the mind developed to date, might be considered a mentalizing treatment *par excellence*. Yet the applications of a clinical focus on mentalizing extend far beyond psychoanalysis and psychodynamic psychotherapy (Allen and Fonagy 2006a). Moreover, a focus on mentalizing *per se* subtly—and not so subtly—influences psychoanalytic practice (Holmes 2006; Munich 2006). Two broad shifts stand out (Bateman and Fonagy 2004, 2006). First, mentalizing interventions tend to be experience-near, emphasizing relatively conscious (and preconscious) mental states as well as the here and now. Second, a focus on mentalizing gives priority to process over content, as Lecours and Bouchard (1997) also observed: "This model is more concerned with the way in which the experience is transformed and with the shape of its expression than with its content, which is usually more readily taken into consideration in clinical practice" (p. 861). As we will continue to elaborate throughout this book, this process orientation is consistent with construing treatment as promoting *attention* to mentalizing and thereby enhancing *skill* in mentalizing. Nevertheless, we have no inclination to eschew the importance of mental content: every process requires content, and we must be concerned with the mental contents in relation to which mentalizing skill is impaired—especially those mental contents associated with conscious and unconscious conflicts in attachment relationships.

To reiterate, from the standpoint of its origins, our focus on mentalizing appears closer to psychoanalysis and psychodynamic psychotherapy than to any other school of treatment to the extent that the focus remains on the relationship and interaction between the therapist and the patient. Yet emphasizing relatively conscious, here-and-now mental processes aligns us more closely with a range of post-psychoanalytic therapeutic approaches. Some of the work we present in this book, for example, might be viewed as equidistant between psychodynamic psychotherapy and cognitive therapy. More aware of similarities than differences, we find it instructive to view established treatment approaches through the lens of mentalizing. Developing techniques to enhance mentalizing has required that we become not only more aware of interventions from different therapies that *promote* mentalizing but also sensitive to types of intervention that might unwittingly *undermine* mentalizing. Moreover, apart from the theoretical approach, inasmuch as levels of mentalizing skills vary among individuals (partly as a function of psychiatric condition), interventions must be tailored carefully to the patient's abilities.

Our conviction that clinicians of all persuasions have much to gain from a deeper understanding of mentalizing is the *raison d'être* of this book. To illustrate, we here apply the perspective of mentalizing to a broad spectrum of influential schools of therapy: cognitive therapy, interpersonal psychotherapy, and client-centered therapy.

Cognitive Therapy

The techniques of cognitive therapy (Beck et al. 1979) actively and systematically—if not deliberately—promote mentalizing (Björgvinsson and Hart 2006). Beck and colleagues' fundamental intervention of drawing patients' attention to *automatic* negative thoughts and their influence on mood plainly exemplifies mentalizing in relation to the self. In short, cognitive therapy enhances awareness of how one's mind works. Reflecting on fleeting and habitual thought patterns exemplifies mentalizing in the sense of mental elaboration—in effect, making the preconscious more fully conscious. Taking an empirical attitude toward the validity of one's thoughts and challenging global negative thinking exemplifies the mentalizing stance in the sense of promoting curiosity and inquisitiveness and—above all—flexibility in thinking (Allen 2006a). As Björgvinsson and Hart (2006) note, thought records documenting situations that trigger automatic negative thoughts in conjunction with emotions promote "alternative ways of thinking about events, reinforcing the experience of multiple mental perspectives" (p. 163). Thus, as they summarize, "cognitive therapy provides highly structured ways of practicing mentalizing" (p. 169). To illustrate, Table 1–4 lists some reminders that our cognitive therapist colleague John Hart wrote down for one of his anxiety-ridden patients; these reminders are prompts to mentalize.

A relatively recent innovation in cognitive therapy for depression comes even closer to an explicit focus on mentalizing by incorporating mindfulness training into the treatment process (Segal et al. 2002). Although mindfulness is not identical to mentalizing, the concepts overlap (see Chapter 2, "Mentalizing"). Mindfulness training emphasizes process over content; that is, it does not aim to change the content of depressive thinking but rather aims to change the patient's *relationship* to thoughts and feelings—in Bogdan's (2005) terms, cultivating a sense of the representingness of thoughts and feelings. Specifically, patients are encouraged "to 'allow' difficult thoughts and feelings simply to be there, to bring to them a kindly awareness, to adopt toward them a more 'welcome' than a 'need to solve' stance" (Segal et al. 2002, p. 55). Mindfulness promotes mentalizing skill in the sense of enhancing awareness of thoughts and feelings, and it promotes a mentalizing stance by drawing attention to the unceasing flux in mental states. Crucially, mental *states* change—a phenomenon that escapes the attention of depressed patients. Mindfulness can provide some detachment, for example, as patients learn to identify "the-mental-state-in-which-I-view-myself-as-utterly-worthless" (Segal et al. 2002, p. 31).

Encouragingly, there is some evidence that cognitive therapy (Segal et al. 1999) and mindfulness-based cognitive therapy in particular (Segal et al. 2002) promote resilience in the form of relapse prevention. From our perspective (Allen 2006a), this treatment approach amelio-

---

TABLE 1–4. MENTALIZING TIPS FROM A COGNITIVE THERAPIST

- Anxiety is not lethal.
- Anxiety does not equate with personal weakness.
- Thoughts are thoughts and not facts.
- Emotions are not direct reflections of reality.
- When I get anxious, I have more anxious thoughts.
- If I am more anxious, it does not make the world more dangerous.
- Controlling anxiety causes more anxiety.
- I must be willing to experience anxiety to lower anxiety.

---

rates cognitive vulnerability to depression by interrupting the potential spiral from depressed *feelings* to depressive *illness*. Mentalizing affords some detachment by helping the patient to adopt multiple perspectives on a given situation (e.g., "At first I thought she didn't greet me because she was blowing me off, but then it occurred to me that she might have been preoccupied with her upcoming exams"). Thus mentalizing counters the proclivity to ruminate, which is liable to entrench the person in a depressed mood and, over time, generate depressive illness (Ingram et al. 1998).

As we will elaborate in the next chapter, cognitive therapy comes closest to mentalizing in its concern with *metacognition:* thinking about thinking (Wells 2000). In this domain and others, cognitive therapy has the advantage of offering highly structured and evidence-based techniques that, from our standpoint, facilitate mentalizing (Björgvinsson and Hart 2006). Not incidentally, metacognitive capacities play a central role in secure attachment and vice versa (Main 1991). Accordingly, from the perspective of attachment theory, the quality of the patient-therapist relationship is central to the process of mentalizing in cognitive therapy. Moreover, viewed from the perspective of developmental psychopathology, the cognitive distortions evident in depression often have roots in traumatic attachment relationships (Allen 2006a).

Interpersonal Psychotherapy

Interpersonal psychotherapy originally was developed as an evidence-based treatment for depression (Klerman et al. 1984) and subsequently has been extended to a wider range of psychiatric disorders (Weissman et al. 2000). Interpersonal psychotherapy focuses on the interpersonal context in which psychiatric disorders develop as well as the impact of these disorders on interpersonal relationships. Interpersonal psychotherapy promotes active problem solving in relationships, focusing particularly on attachment relationships. In short: interpersonal psychotherapy "tries to change the way the patient thinks, feels, and acts in problematic interpersonal relationships" (Klerman et al. 1984, p. 15). Hence interpersonal psychotherapy implicitly draws attention to mentalizing in relation to *others'* mental states while also promoting *self*-awareness with an eye toward interpersonal problem solving in the here and now.

Several core domains of interpersonal psychotherapy techniques promote mentalizing; these domains include encouragement of affect, clarification, communication analysis, and use of the therapeutic relationship (Weissman et al. 2000). At the risk of belaboring the obvious, we draw attention in Table 1–5 to some ways in which these techniques encourage mentalizing.

Conjoint treatment for patients with marital disputes is a natural extension of interpersonal psychotherapy. Some examples of what would be standard interventions in marital therapy (Weissman et al. 2000, p. 239) highlight the requirement to mentalize in the therapy as well as the potential for the therapy to enhance mentalizing capacity:

- "Did you understand what your wife just said?… Well, I didn't either."
- "You say 'Yes,' but you don't look like you agree."
- [To the husband:] "Does your wife know that this makes you unhappy?… How does she know?" [To the wife:] "Did you know that that was upsetting to your husband?"
- "Did you know that [s]he felt so strongly about that?"
- "I'm concerned: anyone would be upset by that. You say you aren't upset. What's stopping you from feeling that way?"

All these would be plausible mentalizing interventions; we merely contend that explicit attention to mentalizing provides a useful framework for the process. We find that conscious attention to mentalizing sharpens our focus as therapists. Moreover, educating participants about mentalizing can enhance their collaboration in the process (see Chapter 10, "Psychoeducation").

Client-Centered Therapy

In the 1940s, Rogers (1951) began developing "nondirective" or "client-centered" therapy as a relationship-focused alternative to psychoanalysis. Rogers initially developed and promoted client-centered therapy in part with the desire to create a treatment method that could be learned

TABLE 1–5. MENTALIZING-PROMOTING INTERVENTIONS IN INTERPERSONAL PSYCHOTHERAPY

Goal of intervention	Specific techniques and comments
Encouragement of affect encompasses ways of helping patients understand, regulate, and express their feelings, with the assumption that psychotherapy entails *emotional learning*.	The patient is encouraged to express directly what have been painful, unacknowledged, or suppressed feelings; the therapist's tacit or explicit acceptance of such feelings facilitates such expression. In addition, emotionally constricted patients are helped to express a wider range of feelings more directly in relationships, whereas emotionally labile patients are helped to contain affects or to delay expressing them until they are calmer. This domain of interpersonal psychotherapy techniques is particularly pertinent to what we call *mentalizing emotion*.
Clarification entails restructuring patients' material and providing them with feedback to enhance their awareness of what they are communicating.	Clarifications include rephrasing what a patient has said or asking the patient to do so; drawing the patient's attention to logical implications of what has been said; and calling attention to contradictions or contrasts that the patient has failed to notice. The process of clarification, ubiquitous in psychotherapy, entails negotiating meanings; accordingly, clarification makes the patient aware of what is in the therapist's mind, often with the effect that the patient must clarify what is in his or her mind so as to be adequately understood by the therapist. Hence the process of clarification requires active and reciprocal mentalizing effort on the part of the therapist.
Communication analysis enables the patient to learn to communicate more effectively by reviewing detailed accounts of problematic conversations with significant others.	In general, problems in communication stem from one or both partners' failure to correct distorted perceptions and faulty assumptions—in our terms, *mentalizing failures*. Communication failures often stem from lack of explicitness or clarity; indirect nonverbal communications often lead to mistaken assumptions about effectively having communicated something to the partner or having been understood properly by the partner. Therapists also focus on silences or other ways of closing off communication. All these interventions invite the patient to consider the partner's point of view and also promote self-awareness in the process.

TABLE 1–5.   MENTALIZING-PROMOTING INTERVENTIONS IN
INTERPERSONAL PSYCHOTHERAPY *(continued)*

Goal of intervention	Specific techniques and comments
Use of the therapeutic relationship is especially germane to interpersonal psychotherapy as a model for the impact of the patient's interpersonal style on others. In particular, the therapy relationship presents an opportunity to learn to express negative emotions forthrightly.	Patients are encouraged explicitly at the beginning of therapy to express whatever negative feelings might arise about the therapist or the therapeutic process. The expression of such feelings sets the stage for negotiating and for clarifying distorted perceptions and interpretations. This therapeutic process exemplifies what we call *mentalizing the transference*.

relatively quickly by a wide range of practitioners, that is, without the extraordinarily long apprenticeship that the practice of psychoanalysis required. Rogers also made a major contribution to the field of psychotherapy in being a strong voice for research on the process and, quite boldly, focusing on therapists' empathic characteristics in particular—indeed, researching what we could call their mentalizing capacities.

As we also do, Rogers (1951) downplayed the value of "verbalized insight" (p. 15) and focused instead on the therapist's skill, the relationship climate, and the interactive process. As is well known, the cornerstone of client-centered therapy is *empathy,* and the central intervention is *clarification:* "As material is given by the client, it is the therapist's function to help him recognize and clarify the emotions which he feels" (p. 27). All this requires mentalizing as we construe it:

> This formulation would state that it is the counselor's function to assume, in so far as he is able, the internal frame of reference of the client, to perceive the world as the client sees it, to perceive the client himself as he is seen by himself, to lay aside all perceptions from the external frame of reference while doing so, and to communicate something of this empathic understanding to the client. (p. 29)

Continuing in this vein, Rogers (1951) proposed that the therapist "must concentrate on one purpose only; that of providing deep understanding and acceptance of the attitudes consciously held at this moment by the client as he explores step by step into the dangerous areas which he has been denying to consciousness" (p. 30). Foreshadowing

Bowlby—and the patient who remarked that one wouldn't want to go into a scary mental place alone—Rogers recognized that this exploration of "dangerous areas" was made possible by the emotional warmth of the relationship, the therapist's acceptance of the client's experience, and the feeling of safety this relationship climate provides. Rogers also emphasized the importance of the therapist's attitude; consistent with a mentalizing stance, he advocated that empathic comments be conveyed with a sense of tentativeness, namely, "If I understand you correctly...." (p. 28).

Rogers countered the common misconception that his "nondirective" therapy entailed passivity on the part of the therapist; on the contrary, he emphasized the sheer *difficulty* of the therapist's task. One would be hard pressed to challenge Rogers' view that the capacity to empathize is the therapist's core skill—and empathy is a cornerstone of mentalizing (see Chapter 2, "Mentalizing"). Yet empathy is only one side of mentalizing—the other side being self-awareness, which is also central to the effective conduct of psychotherapy (as psychoanalysis brought to the fore in the context of countertransference).

To summarize, in client-centered psychotherapy, empathy is required to establish a relationship climate of security, to apprehend the client's experience from the client's perspective, and to communicate that awareness back to the client. In the process, the client also develops greater mentalizing capacity. Unsurprisingly, Rogers concluded that "the best therapeutic relationship may be related to good interpersonal relationships in general" (p. 53). From our standpoint, a secure attachment relationship that promotes mentalizing is indeed the best model for close relationships.

As we will explicate in this book, empathizing is not simple, and, as Rogers recognized, it is not easy. Mentalizing should not be equated, for example, with warm and compassionate sympathy. For example, in a state of obvious distress, a patient might tell her therapist that, the day before, she had inadvertently walked in on her husband while he was in their bed with another woman. With great tenderness, the therapist might say to the patient, "You must have felt terribly betrayed, hurt, and sad." This highly sympathetic response is a *nonmentalizing* intervention, to which the word "must" is a tip-off. The patient might legitimately respond indignantly: "No!! I was outraged and felt vindicated: I finally caught the lying bastard red-handed!" The therapist would have done better to maintain an inquisitive and curious mentalizing stance, not making assumptions. As we will discuss in detail in Chapter 3 ("Development"), attachment research is demonstrating that affect regulation stems from being accurately mentalized, not from warmth or benevolence alone. Perhaps we should visualize psycho-therapy as being less like lounging in a warm bath and more like swim-ming in a cool, crystal-clear lake. Warmth is easier; clarity is harder.

Thus, from a mentalizing perspective, accurate empathy in the Rog-erian sense is a necessary but insufficient basis for the stimulation of full mentalizing. The empathic and nondirective therapist creates a trusting milieu in which mentalizing can develop. Yet the therapist's empathic stance is only one component of a mentalizing stance and just the plat-form for a series of more active interventions that are necessary for mentalizing to flourish (see Chapter 6, "Mentalizing Interventions"). Our intermingling of more directive aspects of therapy, to promote mentalizing, with the traditional nondirective components is consistent with the burgeoning research literature suggesting that greater effec-tiveness is associated with more focused interventions (Roth and Fon-agy 2005).

Recapitulation

We construe the gist of mentalizing as attending to mental states—hold-ing mind in mind. Mentalizing pertains to self *and* others: mentalizing is part and parcel of self-awareness and is thus essential to self-regula-tion, including coping with strong emotions; mentalizing in relation to others is crucial for healthy interpersonal relationships, and especially for developing and maintaining secure attachment relationships. In ad-dition, we have argued that mentalizing is fundamental to *all* forms of psychotherapeutic treatment; ultimately, the success of any treatment will depend on the mentalizing capacity of both the patient and the therapist. Hence we also have acknowledged a catch-22: patients whose mentalizing capacities are significantly and consistently impaired will have difficulty making use of treatment; in such instances, particular focus on building mentalizing capacities will be crucial (e.g., see Chapter 9, "Borderline Personality Disorder").

Because it is fundamental to all forms of therapy, a treatment ap-proach that highlights mentalizing cannot be novel. Yet because it is of such fundamental importance, keen attention to mentalizing is war-ranted throughout mental health treatments. Accordingly, we believe that *therapists of all persuasions* can benefit from a solid understanding of mentalizing and, furthermore, that *patients* also can benefit from this understanding—*regardless of the type of treatment in which they are en-gaged*. We have written this book to promote such understanding.

While we claim no innovation, we believe that clinicians and pa-tients have much to gain from *refining* their understanding of mentalizing and its significance. Mentalizing may be commonplace, but it is not simple and it is not easy. We have noted that mentalizing is not an all-or-none phenomenon; it is a matter of degree. As we will discuss in the next chapter, mentalizing is not only a matter of degree but also a multifaceted concept, so we have much work yet to do in articulating its various facets. To take a common example, an individual might be more capable of mentalizing with respect to others than the self—or vice versa. Or an individual may be better able to mentalize in some emotional states or in some relationships than in others.

We have identified how the perspective of mentalizing can be applied to a wide range of therapeutic approaches beyond psychoanalysis, as illustrated by cognitive therapy, interpersonal psychotherapy, and client-centered therapy. Yet this book would be pointless if we were merely tossing a new concept into the mix. We believe that a focus on mentalizing is genuinely enriching by virtue of its foundation in developmental research and developmental psychopathology—the legacy of its origins in psychoanalysis and attachment theory (see Chapter 3, "Development"). To take one example, Rogers put empathizing center stage, but his work long antedated the developmental research now at our disposal that exemplifies just how one does this. Hence we can use our knowledge of developmental psychopathology to refine our understanding of the relationship conditions that inhibit and promote mentalizing; this developmental work is our best guide to facilitating mentalizing in treatment, regardless of the clinician's theoretical persuasion.

We also believe that our focus on mentalizing holds promise for refining our treatment efforts through research, as we are aspiring to do in different applications that will be summarized later in this book (Part II, "Practicing Mentalizing"). As Roth and Fonagy (2005) stated it, we are following the principle that "treatment should reflect what we know about the processes that directly bear on the onset and course of a clinical problem" (pp. 507–508). As we have just argued, knowledge of developmental processes is especially valuable in this regard, and this knowledge can be put to good use even in treatments that do not concentrate on childhood origins of current life problems. As Roth and Fonagy concluded from their review of the vast array of contemporary treatment research, "The promise of identifying key, mutative psychological processes is especially attractive given its potential to bring order to the current proliferation of therapeutic approaches, and to identify what is, or is not, both effective and common across orientations" (p. 508).

In sum, without desire to create another new brand of therapy, we construe focusing on mentalizing in treatment as a research-informed approach to providing essential *developmental help* (Fonagy and Target 1997a; Hurry 1998). From our perspective, as optimal development in secure attachment relationships does, successful mentalizing treatment accomplishes no less than *enhancing individuals' freedom to think and feel,* in solitude and in close relationships.

Key Clinical Points

- *Mentalizing* entails attending to mental states in oneself and others, coupled with the implicit or explicit awareness that these mental states are representations of reality from one of many possible perspectives.

- *Mentalizing interventions* aim to 1) encourage greater attention to mental states in self and others, 2) cultivate awareness of multiple perspectives, and 3) increase mentalizing capacity, especially under conditions of emotional arousal.

- *Mentalizing begets mentalizing* and non-mentalizing begets non-mentalizing. While endeavoring to improve patients' mentalizing, therapists must be equally attentive to their own mentalizing, and especially to mentalizing failures that unwittingly undermine patients' mentalizing.

- *Mentalizing is a common factor* in psychotherapeutic interventions. Different treatment modalities conducted from diverse theoretical orientations all can promote mentalizing and can do so best when clinicians are attentive to it in themselves and their patients. Mentalization-based treatment may be conceived as falling somewhere between traditional psychodynamic and cognitive-behavioral approaches.

PART I

Understanding Mentalizing

Chapter 2

Mentalizing

As readers might have begun to surmise, "mentalizing" reflects a variety of mental processes, and we begin this chapter by articulating its many facets. Then we contrast mentalizing with several related terms, in part to make the case that there is no other concept for mentalizing but *mentalizing*. Finally, because emotion is so central to mentalizing, we conclude the chapter with a discussion of mentalizing emotion.

Facets of Mentalizing

One point alone underscores the sheer complexity of mentalizing: in construing mentalizing as attending to "mental states," we are encompassing a huge territory of mental states, including everything ranging from ordinary phenomena like needs, desires, feelings, thoughts, beliefs, fantasies, and dreams to pathological processes such as panic attacks, dissociative states, hallucinations, and delusions. But this is just the beginning; Table 2–1 provides a quick overview of the various facets of mentalizing discussed next. Specifically, we will distinguish between mentalizing explicitly and implicitly, mentalizing in relation to self and others, and mentalizing in various time frames with varying scope. We will also consider two core mental processes involved in mentalizing—attention and imagination—along with their corresponding failures.

Explicit Versus Implicit

Much of what we clinicians encourage in psychotherapy is mentalizing explicitly, for example, putting feelings into words: "When she said that, I thought she was trying to one-up me, and it annoyed me." Explicit mentalizing is symbolic, and painting a picture or composing a song to represent a mental state—as one might do in art therapy—also would count as mentalizing explicitly. Typically, however, language is the medium of choice for explicit mentalizing, and much of mentalizing takes the form of narrative—stories. Holmes (1999) aptly construed psychotherapy as fostering a story-telling function, and he characterized psychological health as depending "on a dialectic between story-making and story-breaking, between the capacity to form narrative, and to disperse it in the light of new experience" (p. 59). At its best, explicit mentalizing is characterized by a combination of accuracy, richness, and flexibility. As the practice of psychotherapy attests, secure attachment is the wellspring for explicating mental states:

> secure attachment is marked by coherent stories that convince and hang together, where detail and overall plot are congruent, and where the teller is not so detached that affect is absent, is not dissociated from the content of the story, nor is so overwhelmed that feelings flow formlessly into every crevice of the dialogue. Insecure attachment, by contrast, is characterized either by stories that are overelaborated and enmeshed… or by dismissive, poorly fleshed-out accounts. (p. 58)

TABLE 2–1.   FACETS OF MENTALIZING

Facet	Aspects
Content of mental states	Needs, desires, feelings, thoughts, hallucinations, etc.
Level of representation	More explicit (narrative) versus more implicit (intuitive)
Object	Self versus others
Time frame	Past, present, or future
Scope	More narrow (present mental state) versus more broad (autobiographical context)

In the context of insecure attachment, Holmes (1999) distinguished three pathologies of narrative capacity, all of which reflect impairments in explicit mentalizing: "clinging to rigid stories; being overwhelmed by unstoried experience; or being unable to find a narrative strong enough to contain traumatic pain" (p. 59). As Holmes states, secure attachment is the key to fostering the narrative capacity required to heal from trauma (see Chapter 7, "Treating Attachment Trauma").

As the foregoing implies, explicit mentalizing is relatively conscious, deliberative, and reflective. But explicit mentalizing is the tip of the iceberg; predominantly, in interpersonal interactions, we mentalize implicitly—automatically and unreflectively. Empathizing, for example, entails to some degree non-consciously mirroring facial expressions and postures; if a therapist were to attempt to do this mirroring based on explicit reasoning, the result would be wooden and stilted. Turn taking in rapid-fire conversation also requires implicit mentalizing, as does perspective taking: we are rightly irritated when someone talks about another person we do not know without taking our ignorance into consideration and providing the needed context. Ideally, we take turns and keep others' perspectives in mind without needing to think explicitly about doing so, and the mental activity required to do this is mind-bogglingly complex (Barker and Givon 2005; Malle 2005).

The difference between mentalizing explicitly and implicitly is captured by a parallel distinction in the realm of memory (Eichenbaum 2002), namely, the distinction between declarative (explicit) and procedural (implicit) memory or, more simply, the difference between knowing *that* and knowing *how*. Explicit memory is what we need for passing the written part of the test for a driver's license; implicit memory is what we need for the driving test itself. Mentalizing implicitly is procedural know-how; mentalizing explicitly is what can be declared in symbolic form.

We construe implicit mentalizing as *intuition*, which Lieberman (2000) defines as "a phenomenological and behavioral correlate of knowledge obtained though implicit learning" (p. 110) and which includes "feelings, judgments, or hunches people have toward other social targets or situations that are often experienced in the absence of a well-articulated reason" (Satpute and Lieberman 2006, p. 89). Implicit learning is based on repeated exposure to patterns of stimuli associated with rewards; it takes place without awareness and without explicit knowledge of what has been learned, much less *how* it was learned. Intuition, grounded in implicit learning, is the basis of our ability to respond appropriately to nonverbal emotional communication, and much of this responsiveness also occurs outside of explicit awareness.

Our implicit-explicit distinction is solidly buttressed by findings in social cognitive neuroscience. Lieberman (2007) summarizes extensive evidence for a dual-process model of social cognition in which automatic-reflexive processes (e.g., emotional responses to subliminal perception of a threatening facial expression) can be differentiated from controlled-reflective processes (e.g., becoming aware of feeling threatened and, on reflection, interpreting the particular situation as being relatively benign). We will be discussing a number of brain regions implicated in different facets of mentalizing in Chapter 4 ("Neurobiology"); here we merely note that different brain regions are active in implicit and explicit mentalizing (Satpute and Lieberman 2006).

It is difficult to draw a bright line between implicit and explicit mentalizing, as it is hard to make a sharp distinction between what is intuitive and automatic and what is conscious and reflective. As we discussed in the Introduction (Chapter 1), Lecours and Bouchard (1997) described a hierarchy of mentalizing in terms of the degree of mental elaboration. Karmiloff-Smith (1992) made a similar point in her concept of *representational redescription:* "a process by which implicit information *in* the mind subsequently becomes explicit knowledge *to* the mind" (p. 18, emphasis in original). When we are mentalizing, we are continually moving back and forth between more implicit and more explicit processes. Typically, as long as matters proceed smoothly, we need not explicate. When something goes awry, however, mentalizing explicitly is in order—as when we become puzzled by our own behavior or someone else's: "How could I have done that?"; "What could she have been thinking?"

As the work of psychotherapy exemplifies, we engage patients in mentalizing explicitly for the sake of interpersonal and intrapersonal problem solving. Engaging in explicit mentalizing exploits the more general phenomenon of the adaptive function of consciousness. Implicit mentalizing, being in the realm of the mental, is a conscious process but reflects what has been called lower-level consciousness, that is, basic awareness. In contrast, explicit mentalizing entails higher-order consciousness, which entails self-awareness (Edelman 1989). Higher-order consciousness allows us to cope with novelty and to engage in flexible problem solving (Baars 1988).

Engaged in "talk therapy," we clinicians and our patients are self-consciously attending to mentalizing explicitly; we are routinely making the less conscious more conscious by mentalizing. Yet we should not construe psychotherapy as solely devoted to explication. On the contrary: we also employ explicit processes (higher-order consciousness) to draw attention to the implicit domain, most importantly, attending to feelings in oneself and others, with the intention that this attentiveness will become increasingly automatic and intuitive as reflective processes gradually become transformed into reflexive processes (Satpute and Lieberman 2006). As Karmiloff-Smith (1992) stated, development proceeds both ways, from implicit to explicit and vice versa:

> Development and learning, then, seem to take two complementary directions. On the one hand, they involve the gradual process of proceduralization (that is, rendering behavior more automatic and less accessible). On the other hand, they involve a process of "explication" and increasing accessibility (that is, representing explicitly information that is implicit in the procedural representations sustaining the structure of behavior). Both are relevant to cognitive change. (p. 17)

Self Versus Others

Admittedly, in combining mentalizing implicitly and explicitly with mentalizing in relation to self and others, we encompass an extremely wide territory of mental activity. Plainly, adaptation requires both self-awareness and other-awareness; as we discuss in this section, there are fundamental similarities that justify applying "mentalizing" to both domains as well as important differences between them.

In individual psychotherapy, we tend to highlight self-awareness, or mentalizing the self; yet, given the pervasive focus of psychotherapy on relationships, we frequently promote mentalizing of others (e.g., "What do you think he might have been feeling after you said that?"). We consider this dual, self-other focus to be a major clinical advantage of the concept of mentalizing as contrasted, for example, with empathizing: the double aspect helps us to keep in mind the necessity to balance our therapeutic attention between self and others, with the balance varying according to the domain of the patient's greatest difficulty at a given moment. Couples therapy, family therapy, and group therapy provide a natural forum for promoting mentalizing in relation to others; and transference focus in individual psychotherapy also does so, for example, in examining the patient's perceptions of what the therapist is feeling (see Chapter 6, "Mentalizing Interventions").

The basis of our capacity to mentalize others has occupied philosophers for centuries as the problem of knowing the existence of other minds (Stueber 2006); it has concerned psychologists in recent decades largely under the rubric of "theory of mind" (Goldman 2006; Malle 2004), which we will discuss in the next section of this chapter. Through developmental research, psychology has made an enormous contribution to the problem of how we come to know other minds, as we will discuss in Chapter 3 ("Development"). In this section, we focus on the equally challenging problem of how we know our own mind—mentalizing the self. This discussion will rely heavily on philosopher Richard Moran's (2001) insightful work on self-knowledge, which gets to the crux of how we promote mentalizing—and how we can unwittingly undermine it—in psychotherapy. We will discuss the initial development of a mentalized sense of self later; in this section, we are concerned with the ongoing elaboration of the self through mentalizing. First, however, we state our rationale for applying the same term, "mentalizing," to self and others.

We are able to mentalize in relation to self and others on the basis of our fundamental like-mindedness. As Moran (2001) cogently argued, "Terms that describe some state of mind must be applicable without change of meaning…in the first-person and third-person cases" (p. 160). We understand a belief as being true or false whether I hold it or you hold it. We understand shame as being a response to social transgression whether I feel it or you feel it. Crucially, as we will discuss later, our like-mindedness is grounded in the intrinsically interpersonal nature of our mental development, the social basis of our like-mindedness. The social basis of mentalizing also ensures that we apply similar mental state concepts and language to self and others. Notably, evidence from neuroscience, which we will discuss at greater length in Chapter 4 ("Neurobiology"), also implies some uniformity in mentalizing with regard to self and others, at least insofar as overlapping brain areas are implicated. Lieberman (2007), for example, distinguishes between internally focused and externally focused processes in interpreting the behavior of self and others. *Internally focused* processes entail attention to the "interior psychological worlds" of self and others, whereas *externally focused* processes entail attention to "external, physical, and most often visual characteristics of other individuals, oneself, or the interaction of the two" (p. 18.21). Gross patterns of brain activation do not vary as a function of directing attention to self versus others but rather as a function of directing attention to the inner versus the outer world: internal focus, whether directed to self or others, is associated with greater activation in a medial frontoparietal network; whereas external focus directed to self or others is associated with greater activation in a lateral frontotemporoparietal network. Yet, notwithstanding the self-other overlap, the means by which we acquire self-knowledge and knowledge of others sometimes differs profoundly in a way that bears directly on the conduct of mentalizing-focused psychotherapy.

Moran recognizes that no source of self-knowledge is infallible, as a century of psychoanalytic practice attests. Given this caveat, he usefully distinguishes two forms self-knowledge, objective and subjective, reflecting the third-person versus first-person perspectives. Our knowledge of other minds—employing our theory-of-mind ability to mentalize others—is based on observation and inference. We observe behavior (opening the refrigerator) and infer mental states (intending to obtain food to assuage hunger). These theory-of-mind abilities also can be employed to acquire knowledge about the *self* from a third-person perspective, for example, by reflecting on the meaning of behavior and drawing inferences about the self (e.g., noticing that you are trembling and talking faster than usual and inferring on that basis that you must be more anxious than you had realized).

Here we are concerned not only with the overlap between mentalizing others and the self from the objective, third-person perspective but also with the way in which mentalizing the self from the subjective, first-person perspective is a radically different process. This difference has considerable therapeutic import: mentalizing the self from the objective perspective tends to be relatively shallow, whereas mentalizing from the subjective perspective comprises mentalizing in the fullest sense. Moran (2001) aptly titled one of his chapters "Making up Your Mind." Ideally, in our view, mentalizing in psychotherapy entails making up one's mind—actively constructing it. This phrase captures the early psychoanalytic spirit of the concept as we discussed it in Chapter 1 ("Introduction"): mental*izing* entails transforming the non-mental into the mental and, beyond this, mental elaboration. We might picture mentalizing as a flowering of mental activity that makes up the mind.

We begin the subjective-objective contrast by elaborating the objective form of self-knowledge that parallels knowledge of others, what Moran calls *attributional* knowledge of oneself. As Moran explicated, you can know yourself as if from a third-person perspective, akin to the way you know others. That is, you can acquire self-knowledge as a spectator—through perception, evidence, and inference—in short, by examining the facts. For example, despite your current fervent desire to quit smoking, you might be pessimistic about your prospects for doing so, given your empirical knowledge of your multiple failed attempts to do so in the past. More germane to our clinical concerns, consider the following scenario:

> A patient in psychodynamic psychotherapy is reflecting on her increasing feeling of social isolation. She is talking about a friend whom she "absolutely adores" and yet seems to be avoiding, about which she is starting to feel guilty. She mentions how her friend has been "really stressed out" for quite some time and has been asking the patient to do a lot of "favors" for her, some of which have been extremely inconvenient for the patient to do.

The psychotherapist infers that the relationship has become one-sided and that the patient—whom the psychotherapist knows to be characteristically self-sacrificing—is being exploited and is becoming resentful. Accordingly, the psychotherapist gives the patient an intellectually compelling interpretation about her resentment, which the psychotherapist believes the patient to be repressing. In response, the patient merely shrugs and says, "You must be right," then immediately changes the subject. With persistence on the part of the therapist, the patient might come to *believe* the interpretation on the sheer strength of the evidence that the psychotherapist marshals, even though she cannot *feel* her resentment.

Would such an interpretation be of any help? In believing that she is resentful without feeling the resentment, the patient would be taking a theoretical or speculative stance toward her state of mind, *attributing* it to herself without making up her own mind about it. The patient's putative resentment would remain impersonal and alien—unmentalized or, perhaps, mentalized in a relatively shallow way. No doubt, objective external data, much of which is accessible to others as well as ourselves, comprise an important domain of our self-knowledge. Yet, as the example of repressed resentment illustrates, without the first-person subjective perspective, something radical can be missing.

As Moran explains, in addition to objective self-knowledge, we also have immediate and transparent self-knowledge that is *not* based on perception, inference, or evidence. An acquaintance who lends you money and asks for assurance that you will repay it will not be reassured if you reply on the basis of objective evidence, as if from a third-person perspective, "I believe I'll pay you back, because I have typically paid back my debts in the past." Your acquaintance wants a commitment, not an evidence-based prediction. You must make up your mind about it, in the course of which you would know your own mind.

How does one mentalize in this fullest, subjective sense of mentalizing? Our commonsense notion of introspection—looking inside—is misleading here. Moran (2001) argues that we should avoid "a picture of self-knowledge as a kind of mind-reading as applied to oneself, a faculty that happens to be aimed in one direction rather than another" (p. 91). Mindreading is too easy. Mentalizing fully entails the exercise of agency in the form of hard mental work: deliberating, considering, reflecting, debating, and deciding—often in emotionally fraught mental territory that entails elaborating and grappling with conflicts. Taking seriously the idea of making up one's mind, we might think of mentalizing as self-discovery through the process of self-creation. From this perspective, your mental life is partly self-constituted; in making up your mind about how you feel, you influence how you feel: "for someone to interpret his own response as, say, either righteous indignation or as mere peevishness *constitutes* his state as being of a different kind" (Moran 2001, p. 38, emphasis in original).

Counterintuitively, as Moran explains, in knowing your own mind, you often look outward, not inward. To varying degrees, your knowledge about your attitudes, beliefs, feelings, commitments and such stems from the intentionality of mental states as described in Chapter 1 ("Introduction"); mental states are *about* something. You know what you believe not by introspection but rather by attending to the object of your belief. You determine if you believe it is raining not by introspection but by looking out the window. You know what you feel by attending to what your feelings are about—the jammed garage door that prevents you from getting to work on time. You judge the level of your commitment to repay the loan on the basis of the reasons you have for following through, not least, that you have promised to do so:

> a person may have a purely predictive basis for knowing what he will do, but in the normal situation of free action it is on the basis of his decision that he knows what he is about to do. In deciding what to do, his gaze is directed "outward," on the considerations in favor of some course of action, on what he has most reason to do. Thus his stance toward the question, "What am I going to do now?" is transparent to a question about what he is *to do*, answered by the "outward-looking" consideration of what is good, desirable, or feasible to do. (Moran 2001, p. 105, emphasis in original)

Again, acquiring self-knowledge from the subjective perspective is self-constructive; self-awareness and a sense of ownership are inherent in the process of coming to believe and to feel. Alternatively, idle verbalizing of intellectual insights—attributions from the third-person perspective—is indicative of mentalizing only in the most superficial sense. Moran (2001) characterizes the therapeutically "educated neurotic" as someone who can "confidently ascribe some repressed attitude to himself" (p. 86). Yet he adds:

> clearly something is wrong if he cannot consciously avow the…attitude and can only ascribe it to himself on the evidence.…it would still make sense to say that the original attitude of resentment remains *under repression*, even with the person's own ability to report on it…. What's missing, on this view, is the person's *endorsement* of the attitude he ascribes to himself, the ordinary ability to declare oneself. (p. 86) [Moran continues, pointing out] the crucial therapeutic difference between the merely "intellectual" acceptance of an interpretation, which will itself normally be seen as a form of resistance, and the process of working-through that leads to a fully internalized acknowledgement of some attitude which

make a felt difference to the rest of the analysand's mental life. This goal of treatment, however, requires that the attitude in question be knowable by the person, not through a process of theoretical self-interpretation but by avowal of how one thinks and feels. (pp. 89–90, emphasis in original)

To summarize, we construe the self-constituting agency manifested in making up one's mind as mentalizing the self in the fullest sense. Moving from a third-person "intellectual insight" to a first-person "emotional insight" is what we will call in the final section of this chapter *mentalizing emotion*. The intellectual insight of the "educated neurotic" is what we will call *pseudo-mentalizing* or mentalizing in the pretend mode. Thus we characterize a therapist's merely explaining how a patient's mind is working as a non-mentalizing intervention (see Chapter 6, "Mentalizing Interventions").

If they lead only to unmentalized self-attributions, psychotherapeutic interpretations of unconscious mental contents can be harmful, abetting self-alienation. Fonagy and colleagues (2002a) have shown how a distorted third-person perspective on the self, whether internalized from parents or psychotherapists, can lead to an unintegrated alien presence in the self—a self-alienating process that Moran calls *estrangement*. In contrast, psychotherapists can help patients literally make up their own mind through mentalizing, for example, by making the preconscious more fully and transparently conscious, taking ownership, and *changing what they actually think and feel* in the process. This is what we mean by mentalizing in the sense of mental elaboration, and Moran's discussion underscores the patient's active role in the process. Agency is essential to therapy: in making up one's mind, one changes one's mind, and vice versa.

Time Frame and Scope

Predominantly, mentalizing—whether in relation to self or others—pertains to the present, that is, to current mental states. Interactions with others and self-regulation depend on mentalizing in the present. Yet, as much of psychotherapy exemplifies, making sense of past mental states also can be helpful, given the not infrequent superiority of hindsight. For example, patients can benefit from reflecting on their own mental states that led up to impulsively self-destructive behavior or on both parties' mental states in an interaction that led to a blowup. In psychotherapy we term this process a "Rewind and Explore," that is, going back to the point at which mentalizing was lost. Of course, the value of such reflection is to transform hindsight into foresight, that is, to learn from the past so as to become more skillful in the future in mentalizing with respect to current mental states in oneself and others.

In addition, we can mentalize in relation to the future, endeavoring to anticipate, for example, how a spouse might respond to a proposed separation. We also mentalize in relation to the future in anticipating our own mental states (e.g., thinking about how we will feel if we do something), although our capacity to do so accurately is more limited than we generally assume (Gilbert et al. 2002)—especially when, from a relatively calm state, we are predicting how we will respond in an emotional state (Van Boven and Loewenstein 2005).

The narrowest scope of mentalizing would be to focus on a state of mind at a given moment: "What I just said seems to puzzle you; what are you thinking?" Yet in psychotherapy, we often strive to expand the scope of mentalizing beyond a given moment, articulating the intrapsychic and interpersonal surround of current mental contents. We expand on mental states by articulating reasons for beliefs, feelings, and actions. We also expand on a particular emotional state by exploring the possibility of other feelings—for example, looking for resentment in the background of guilt feelings or thinking about the possibility of fear in the background of anger. Indeed, the therapeutic question "And *what else* did you feel?" is often appropriate in a wide range of contexts. Yet in making this inquiry, we therapists must maintain our own mentalizing abilities and understand not just what is in or on the patient's mind but also his or her current mentalizing capacity and state of mind. Thus, when our patients answer that they felt nothing else, they might be exemplifying their limited current capacity to reflect and not their state of mind at the time of the events they are describing. They might be able to mentalize the moment but not expand within a wider time frame, and only when their state of mind changes (e.g., when they feel safer in the relationship) will they be able to reflect more extensively.

Emotions and the stories surrounding them are layered, and emotionally significant events often have a narrative that extends deeply into the whole autobiography. Using the metaphor of the autobiography, Wittgenstein alluded to how little we know from a momentary state of mind: "Even if I were now to hear everything that he is saying to himself, I would know as little what his words were referring to as if I read *one* sentence in the middle of a story" (quoted in Monk 2005, p. 105, emphasis in original). Indeed, we only understand current mental states—our own or others'—in contexts of varying degrees of breadth. Much of what we do in psychotherapy is in the service of expanding the context—in effect, going from one sentence to the broader autobiographical story, gradually developing a multifaceted representation that symbolically links the experience to an ever-expanding personal understanding.

Mental Processes and Mentalizing Failures

In clinical practice, we prefer the verb "mentalizing" to the noun "mentalization," so as to emphasize the *activity:* mentalizing is mental action, something we *do,* more or less skillfully or artfully (Allen 2003). Further underscoring the sheer complexity of mentalizing at implicit and explicit levels, numerous cognitive operations come into play—for example, perceiving, recognizing, responding, mirroring, remembering, interpreting, and explaining. Here we focus on two important domains of cognitive activity in mentalizing: attention and imagination, and we consider common failures of mentalizing in relation to these two mental processes.

Attention and Imagination

From an evolutionary perspective, de Waal (2006) observed:

> Responsiveness to the behavioral states of conspecifics ranges from a flock of birds taking off all at once because one among them is startled by a predator to a mother ape who returns to a whimpering youngster to help it from one tree to the next by draping her body as a bridge between the two. (p. 25)

From such observations, de Waal concluded: "The *selection pressure on paying attention to others* must have been enormous" (p. 25; emphasis added).

We cannot overstate the role of attention in mentalizing—which we define most briefly as attending to mental states—and much of what we clinicians do in psychotherapy or psychoeducation is intended to influence attention. Insofar as mentalizing is mental action, attention provides our main leverage. Implicitly or explicitly, we are continually urging our patients to *pay attention* to what they or others are doing, thinking, and feeling: a psychotherapist's raised eyebrow can be a subtle exhortation to pay attention to the import of what one just said, to think about it and to elaborate—in short, to mentalize.

As Fonagy (2006) has highlighted, often enough, mentalizing is not easy; as Posner and Rothbart (1998) characterized it, it requires *effortful control* of attention. We capture the effortful nature of mentalizing in the metaphor of "pushing the pause button" in the throes of unbearable emotional states by becoming self-aware for the sake of emotion regulation and constructive coping (Allen 2005). Yet effortful control is essential in accurate mentalizing in a more subtle and pervasive way. Our default mode in interpreting others' mental states is egocentrism: unthinkingly, we assume that others share our perspective, knowledge, and attitudes (Decety 2005). Here is a humbling perspective: "the egocentrism observed in three-year-old children and in individuals with frontal brain damage is also present in normal adults" (Barr and Keysar 2005, p. 273). Alternatively, we can take the easy road by stereotyping (Ames 2005). Thus, to consider another person's different point of view requires *effort:* inhibiting the egocentric or stereotypical perspective, attending to another perspective, and juggling different perspectives in working memory; these are cognitive executive functions.

Accordingly, developmentalists debate whether mentalizing capacities depend on executive functions (Moses 2005) or vice versa (Perner and Lang 2000); plainly, the two are intertwined. Mentalizing is mental work: in mentalizing, for example, we must remain aware that thinking and feeling something does not make it so. Bogdan (2005) aptly termed this implicit awareness "a *mental* sense of self-representingness" (p. 203, emphasis in original). Hence in the mentalizing mode, we have at least an implicit sense that the world is not necessarily as we experience it to be and, not infrequently, we must work actively at this distinction ("Is this true, or just my imagination?"). Thus, in mentalizing we reappraise our experience, and psychotherapy fosters this capacity for reappraisal.

Given the relation between attention and mentalizing as well as the relation between attachment and mentalizing, it is worth noting that attachment and attention are directly related: stress impairs attention, and attachment regulates stress. Moreover, as we will discuss in Chapter 3 ("Development"), joint attention between infants and caregivers plays a pivotal role in mentalizing, and research demonstrates a link between secure attachment and attention in childhood. Belsky and Fearon, for example, observed a specific link between early attachment relationships and the organization of attentional systems (Belsky and Fearon 2002; Fearon and Belsky 2004). Their study of nearly 1,000 children showed a positive relationship between quality of infant-mother attachment at 14 months and attentional performance on a Continuous Performance Test at 54 months. Relative to their insecure counterparts, children with secure attachment appeared to be protected from the effects of cumulative social contextual risk (and male gender) on attentional performance. Other research also links attachment to attention. For example, infants with disorganized attachment show difficulty coordinating their social attention in interactions with their caregiver (Schlomerich et al. 1997), and cocaine-exposed children showing disor-

ganized attachment with their mother at 12 months demonstrate exceptional dysfunctions of social attention coordination—dysfunctions that
are generalized insofar as they are evident in interactions not only with
the attachment figure but also with experimenters (Claussen et al.
2002). Finally, severe problems in attention have been observed in late-
adopted Romanian orphans with profound attachment disorganization
(Chugani et al. 2001; Kreppner et al. 2001).

Imagination is also central to mentalizing, although we are challenged to play with possibilities imaginatively while also grounding
our imaginings in reality (Allen 2006b). As we will discuss later in this
chapter, empathy requires not only a relatively automatic emotional resonance but also active imagination that draws on memory, as one brings
to mind relevant experiences evocative of pertinent feelings. More generally, entertaining different perspectives on what another person might
believe, think, and feel requires imaginative activity. Indeed, even entertaining different perspectives on one's own emotions requires imagination. In psychotherapy, for example, we invite patients to imagine what
else they might have felt in a given situation if they had allowed themselves to do so (e.g., feeling frightened in addition to feeling angry).

Mentalizing Failures and Costs

Broadly, mentalizing can be impaired in three different ways: one can fail
to mentalize; one can mentalize in a flawed or distorted fashion; and one
can misuse mentalizing, for example, to manipulate, exploit, or torment
others (Sharp 2006). We address the first two impairments here and the
third in the context of psychopathy (see Chapter 4, "Neurobiology").

Failing to mentalize not only involves a failure to attend to mental
states but also may involve an unwillingness or inability to engage in
the imaginative activity required. Fonagy and colleagues (1997c) give a
striking example from their interview measure of mentalizing capacity
(reflective functioning): "*Interviewer:* Why do you think your parents
behaved as they did? *Subject:* How do you expect me to know? You tell
me, you are the psychologist!" (p. 17). Here is a glaring instance of lack
of imaginative capacity: "*Interviewer:* Do you think your childhood experiences have influenced you in any way? *Subject:* I can't think of anything... What I learnt from my childhood experiences? Nothing that I
can think of at the moment" (p. 20).

Yet mentalizing also can go awry when imagination is unrestrained,
as paranoid processes best illustrate. Through paranoid projections—
at worst, demonizing—perceptions and interpretations of others' intentions can be grossly distorted yet treated as utterly real. At a less

flagrantly distorted level, depressive thinking notoriously skews perceptions and interpretations of others' mental states as well as one's own (Beck et al. 1979). A striking example of depressive thinking prompted us to introduce a new colloquialism for distorted mentalizing into the lexicon. The senior author and his family went to see the movie *Sideways,* and all were captivated by a scene in which one of the main characters, Miles (Paul Giamatti), is bemoaning his failure to get his novel published; even his agent has given up on him. Sitting under a bridge with his cohort, he laments: "Half my life is over and I have nothing to show for it—Nothing!" He muses about his insignificance: "I'm a thumbprint on the window of a skyscraper." Then the line that grabbed our collective attention: "I'm a smudge of excrement on a tissue surging out to sea with a million tons of raw sewage!" Reflecting on this memorable line during the drive home from the movie, the author's daughter, Yvonne Allen (a speech and language pathologist), declared that Miles was *excrementalizing*—mentalizing, but doing a crappy job of it. Patients readily grasp the point when we use this term to capture distorted mentalizing, particularly in the context of trashing oneself in depressive states.

The phenomenon of distorted or inapt mentalizing relates to a common question: can one mentalize too much? Often when patients raise this question in psychoeducational groups (Haslam-Hopwood et al. 2006), they are confusing mentalizing with rumination, a decidedly unproductive form of self-focused thinking (Nolen-Hoeksema 2000). Yet there is another form of excessive mentalizing, namely, hypervigilance about mental states. Such hypervigilance might arise, for example, from a child's alertness to the possibility of a parent's abusive behavior or from the child's persistent efforts to cheer up a parent who is continually on the brink of lapsing into a depressive mood. As we will note in Chapter 3 ("Development"), one of the main benefits of a secure attachment relationship is the opportunity to *relax* mentalizing, inasmuch as the feeling of security obviates the need to mentalize.

We should also introduce a caveat that, as much as we advocate it, accurate mentalizing is not always to the obvious advantage of the mentalizer. Ickes and colleagues (2005) offer the truism, "sometimes the truth hurts" (p. 310). These researchers marshal evidence that empathic accuracy stabilizes close relationships when the partner is engaged in benevolent and non-threatening thinking and feeling. On the other hand, when one's partner is thinking and feeling in ways that potentially threaten the relationship (e.g., feeling romantically attracted to someone else), accurate empathy can destabilize the relationship. As Ickes and colleagues put it,

According to our model, when relationship partners enter a situation, each individual first determines whether the current situation is likely to present a *danger zone* for the relationship. The danger zones for relationships are insights that would threaten the relationship if the individual perceivers accurately inferred their partner's actual relationship-threatening thoughts and feelings in that particular situation. (Ickes et al. 2005, p. 312, emphasis in original)

In such contexts, switching off mentalizing or, as Ickes and colleagues put it, "motivated inaccuracy," might serve to preserve the relationship. The alternative, as the authors state, is being "sadder but wiser" (p. 316). The notion that mentalizing can be painful will hardly be lost on psychotherapists; helping patients mentalize in emotionally painful contexts is precisely what our clinical work often entails, and some sense of security in the *treatment* relationship—itself fostered by mentalizing—is essential for this work to take place.

Thus we might construe psychotherapy as countering mentalizing failures by directing attention, promoting flexible thinking, and encouraging imagination, while aspiring to keep the imaginative thinking grounded in reality. Psychotherapy, by involving another mind in the person of the therapist, also promotes objectivity and thus restrained imagination—for example, by questioning emotionally skewed interpretations and, most importantly, by encouraging direct communication (e.g., "Perhaps instead of assuming that you know what she is thinking, you might ask her to clarify what she meant by that statement"). Of course, becoming sadder but wiser is always a possible outcome. To reiterate: mentalizing may be basic to our human nature, but it is anything but simple, easy, and painless.

Overlapping Terms

Inasmuch it is fundamental to our humanity, what we are calling mentalizing can hardly be a novel concept. Fittingly, many terms have been employed to cover various aspects of this territory, although none has exactly the same boundaries as mentalizing. In the first part of this chapter, we have begun to clarify the complex concept of mentalizing by delineating its various facets. Here we continue to clarify mentalizing by articulating its relations to similar concepts, addressing the frequently asked question, "How does mentalizing differ from...?" More importantly, the rich scholarly work conducted under the rubrics of these related terms will serve to illuminate what we are calling mentalizing. Table 2–2 provides a glimpse of the array of overlapping terms and the distinguishing features of mentalizing that we discuss next.

Mindblindness

The concept of mentalizing can be sharpened by contrast with its antithesis, *mindblindness*, a term Baron-Cohen (1995) introduced to highlight the core deficit in autism:

> Imagine what your world would be like if you were aware of physical things but were blind to the existence of mental things. I mean, of course, blind to things like thoughts, beliefs, knowledge, desires, and intentions, which for most of us self-evidently underlie behavior. Stretch your imagination to consider what sense you could make of human action (or, for that matter, any animate action whatsoever) if, as for a behaviorist, a mentalistic explanation was forever beyond your limits. (p. 1)

Autism entails relatively stable mindblindness of varying degrees of severity, stemming from neurobiological impairment (see Chapter 4, "Neurobiology"). Yet we can usefully stretch the term "mindblindness" to encompass the functional, context-dependent, transient impairments

TABLE 2–2. DIFFERENTIATING "MENTALIZING" FROM OVERLAPPING TERMS

Term	Distinctions
Mentalizing	Attending to mental states in self and others, and interpreting behavior accordingly
Mindblindness	Antithesis of mentalizing; employed originally to characterize autism
Mindreading	Applies to others and focuses on cognition
Theory of mind	Focuses on cognitive development and provides a conceptual framework for mentalizing
Metacognition	Focuses primarily on cognition in the self
Reflective functioning	Operationalizes the general level of mentalizing
Mindfulness	Focuses on the present and is not limited to mental states
Empathy	Focuses on others and emphasizes emotional states
Emotional intelligence	Pertains to the mentalizing of emotion in self and others
Psychological mindedness	Characterizes the disposition to mentalize, broadly defined
Insight	Mental content that is the product of the mentalizing process

of mentalizing associated with developmental psychopathology. All of us, to varying degrees, are prone to *dynamic mindblindness* under some circumstances (Allen 2006b).

> On the eve of discharge from an inpatient program for treatment of trauma, depression, and substance abuse, Anne came into her final psychotherapy session saying she had just had a "bizarre" interaction with her father over the telephone. In the previous two weeks, she had been working productively on establishing boundaries with him, telling him directly when she felt he was being overly controlling of her actions, and he had responded thoughtfully to her self-assertion. Importantly, she was able to see his point of view and to address his concerns. Just prior to the session, however, he had warned her sternly about staying away from her friend who had been engaging in criminal activities that had contributed to Anne's arrest for drug possession.
>
> Anne came to the session infuriated by her father's "totally inappropriate" and "controlling" behavior, and she gave numerous justifications for seeing her friend immediately after discharge. She was unable to attend to the basis of her father's concern, or of her own insistence on reconnecting with her friend immediately. As the therapist explored the history of Anne's relationship with her friend, its potential grave dangers and the reasons for her father's alarm came to light. Moreover, Anne was able to recognize the hostile defiance in her impulsive inclination to see her friend. Furthermore, she was able to see some basis for her current hostility toward her father in her adolescent relationship with him as well as recognize that her self-destructiveness had roots in her identification with her mother's long history of reckless behavior.

Anne, who was typically highly reflective even in the midst of emotional states, had become temporarily mindblind with respect to her father and her own motivation; in the course of the session, she was able to mentalize. Notably, however, in initially identifying the interaction as "bizarre" and presenting it for discussion, she demonstrated some nascent mentalizing capacity, which the therapy then cultivated.

Mindreading

In Baron-Cohen's (1995) terms, mindblindness is a failure of *mindreading,* which is "simply the best way to make sense of the actions of others" (p. 21). Baron-Cohen articulated various components of the "mindreading system" in his modular conception of the development of theory of mind, a line of research that we will describe in the next subsection. The term "mindreading" is used throughout the theory-of-mind literature (Ames 2005; Barr and Keysar 2005) to refer to "the human activity of inferring other people's mental states" (Malle 2005, p. 26). Notably, in his fine synthesis of the theory-of-mind literature, Goldman (2006) explicitly uses the terms "mindreading" and "mentalizing" interchangeably. Yet mentalizing differs from mindreading in two respects: first, mentalizing pertains to self as well as others, whereas mindreading is used in relation to others; second, as Baron-Cohen (2005) observed, mindreading implicitly leaves out emotion, which is a central facet of mentalizing. Perhaps in conjunction with its connotations of mental telepathy, we often caution patients about "mindreading" (i.e., as evidenced in distorted interpretations of others' mental states based on unquestioned assumptions). Thus we might think of mentalizing as *mindreading with caution,* tempered by the stance of open-mindedness and inquisitiveness.

Theory of Mind

We examined the roots of mentalizing in attachment theory in Chapter 1 ("Introduction"); here we consider its equally deep roots in developmental psychology under the rubric of "theory of mind"—ironically, a phrase first introduced into the literature in the context of understanding social cognition in chimpanzees (Premack and Woodruff 1978). This domain of research has been teasing out the process and the steps by which infants and young children come to an understanding of mental states and their relation to behavior—the territory of mentalizing. Although we will be considering development more broadly in the next chapter, here we will capture the highlights of theory-of-mind research, which focuses largely on *cognitive* development pertinent to mentalizing. Much of the impetus for developing theories of theory-of-mind acquisition stems from efforts to understand autism, where the failure to develop a theory of mind is most conspicuous (Baron-Cohen et al. 2000).

The hallmark of having developed a full-fledged theory of mind in childhood is passing false-belief tests (Wimmer and Perner 1983); accordingly, Sharp (2006) dubbed this developmental milestone "theory-of-mind graduation day" (p. 105). A child's capacity to interpret relevant behavior as based on false beliefs is of monumental importance in signifying his or her explicit comprehension of the representational nature of mental states (Perner 1991). Here is the critical exam:

> Maxi is helping his mother to unpack the shopping bag. He puts the chocolate into the GREEN cupboard. Maxi remembers exactly where he put the chocolate so that he can come back later and get some. Then he leaves for the playground. In his absence his mother needs some chocolate. She takes the chocolate out of the GREEN cupboard and uses some of it for her cake. Then she puts it back not into the GREEN but into the BLUE cupboard. She leaves to get some eggs and Maxi returns from the playground, hungry.
>
> *Test Question:* "Where will Maxi look for the chocolate?" (Perner 1991, p. 179)

Children who have failed to develop a representational theory of mind will equate Maxi's beliefs with their own knowledge of the situation; they will answer that Maxi will look in the blue cupboard. Children who have acquired a theory of mind will infer that Maxi falsely believes that the chocolate remains in the green cupboard and will expect him to look there. As measured by this criterion, most children fail before age three and most pass by age four (Wellman and Lagattuta 2000). Of course, theory of mind does not spring forth *de novo* at age four (Baron-Cohen et al. 2005; Wellman and Lagattuta 2000), and research on nonverbal forms of false-belief tasks that do not rely on explicit (linguistic) mentalizing indicate that 15-month-old infants implicitly distinguish between true and false beliefs as determinants of behavior (Onishi and Baillargeon 2005).

Theory-of-mind research addresses not only the development of mentalizing capacities but also the psychological processes that enable us to mentalize in adulthood—as we conduct psychotherapy, for example. Researchers have proposed contrasting theories to account for the development and employment of theory of mind; Table 2–3 provides an overview of the three main contenders: modularity theory, theory-theory, and simulation theory.

According to *modularity theory,* theory of mind develops from the sequential articulation of various component brain-based competencies (modules). Baron-Cohen (1995), for example, distinguished four modules: 1) an Intentionality Detector (ID) as "a perceptual device that interprets motion stimuli in terms of the primitive volitional mental states of goal and desire" (p. 32); 2) an Eye-Direction Detector (EDD) that "detects the presence of eyes or eye-like stimuli...computes whether eyes are directed toward it or toward something else, and...infers from its own case that if another organism's eyes are directed at something then that organism sees that thing" (pp. 38–39); 3) a Shared-Attention Mechanism (SAM) that builds up triadic representations that "specify the relations among an Agent, the Self, and a (third) object" (p. 44); and, finally, 4) a Theory-of-Mind Mechanism (ToMM), namely, "a system for inferring the full range of mental states from behavior.... It has the dual function of representing the set of epistemic mental states and turning all this mentalistic knowledge into a useful theory" (p. 51) (Baron-Cohen 1995; Baron-Cohen and Swettenham 1996). More recently, Baron-Cohen (2005) recognized the need to incorporate emotionality into his modularity view, and he added two more modules: The Emotion Detector (TED), which represents affective states, and The Empathizing SyStem (TESS), which mediates an appropriate emotional response to the perception of emotion in others along with motivation

TABLE 2–3.   THEORIES OF THEORY-OF-MIND DEVELOPMENT

Theory	Propositions
Modularity theory	Theory-of-mind abilities develop sequentially from the activity of a set of innate cognitive modules, each of which mediates a component capacity (e.g., detecting intentional behavior and direction of eye gaze, sharing attention and, ultimately, constructing a theory of behavior on the basis of mental representations).
Theory theory	Being empiricists akin to scientists or natural psychologists, children develop a set of mental-state concepts and learn their lawful relations so as to explain behaviors; thus they learn to explain observables (overt behavior) on the basis of unobservables (mental states).
Simulation theory	Children develop a set of mental concepts and learn their lawful relations on the basis of their own phenomenal experience; they understand others by simulating others' mental states, employing projection and imagination.

to take corresponding action (e.g., to alleviate the other's pain). This modularity perspective has been highly influential in guiding neuro-biological research on the multiple component processes involved in mentalizing, and we will pursue this line of research further in Chapter 4 ("Neurobiology").

The *theory-theory* of theory-of-mind acquisition holds that children are akin to scientists in gradually developing a theory about mental states so as to explain behavior. Hence children are natural psychologists, developing a "folk-psychological" theory that postulates unobservables (mental representations and the laws that govern them) to account for observable actions. Over the course of development, their theories become increasingly refined and sophisticated (Carruthers 1996). Accordingly, Gopnik and Meltzoff (1997) explicitly liken the theory-theory to the acquisition of scientific knowledge: "the processes of cognitive development in children are similar to, indeed perhaps even identical with, the processes of cognitive development in scientists" (p. 3); moreover, "It is not that children are little scientists but that scientists are big children" (p. 32). Consistent with Gopnik and Meltzoff's view, Goldman (2006) formulated the key premises of theory-theory as follows:

(1) Mental-state concepts are conceptualized in terms of causal laws relating mental states to peripheral events (behavior and external stimuli) and other mental states. (2) Both third-person and first-person attribution proceed by way of law-guided inference from observed peripheral events. (3) Putative laws are acquired "empirically," by means of general-purpose scientizing procedures. (p. 26)

An intuitively appealing alternative to the theory-theory is *simulation theory*; to understand others' minds, we do not make inferences on the basis of theories but rather imagine them as being similar to our own:

> although children's understanding is dependent on a system of mentalistic concepts, of belief, desire, intention, and so on, the...concepts are derived from children's own direct experience of such states. On this view, even young children can introspect their own mental states and are intuitively aware of their own phenomenal experience. They can then understand other people by a process of simulation, using their abilities for pretence which develop early in the pre-school years. That is, the child imagines herself having the beliefs and desires that the other person has, and imagines what she herself would do if she possessed those imagined beliefs and desires...*these are not unobservable states* which children have to posit in some way. Children are aware of these states in themselves and do not have to construct them as "theoretical postulates." (Astington 1996, pp. 184–185; emphasis added)

The question of how well the simulation theory can account for the *development* of theory of mind will continue to be debated. Yet there is little question that, once having acquired a robust theory of mind, we adults use simulation in mentalizing; moreover, a strong case can be made that simulation—empathy—is fundamental to mentalizing (Stueber 2006). Hence insights from simulation theory are pertinent to the conduct of psychotherapy.

Goldman (2006) has developed a comprehensive version of simulation theory, based on the concept of mental simulation, namely, "the simulation of one mental process by another mental process" (p. 37). A paradigm case for simulation theory is the process by which one person predicts another person's decision. Here is the general model:

> an attributor goes about this task by imaginatively putting herself into the target's shoes. She pretends to have the same initial states—for example, the same desires and beliefs—and then makes a decision given those initial, pretend states. Having made a decision in the pretend mode, the attributor predicts that this is the decision the target will make. (p. 19)

As Goldman (2006) explains, this is a *simulation-plus-projection* model: "a mindreader commonly takes one of her own first-order (pretend) states and imputes it (as a genuine state) to the target" (p. 40). Usefully, the simulation-plus-projection model allows for ubiquitous egocentric biases to influence mentalizing: there is always the danger that the simulated (pretend) states are excessively colored by the subject's own mental states. Accordingly, as we noted earlier in this chapter, accurate simulation requires a cognitively effortful process of imagining the target's mental states that differ from one's own while *"quarantining* one's own genuine states that don't correspond to states of the target, that is, keeping such states from intruding into the simulation" (Goldman 2006, p. 41; emphasis in original). This quarantining process entails "inhibiting the self-perspective" (p. 170). Without such inhibition, simulation will be inaccurate: "If leakage or quarantine failure is rampant, egocentric biases will also be rampant" (p. 41). Thus accurate mentalizing of others entails two distinct processes: first, inhibiting one's own perspective; second, inferring another person's perspective. Samson and colleagues (2005) present neuropsychological evidence that these two facets of mentalizing depend on distinct neural processes.

We clinicians should keep in mind that egocentrism is the default mode for all of us. Hence it is part of our responsibility as psychotherapists to be mindful of potential quarantine failures—failing to prevent our own mental states from unduly coloring our inferences about our patient's mental states. This quarantine problem is one way of construing the challenges of working productively with countertransference. That is, to use countertransference effectively, psychotherapists must keep in mind the distinction between their own mental states and the mental states of their patients, inhibiting their natural human tendency to equate the two automatically and to make inferences accordingly. Deliberately maintaining the mentalizing stance of "not knowing" counters this natural tendency (see Chapter 6, "Mentalizing Interventions").

Notably, Goldman (2006) distinguishes between low-level (automatic) and high-level (controlled) simulation, akin to our implicit-explicit distinction. We discuss automatic mirroring processes in Chapter 4 ("Neurobiology"); here we focus on high-level simulation, which requires what Goldman (2006) calls *enactment imagination* ("E-imagination"): "When I imagine feeling elated, I do not merely suppose *that* I am elated; rather, I *enact*, or *try* to enact, elation itself" (p. 47; emphasis in original). Goldman elaborates: "If high-level mindreading is substantially simulationist, mentalizers must ... E-imagine many types of mental states, including beliefs, desires, plans, and hopes" (p. 151). Goldman (2006) makes a crucial point about the integration of implicit and explicit processes in simulating others' mental states, namely, that implicit simulation does not necessarily lead to explicit simulation: "A mirroring event is a *potential* launching pad for an act of (accurate) mindreading, but it's an open question whether, and to what extent, such potential launching pads are actually exploited for mindreading" (p. 133). Working with one's countertransference, for example, entails explicit mentalizing: psychotherapists must explicate their implicit emotional responses and quarantine them when imagining their patients' mental states and deciding how best to respond. This process requires effortful control indeed.

As various integrative efforts attest (Carruthers and Smith 1996; Goldman 2006), these contrasting theories of theory-of-mind acquisition are not entirely mutually exclusive, and they continue to be refined. These theories will continue to be of major interest, because they not only address how we *develop* mentalizing but also how we *do* it (Goldman 2006; Malle 2004; Malle and Hodges 2005)—a matter of no small importance to us psychotherapists and to our patients. Furthermore, this theory-of-mind literature overlaps a huge body of research in social psychology subsumed under the rubric of *social cognition*, defined as "the study of the mental processes involved in perceiving, attending to, remembering, thinking about, and making sense of the people in our social world" (Moskowitz 2005, p. 3).

For present purposes of clarifying terminology, we note three distinctions between "mentalizing" and "theory of mind." First, the theory-of-mind literature primarily addresses the *cognitive* development of mentalizing capacities as they begin evolving in the latter part of infancy and come to fruition in early childhood, by which time the capacity to interpret behavior on the basis of explicit understanding of the representational nature of mind has developed. As we have noted repeatedly, we are interested in *emotional* as well as cognitive aspects of mentalizing. Accordingly, taking the same path in finding the terms, "mindreading" and "theory of mind," to be too narrow, Baron-Cohen (2005) has emended his modular view of theory of mind to include an Emotion Detector as well as an Empathy System. Second, in addition to being aimed primarily at cognition, theory-of-mind research is narrower than mentalizing in focusing primarily on interpreting others and not the self, although Goldman (2006) also has tied the process of self-attribution into the theory-of-mind literature. Third, theory of mind—however acquired and comprised—is the ever-evolving *product* of developing mentalizing *activity,* and we are primarily concerned with the latter. In accord with Malle (2004), we construe theory of mind as our folk-psychological *conceptual framework* for explaining behavior in terms of mental states; hence the activity of mentalizing *employs* our theory-of-mind framework as well as contributing to its development and refinement.

Metacognition

Upon initial exposure to the word, many persons equate "mentalizing" with thinking. Of course, mentalizing explicitly entails thinking, deliberation, and reflection; but we restrict the scope of mentalizing to thinking (and feeling) about *mental states*. Moreover, mentalizing implicitly does not entail reflective thinking but rather is intuitive and relatively automatic. Hence explicit mentalizing pertains only to one domain of thinking, and implicit mentalizing extends beyond thinking in its deliberative sense. We construe metacognition as a specific domain of thinking that falls within the scope of mentalizing. Here we summarize four lines of work on metacognition: theories of cognitive processes, applications to cognitive therapy, psychotherapy research on personality disorders, and manifestations in attachment narratives.

Metacognition can be defined simply as "cognition about cognition" (Smith et al. 2003, p. 318) or "knowing about knowing" (Koriat 2000, p. 149). More specifically, Wells (2000) defined metacognition as "any knowledge or cognitive process that is involved in the appraisal, monitoring or control of cognition" (p. 6). Metacognition has a straightforward pragmatic function; simply put, "some minds contain a cognitive executive that looks in on thought or problem solving to see how it is going and how it might be facilitated" (Smith et al. 2003, p. 318). This is mentalizing in the sense of knowing how your mind works.

Although "meta*cognition*" connotes thinking about thinking, Jost and colleagues (1998) cogently argued for an "expansionist" view that would encompass thinking not only about thinking but also thinking about emotions and motives in others as well as oneself—a view that brings "metacognition" into line with "mentalizing." Moreover, they argued that metacognition, as part of folk psychology, is intrinsically social, a point we will elaborate in relation to mentalizing in Chapter 3 ("Development").

Central to understanding metacognition in the narrower sense is the distinction between object-level and meta-level processing (Nelson 1996). *Object-level* processing entails focus on the task at hand (e.g., carrying on a conversation); whereas *meta-level* processing entails focus on the cognitive processes involved in the task at hand (e.g., thinking about your inability to get a point across). In addition, metacognition encompasses both knowledge and regulation (Fernandez-Duque et al.

2000). Metacognitive *knowledge* includes knowledge about your cognitive abilities (e.g., you're better at language than math) and about cognitive strategies (e.g., you need to make a note to ensure remembering something that you must do). Metacognitive *regulation* serves to coordinate cognition and includes two intertwined facets (Koriat et al. 2006): cognitive *monitoring* (e.g., becoming aware that you are failing to make your point in conversation) and cognitive *control* (e.g., taking time to think and presenting your argument in more detail).

Metacognition capitalizes on the reflexive nature of consciousness, and the distinction between cognition and metacognition parallels the distinction we have drawn between implicit and explicit mentalizing. Exerting conscious control in the metacognitive mode is consistent with our emphasis on the adaptive flexibility afforded by mentalizing explicitly. We shift to the metacognitive (explicit mentalizing) mode in the face of uncertainty, novelty, error, conflict, and emotion—all of which are ubiquitous in interpersonal interactions. Accordingly, metacognition requires inhibitory control (what we call the pause button) and effortful attention (Fernandez-Duque et al. 2000; Posner and Rothbart 1998). Especially important clinically, focusing and shifting attention is crucial for emotion regulation.

> A patient who experienced rapid changes in emotions suddenly became convinced that the therapist didn't like her, and she started shouting, saying that, being treated so badly, she wasn't going to stay in therapy. As she got up to leave, the therapist immediately tried to focus on her current mental experience by asking if there was anything that she, the therapist, had done to make the patient suddenly feel this way. In doing so, the therapist not only focused on the interpersonal context that might have stimulated the sudden mood shift but also tried to move the attention from a primarily internally focused experience to a more explicit or external focus—a move from the immediacy of the impulse to an appraisal of the experience. This movement between internal and external explication and understanding of mental states is crucial in a therapy that focuses on mentalizing.

Plainly, making such shifts in attention is not easy; to reiterate, doing so requires *effortful* control—and practice. Adapting research on metacognition to cognitive therapy, Wells (2000) has developed interventions for basic attention training as well as for refocusing attention. The clinical need for attention refocusing underscores a crucial caveat regarding the promotion of mentalizing: *attending to one's own mental states sometimes can be counterproductive.* As Wells (2000) reviews, extensive research on patients with anxiety disorders indicates that self-focused attention is liable to increase anxiety. For example, the person with social phobia who focuses on increasing heart rate or blushing in a social situation is liable to experience an escalation of anxiety into a panic attack. Furthermore, mentalizing in a way that proves maladaptive, socially phobic patients might concentrate on imagining how they appear to others (e.g., imagining that they are the focus of others' attention). Refocusing attention entails a shift in mentalizing strategy, namely, directing attention to the external situation, that is, the social task, which includes attending to *others'* mental states instead of one's own:

> it is likely that external focusing shifts attention onto social information that is capable of disconfirming negative beliefs. In particular, if the patient believes that he/she is the centre of everyone's attention, shifting to external focused attention on other people offers a means of disconfirming this belief. Furthermore, external attention is likely to reduce awareness of anxiety symptoms and may also disrupt other unhelpful self-focused coping strategies that could deleteriously affect performance and prevent belief change. (Wells 2000, pp. 149–150)

Wells's (2000) approach to the treatment of generalized anxiety disorder—a condition characterized primarily by excessive worry—illustrates the potential value of shifting the focus of cognitive therapy from cognitive content (i.e., correcting cognitive distortions) to metacognitive processes (i.e., mentalizing). Wells focuses interventions on worry about worry (e.g., "My worrying will drive me crazy"), which includes two broad forms of negative metacognitive beliefs about worry, namely, that worry is uncontrollable and that it is potentially dangerous. Such beliefs increase anxiety and consume attentional resources that would be better devoted to problem solving. Notably, positive metacognitive beliefs about worry (e.g., "Worrying keeps me prepared and safe") also abet worrying and thereby anxiety. Metacognitive interventions draw patients' attention to the advantages and disadvantages of worrying and also include strategies for interrupting worrying (e.g., postponing worrying to a specified time). Working with patients on the metacognitive level promotes effective coping with worrying and then frees patients to move from ruminating to problem solving. An initial report of treatment effectiveness is promising (Wells and King 2006).

As exemplified in Wells's (2000) clinical practice, the metacognitive approach puts cognitive therapy squarely in the domain of mentalizing and has much to offer: adaptive and maladaptive cognitive strategies are explicated at a fine-grained level, and the approach includes numerous practical strategies for enhancing metacognitive knowledge and regulation. Although much research on metacognition focuses on cognitive processes (e.g., learning and memory strategies), the "expansionist" view of metacognition (Jost et al. 1998) encompasses emotion, and Wells's (2000) clinical applications are intended to facilitate emotion regulation. Yet, as Wells promotes them, metacognitive interventions are employed when the person is not in the throes of anxiety or worrying. By contrast, we aspire to promote mentalizing (metacognition) while in the midst of the emotional state.

A group of psychotherapy researchers in Rome is conducting groundbreaking work on individual differences in metacognition as they relate to treatment of personality disorders (Semerari et al. 2003). This group's Metacognitive Assessment Scale teases apart different facets of metacognition; it evaluates these facets separately for the two domains of self and others; and it includes a third domain of mastery. For the two domains of understanding one's own and others' mental states, the Metacognitive Assessment Scale distinguishes four facets of metacognitive activity: *identifying* mental states and making distinctions among them; *differentiating* subjective mental representations from objective reality; *relating* mental states to each other and to behavior; and *integrating* metacognitive knowledge into abstract narratives. The domain of others' mental states includes the additional facet of *decentering*: recognizing the separateness of others' mental states from one's own. The third domain of *mastery* assesses the complexity of the individual's metacognitive regulation and control strategies (e.g., the capacity to modify one's mental states by means of attention, inhibition, and reflection). Multifaceted assessment of individuals' metacognitive successes and failures in the psychotherapy process shows promise for differentiating among personality disorders, tracking progress and outcomes of psychotherapy, and—most importantly—shaping therapeutic interventions (Dimaggio et al. 2007). A distinctive strength of Dimaggio and colleagues' therapeutic approach is their systematic focus on specific facets of impaired mentalizing as reflected in particular personality disorders.

We are giving extensive play to the tight links between mentalizing and secure attachment throughout this book, and it is of more than historical interest that Main (1991) introduced this line of thinking under the rubric of "metacognitive monitoring" in attachment-related discourse. As we will discuss at length in Chapter 3 ("Development"), Main reviewed evidence that parents' secure attachment to their own parents is associated with their infants' security of attachment to them and, moreover, to their infants' subsequent representational (mentalizing) capacities. Paralleling the cognitive therapy literature, Main (1991) distinguished between representational and metarepresentational processes as the difference between "*thinking vs. thinking about thought,* or, at a deeper level, possessing a mental representation of an experience vs. being able to reflect on its validity, nature, and source" (p. 128, emphasis in original). Parental security of attachment, assessed by the Adult Attachment Interview (Main and Goldwyn 1994), is not based on the actual nature of the childhood relationships of the parent with his or her own parents but rather on the adult parent's capacity to give a *coherent narrative account* of the relationships. Specifically, coherent discourse is truthful, succinct yet complete, relevant, as well as clear and orderly (Main 1991). Thus a parent who had a traumatic childhood would be considered secure if he or she were able to give a coherent account of that experience in the interview, and the capacity to do so requires metacognitive monitoring. Moreover, as Main proposed, through the medium of secure attachment, children of securely attached parents are more likely to develop metacognitive skills.

Reflective Functioning

Main's pioneering work on attachment-related metacognitive capacities led to Fonagy and colleagues' (1997b) more refined operationalization for research purposes, the *reflective-functioning* (RF) scale. This instrument is employed in assessing the quality of mentalizing in the Adult Attachment Interview; ratings are made on a scale ranging from negative RF (antipathy toward mentalizing) to exceptional RF (exceptionally sophisticated and consistent mentalization); Table 2–4 provides general descriptions of the various levels of RF. In contrast to the Metacognitive Assessment Scale (Semerari et al. 2003), the RF scale integrates the assessment of multiple facets into a global rating of the quality of mentalizing in the specific context of attachment narratives.

Mindfulness

Mindfulness, explicated most thoroughly in the Buddhist literature (Hahn 1975), has been defined recently for research purposes as "an enhanced attention to and awareness of current experience or present reality" characterized by "especially *open* or *receptive* awareness and attention" (Brown and Ryan 2003, p. 822, emphasis in original). Hence attention is pivotal to mindfulness, as it is to mentalizing. Yet mindfulness, like thinking, is not restricted to any particular object; one can be mindful of a flower or of one's breathing. To bring the concepts closer together, we might construe mentalizing as *mindfulness of mind* (Allen 2006b). Indeed, part of what we would call mentalizing is included in a research measure of mindfulness, namely, "receptive attention to psychological states" and "sensitivity to ongoing psychological processes" (Brown and Ryan 2003, p. 823).

TABLE 2–4.   LEVELS OF REFLECTIVE FUNCTIONING (RF)

Level	Characteristics
Negative RF	Active, hostile resistance to the mentalizing stance; derogation of reflection; bizarre or frankly paranoid attributions—all in the context of a total absence of any reflection
Lacking in RF	Reflection is totally, or almost totally, absent; banal and simplistic mentalizing; extreme concreteness; clearly inaccurate attributions indicative of failure to reflect
Questionable or low RF	Rudimentary consideration of mental states; relatively superficial and impersonal; generally, references to mental states and their relation to behavior are not specific or explicated; alternatively, over-analytical, unintegrated insights not linked to the individual's experience
Ordinary RF	Common in non-clinical populations; a number of instances of reflection indicating that the individual maintains coherent models of the mind for the self and attachment figures; ability to make sense of experience in terms of thoughts and feelings; somewhat lacking in complexity or subtlety; indications of limited reflection in relation to one key relationship along with adequate reflection regarding other relationships
Marked RF	Consistently maintained reflectiveness evidencing the effort to tease out mental states underlying behavior; detailed understanding of thoughts and feelings of protagonists; originality of thinking about mental states associated with actions; ability to maintain a developmental and intergenerational perspective
Exceptional RF	Rare cases of exceptional sophistication, coupled with consistent maintenance of a reflective stance throughout; integrating several instances of reflectiveness into unified and fresh perspectives; full and spontaneous reflection with respect to a range of relationships across the speaker's life history

Although mindfulness is broader than mentalizing (i.e., pertaining to more than mental states), it is also narrower in being present-centered; by contrast, mentalizing also can be directed to past and future mental states. In addition, mentalizing explicitly is relatively deliberative, whereas mindfulness is construed as "pre-reflective" as well as "perceptual and non-evaluative" (Brown and Ryan 2003, p. 843). Finally, befitting its Buddhist origins, mindfulness sometimes connotes relatively emotionally detached awareness, whereas we place a premium on mentalizing in the midst of intense emotional states. Notwithstanding these conceptual distinctions, the term, "mindfulness" is not only extremely useful in its own right but also aptly captures the *attentive* spirit of mentalizing, that is, *being mindful* of mental states.

Empathy

As we noted in Chapter 1 ("Introduction"), Rogers (1951) made empathy the foundation of client-centered therapy, and psychotherapy of any form without empathy is inconceivable. The domain of empathy is narrower than that of mentalizing inasmuch as empathy refers to awareness of others' mental states; yet, as Baron-Cohen (2003, 2005) defined it, empathy is not only *about* others' emotional states but also entails emotional responsiveness to them:

> Empathizing is the drive to identify another person's emotions and thoughts, and to respond to them with an appropriate emotion. Empathizing does not entail just the cold calculation of what someone else thinks and feels (or what is sometimes called mindreading). Psychopaths can do that much. Empathizing occurs when we feel an appropriate emotional reaction, an emotion *triggered by* the other person's emotion, and it is done in order to understand another person, to predict their behavior, and to connect or resonate with them emotionally. (Baron-Cohen 2003, p. 2, emphasis in original)

Put crudely, empathizing is half of mentalizing; in promoting mentalizing with patients, we often advocate empathy for the self as well as for others. Yet, even in relation to others, empathy goes beyond mentalizing insofar as it includes an appropriate emotional response to what is mentalized (ordinarily, a sympathetic or compassionate emotional response). To put these two concepts together, we often advocate aspiring to mentalize empathically with respect to self and others.

Preston and de Waal (de Waal 2006; Preston and de Waal 2002) proposed a comprehensive model of empathy that has a number of points of connection with mentalizing. Specifically, they proposed a Perception-Action Model in which empathy is based on subject-object state matching. This model is noteworthy for incorporating attention, that is, "*attended* perception of the object's state *automatically* activates the subject's representations of the state" (Preston and de Waal 2002, p. 4; emphasis added). These automatically activated representations are the basis of empathy and, as we will discuss in Chapter 4 ("Neurobiology"), research on mirror neurons (activated not only when observing another's actions but also when performing the same actions) is pointing to one neurobiological substrate of empathy (Gallese 2001; Rizzolatti and Craighero 2004).

Paralleling our distinction between implicit and explicit mentalizing as well as our view that mentalizing entails mental elaboration (Lecours and Bouchard 1997), Preston and de Waal (2002) proposed a hierarchy of empathic responses. Emotional contagion (Hatfield et al. 1994), a precursor to empathy, includes subject-object state matching but lacks the subject-object differentiation essential for true empathy. Empathy proper entails mentalizing in combining self-awareness with other-awareness as well as including emotion regulation. In this sense, empathy can be implicit (intuitive and automatic). Yet what Preston and de Waal call *cognitive empathy* requires explicit mentalizing, that is, working actively with imaginative representations of shared experience. More specifically, de Waal (2006) notes that higher level empathy requires cognitive empathy in the sense of "understanding the reasons for the other's emotions" as well as mental state attribution in the sense of "fully adopting the other's perspective" (p. 39). To reiterate an earlier point, this view of empathy exemplifies the cardinal roles of attention and imagination in mentalizing.

Preston and colleagues (2007) employed neuroimaging findings to clarify the process of cognitive empathy in a way that has direct bearing on the challenge of mentalizing in psychotherapy. Owing to extensive prior research, the range of brain regions activated in conjunction with emotional feelings is well known. These investigators compared patterns of brain activity in these regions in two conditions: first, when participants vividly imagined a personally emotional experience and re-evoked the associated feelings (of anger or fear) and, second, when they imagined themselves in a situation that another person had experienced and, similarly, strived to evoke strong feelings. Thus the study compared responses to personal and non-personal situations (and included emotionally neutral situations as a control). Moreover, in one experimental condition, participants were asked to choose a non-personal situation to which they could *relate most*; in another condition, participants chose a non-personal situation to which they could *relate least*.

When participants in Preston and colleagues' study were imagining another person's emotional situation to which they could relate most, not only did the intensity of their emotion match the level of emotion they felt while imagining their own personal emotional experience but also there was almost complete overlap in patterns of brain activation—hence a matching of emotional experience and brain activity between self and (imagined) other. When imagining a non-personal situation to which they could relate least, however, not only was their emotional experience less intense but also there were substantial differences in patterns of brain activation; additional brain regions were recruited when participants had to put themselves in the shoes of a highly different other.

Preston and colleagues proposed that aspiring to empathize with another person's different experience requires greater perspective taking and active imagination (i.e., a high level of cognitive empathy). When our own representations of emotional situations closely match those of another person, including a patient, we can empathize relatively fully and effortlessly; using Goldman's (2006) model, simulation plus projection yields accurate empathy. When we do not have a closely matching personal representation, however, we are more likely to need to "quarantine" our own experience, inhibiting the self-perspective. In this case, we need to engage in the effortful attentive work required to adopt a different perspective. Moreover, when we lack similar experience, our empathic feelings are likely to be more muted, for better or for worse.

Emotional Intelligence

Closely related to empathy (and what we will discuss later in this chapter under the rubric of mentalizing emotion) is emotional intelligence. Like intelligence proper, emotional intelligence is multifaceted. Specifically, Mayer, Salovey, and their colleagues (Mayer 2001; Mayer et al. 2000) highlight four broad domains of emotional intelligence: perceiving and expressing emotion, accessing and assimilating emotion in thought, understanding and analyzing emotion, and regulating emotion. Their development of well-designed measures akin to traditional IQ tests has led to a spate of research studies (Barrett and Salovey 2002). In contrast to empathy, emotional intelligence includes emotional competence with respect to oneself as well as others. Thus emotional intelligence comes closer to mentalizing, although it is restricted to emotional mental states, whereas mentalizing pertains to the full range of mental states. Of course, emotional mental states are those of primary interest to clinicians and patients, and promoting mentalizing is tantamount to enhancing emotional intelligence for the sake of enhancing relationships and self-regulation.

Psychological Mindedness and Insight

In contrast to all the terms considered thus far, psychological mindedness was originally employed for the purpose of assessing a prospective patient's amenability to insight-oriented psychotherapy. Hence psychological mindedness refers narrowly to "the ability to identify dynamic (intrapsychic) components and to relate them to a person's difficulties" (McCallum and Piper 1996, p. 52) and somewhat more broadly to

"A person's ability to see relationships among thoughts, feelings, and actions, with the goal of learning the meanings and causes of his experiences and behavior" (Appelbaum 1973, p. 36). As intended, assessments of psychological mindedness have shown some relation to the capacity to engage productively in psychotherapy (Conte et al. 1996).

In its initial formulation, psychological mindedness might be construed as the explicit mentalizing capacity essential for engaging in psychodynamic psychotherapy or psychoanalysis. As such, psychological mindedness would emphasize mentalizing with respect to the self, although the broader definition (Appelbaum 1973) could as well apply to mentalizing others' behavior. Yet the concept of psychological mindedness also has been expanded beyond the psychotherapeutic context, to include others explicitly: "Essentially, psychological-mindedness may be considered a trait which has as its core the disposition to reflect on the meaning and motivation of behavior, thoughts, and feelings in oneself and others" (Farber 1985, p. 170). Moreover, this expanded formulation includes not only explicit mentalizing but also more implicit mentalizing, namely, an experiential-affective mode which involves individuals' "intuitive sensitivity to interpersonal and intrapsychic dynamics...and the capacity to use their own feelings to understand and help others" (Farber 1985, p. 174).

Broadly construed (i.e., as akin to mentalizing capacity), psychological mindedness has been shown to relate to a wide range of phenomena associated with mental health and adaptive functioning (Beitel and Cecero 2003; Beitel et al. 2004, 2005). Whereas the expanded conception of psychological mindedness occupies much of the territory of mentalizing, psychological mindedness has been construed as a trait or broad disposition; in contrast, mentalizing is psychological activity (i.e., mental action). Thus one might construe psychological mindedness as the proclivity to mentalize, especially in the psychotherapeutic context— mentalizing is what psychologically minded individuals are inclined to *do*. Moreover, the developmental processes we review in Chapter 3 ("Development") illuminate how individuals become more or less psychologically minded. In parallel, psychotherapy requires and cultivates psychological mindedness.

In its original formulations, psychological mindedness was closely linked to the capacity to generate *insight* in psychodynamic psychotherapy. No doubt, skillful mentalizing generates insights, inside and outside therapeutic contexts. Yet specific insights are more a by-product of focusing on mentalizing than its primary aim. We emphasize process more than content: by directing attention and encouraging imagination, we aim to enhance mentalizing *activity*—especially in the midst of emotional arousal. The expanded definition of psychological mindedness is essentially the same as our understanding of mentalizing *capacity* or the disposition to mentalize.

Mentalizing Emotion

The word "mentalizing" connotes cognitive and intellectual activity, and thus we must continually remind ourselves that the mentalizing of greatest clinical interest is suffused with emotion. Figuratively, we might think of mentalizing not just as keeping mind in mind but rather as keeping heart and mind in heart and mind. Moreover, mentalizing skillfully is most difficult in the midst of intense emotional states. Thus, mentalizing emotion—what Fonagy and colleagues (Fonagy et al. 2002a; Jurist 2005) have called *mentalized affectivity*—does not mean taking a detached, intellectual stance on one's emotion but rather entails achieving clarity about emotional experience—as one patient in a psychoeducational group cleverly put it, not just thinking clearly but also *feeling clearly*.

To a considerable extent, when we discuss mentalizing in the rest of this book, we will be referring implicitly to mentalizing emotion. Here we set the stage. First, we consider the multifaceted nature of emotion and the varying degrees to which different facets of emotion may be mentalized. Second, we advocate going beyond a narrow focus on identifying "feelings" to appreciating the complex intentional structure of emotions—namely, what they are *about*. Third, we address the centrality of mentalizing to the adaptiveness of emotions. Fourth, with an eye toward psychotherapeutic work, we highlight the importance of mentalizing in the midst of emotional states. Finally, consistent with the intentional structure of emotions, we underscore the role of agency in emotion by presenting emotions as active strategies. Throughout this section, we borrow heavily from philosopher Robert Solomon's (2007) splendid contributions to understanding emotion, inasmuch as his work dovetails so closely with our interest in mentalizing.

Components of Emotion

In its most fundamental (Freudian) sense, mentalizing entails transforming something non-mental into something mental. Considering *emotion* as an umbrella term for a complex package of components unfolding over time (Keltner et al. 2003), part of this dynamic package is mental*ized*. That is, to varying degrees, emotional episodes are experienced and recognized as such. Specifically, emotion involves cognitive appraisals, physiological arousal, action tendencies, and motoric expression (e.g., in posture and in the face)—all *potentially* accompanied by subjective experiences of various sorts. We generally refer to the experiential aspect of emotion as *feeling* (or affect). Clinically, we use the word, "feeling," implicitly to refer to various facets of emotional experience, including sensations, urges, emotional feelings, as well as various emotional thoughts accompanying all these. Our common refrain, "How do you *feel* about that?" is an invitation to mentalize these various facets of emotional experience. Thus we should keep in mind that we use the word, feeling, to allude to a whole complex of emotional experience.

We might say that *feeling* an emotion—in and of itself—is implicit mentalizing: somatic-motoric activation, coupled with interpretations of external events, has been transformed into an emotional mental state. Yet, as Lecours and Bouchard (1997) articulated, mentalizing entails more than transforming the non-mental into the mental; feeling an emotion is only the beginning of an extended process: to a considerable degree, mentalizing entails mental *elaboration*, which is the essence of mentalizing emotion.

Intentionality of Emotion

Intentionality lies at the heart of understanding emotion as a form of mentalizing; we miss the boat if we construe emotion as merely having isolated "feelings" (Solomon 2007). Sartre (1948) gets us right on the boat with one sentence: "Emotion is a certain way of apprehending the world" (p. 52). As intentional mental states, emotional experiences are *about* something. Hence cognition is intrinsic to emotion. This understanding of the cognitive underpinning of emotion dates back to ancient Rome; the Stoic philosopher Epictetus said, "It is not things that disturb people but their judgements about things" (Long 2002, p. 213). Thus emotions have been considered a form of judgment (Nussbaum 2001; Solomon 2004) in the sense of being evaluative responses to situations that are of importance to one's goals and projects. To repeat, these judgments are not detached cognitive appraisals; on the contrary, as Solomon put it, "Emotions are not just *about* (or 'directed to') the world but actively entangled in it…. *emotions are subjective engagements in the world…* a way of cognitively *grappling* with the world" (Solomon 2004, p. 77).

Sartre (1948) and Solomon (2007) go against the grain of the temptation to separate cognition from emotion, as we misleadingly do, for example, when we maintain that a cognitive appraisal triggers an emotional response that is distinct from the appraisal. Cognitive appraisals are better construed as integral components of emotion, inasmuch as emotions are dynamic processes in which the situation which the emotion is about as well as the emotion itself are continually *reappraised* (Ellsworth and Scherer 2003). Moreover, the term "cognitive" appraisal (or judgment) can be misleading if it implies a conscious and reflective process; initial emotional appraisals are often rapid and nonconscious evaluative responses. And we should keep in mind that "cognition" is emotional; as William James maintained, "Not a cognition occurs but feeling is there to comment on it, to stamp it as of greater or less worth" (Richardson 2006, p. 183). We construe *mentalizing* emotion as the dynamic process of continual emotional reappraisal, not only of the evoking situation but also of the emotional responses. Mentalizing is implicated in the maintenance and proliferation of subjective feelings and, most importantly, in elaborating their meanings—what they are about. Moreover, we commonly have emotional responses to our emotions (e.g., feeling afraid of anger), including emotional judgments of our emotions (e.g., feeling guilty about being afraid).

Solomon (2007) has thoroughly integrated cognition into emotion in construing emotions as having an *intentional structure:*

> every emotion type, that is the *kind* of emotion rather than any particular instance or instances of it, can be defined by its *formal object.* This is in a nutshell the intentional structure of the various emotions. So that the formal object of fear is *something dangerous,* the formal object of anger is *something offensive,* and so on. What it is that is dangerous or offensive is, of course, dependent on the situation, the circumstances, and the psychological make-up and subjective state of the individual. But what is built into the very concept of an emotion is that it has such a structure, a formal object that is defined in terms of the *kinds* of things it picks out or perceives in the environment. (p. 161, emphasis in original).

As Solomon articulates it, the intentional structure of emotion encompasses more than "cognitive appraisals" narrowly construed: "emotions also have the power to *constitute* reality in a certain way. They *bestow* value as well as appraise it." Hence, he adds, "The hated person appears as *hateful.* The beloved appears as *lovely*" (p. 162, emphasis in original).

Adaptiveness of Emotion as Mentalized

Many patients who contend with painful affects, especially those who grapple with posttraumatic reexperiencing of unbearable emotional states, understandably wish to avoid or at least squelch their emotions. Our emphasis on mentalizing emotions goes against this avoidant grain. Given the potential painfulness of emotion, in working with traumatized patients we must make a strong case for mentalizing emotion, a case which boils down to the point that emotions are adaptive and, as such, to be cultivated and refined rather than avoided (Allen 2005; Solomon 2007).

Over a century ago, Darwin (1872) began to develop the thesis that emotions have instrumental value, a thesis that became crystallized in the adaptive value of anger and fear in the fight-or-flight response (Cannon 1953). Along with many others, Damasio (1999) has continued to elaborate this thesis in increasingly subtle ways, for example, documenting how gut feelings adaptively steer behavior. Accordingly, a science of intuition is emerging (Lieberman 2000). But our emphasis on the importance of mentalizing emotion goes beyond its direct instrumental value. Emotions not only facilitate adaptive responses on the basis of perceptions; by virtue of their intentional structure, they also *organize* perceptions and judgments. Moreover, emotions have existential value, a spirit Grayling (2002) eloquently expressed in articulating where the Stoics went wrong in their aim of rethinking emotional judgments for the sake of promoting tranquility:

> Although this [Stoic] teaching was designed to help people bear vicissitudes bravely, and in its inspiration is one of the tenderest and most thoughtful of philosophies, it misses a very important point. This is that if one is frugal with one's emotions—limiting love in order to avoid its pains, stifling appetites and desires in order to escape the price of their fulfillment—one lives a stunted, muffled, bland life only. It is practically tantamount to a partial death in order to minimize the electric character of existence—its pleasures, its ecstasies, its richness and colour matched by its agonies, its wretchedness, its disasters and grief. To take life in armfuls, to embrace and accept it, to leap into it with energy and relish, is of course to invite trouble of all the familiar kinds. But the cost of avoiding trouble is a terrible one: it is the cost of having trodden the planet for humanity's brief allotment of less than a thousand months, without really having lived. (pp. 167–168)

Yet in highlighting its instrumental and existential value, we must not idealize emotion's adaptive function; plainly, individual differences loom large, and—for all of us—emotion is only *potentially* adaptive (Parrott 2002), depending in part on the extent to which it is elaborated and regulated through mentalizing.

Taking seriously the intentionality of emotional feelings, Goldie (2004a, 2004b) proposes that we perceive objects or situations as having emotion-proper properties; for example, a piece of rotting meat *is* disgusting or a person's arrogant behavior *is* irksome. As perceptions or judgments (i.e., based on appraisals), emotions are associated with justifying reasons. To the extent that such judgments are fitting, we construe emotional feelings—their quality and intensity—as more or less reasonable. Consistent with Sartre's (1948) philosophy and Damasio's (1999) neurobiological research, Goldie (2004b) maintains that emotions play an epistemic role:

> Our emotional dispositions can, so to speak, *attune* us to the world around us, enabling us quickly and reliably to see things as they really are, and thus to respond as we should. In short, emotions enable us to *get things right.* (p. 255, emphasis in original)

Here Goldie is echoing the psychoanalytic view of affects as adaptive signals; as Rapaport (1967) put it, "affects as signals are just as indispensable a means of reality testing as thoughts. Indeed, they are more indispensable for reality testing in all except successfully intellectualizing and obsessional characters" (p. 508). Plainly, however, depending on the validity of the associated appraisals, emotions can distort as well as clarify. For better or for worse, as Goldie (2004a) writes, "one's emotional feelings tend to *skew the epistemic landscape* to make it cohere with the emotional experience" (p. 99, emphasis in original); depression is a notorious example (Beck et al. 1979). Much of the work of psychotherapy—mentalizing emotion—addresses the perceptions upon which emotions are founded as well as their justifying reasons with an eye toward their reasonableness and their potentially distorted skewing effects on judgments. Thus *rationality is inherent in emotion,* not opposed to emotion. Of course, to say that emotion has a rational structure does not imply that we always reason well: "Emotions are structured by judgments that can be wise or foolish, warranted or unwarranted, appropriate or inappropriate, or right or wrong" (Solomon 2007, p. 181). The main arena in which we are keen to help our patients "get it right" emotionally is that of relationships, and attachment relationships especially.

Mentalizing in the Midst of Emotion

The crux of our view that mentalizing emotion must not be associated with intellectual detachment is this: mentalized affectivity is founded on mentalizing while "*remaining within* the emotional state" (Fonagy et al. 2002a, p. 96, emphasis added), for example, feeling while thinking about feeling. Thus mentalizing emotion may entail maintaining or reactivating an emotional state. To underscore the centrality of emotion in the process, we might best construe mentalizing as *thinking and feeling about thinking and feeling.*

Fonagy and colleagues (2002a) distinguished three elements of mentalized affectivity: identifying, modulating, and expressing affects, core features of which are summarized in Table 2–5.

At the simplest level, *identifying* emotions might entail verbally labeling a *basic emotion* (Ekman 2003) such as fear, anger, sadness, or disgust. Making such identifications is not necessarily easy, and the need to do so is not uncommon. Quite often, at least around their onset, emotions are unformed; one might just feel "emotional" or "upset" or "distressed" (Ellsworth and Scherer 2003), experiencing what Jurist (2005) calls *aporetic feelings*, in which case the person does not know what he or she feels. In such instances, as all psychotherapists and patients know, finding a name for a basic emotion might be no small achievement.

Yet basic emotions come in families, and refined identification of emotions entails capturing the right one in the family. A patient who denies feeling "angry" might readily acknowledge feeling "frustrated," "aggravated," "irked," "irritated," "put out," or even "pissed off." Moreover, rarely does one basic emotion encompass a response to a situation—especially a significant event in a close relationship. Commonly, for example, fear is in the background of anger, and shame comes in the wake of anger. One reason for aporetic (i.e., vague, unformed, and confusing) feelings is the common occurrence of conflicting feelings. Even at the most basic level, for example, one of our patients was helped to clarify his aporetic feelings toward his mother when the therapist made the point that love and hate are often inter-

---

TABLE 2–5.   THREE DOMAINS OF MENTALIZING EMOTION

Domain	Characteristics
Identifying emotions	Labeling basic emotions; identifying shades of emotions; articulating layers of emotions as well as emotional conflicts and ambivalence; and elucidating the meaning of emotions in terms of present and past relationships.
Modulating emotions	Regulating the intensity of emotional states in either a downward or upward direction as well as sustaining a particular level of emotional arousal; entails revaluing emotions in a continual process of reappraisal.
Expressing emotions	Predicated on identifying and modulating emotions (downward or upward), expressing emotions may be done not only outwardly to others but also inwardly to oneself; expressing emotions in attachment relationships also plays a significant role in further identifying and modulating them.

mingled and that the presence of hate does not contradict the fact of love—a possibility that had never occurred to him. Commonly, feelings are complexly textured and layered, and mentalizing emotion entails identifying shades of intermingled emotions.

Yet, as we already have stated, mentalizing emotion goes far beyond identifying feelings; it also entails elucidating their intentional structure, that is, "the capacity to connect to the *meaning* of one's emotions" (Fonagy et al. 2002a, p. 15, emphasis added). Finding meaning is the crux of mental elaboration: fundamentally, mentalizing emotion entails making emotion meaningful. This process will involve elaborating the reasons for emotions in current experience as well as potentially understanding the historical development of emotional responses in a given relationship and in association with prior relationships (i.e., transference in the broadest sense). Quite often, understanding the historical basis of emotional responses is useful in discovering the meaning of unreasonably intense responses, as commonly happens in conjunction with trauma (Allen 2005). Thus, at its most elaborate, emotional meaning will become embedded in complex autobiographical narratives (Holmes 1999).

The second element of mentalized affectivity, *modulating* affects, entails some alteration of the emotional state. Most often, we associate modulation with toning down disruptively intense emotional responses. Indeed, modulation in this sense may be critical to mentalizing emotion, because excessively intense emotion—typified by rage and terror and the fight-or-flight response—is antithetical to mentalizing (Mayes 2000). Accordingly, psychotherapists and patients are continually challenged to create the climate of safety characteristic of secure attachment that will serve to modulate emotion downward sufficiently so as to make mentalizing possible.

Yet modulating also may entail prolonging or even *amplifying* an emotional state—as we often strive to help patients do when we believe that they are minimizing, avoiding, or suppressing emotions. In such instances, modulation upward also is essential for mentalizing emotion, which requires that the patient mentalize while remaining in the feeling. The modulation upward also depends on secure attachment; it is safe to feel only when feelings are likely to be mentalized by the other. Thus, on the one hand, there is much wisdom in Pine's (1984) admonition "Strike while the iron is cold," in the sense of striving for understanding when the patient is not in the throes of excessively intense emotion. Yet, on the other hand, when the iron is *too* cold, the potential to elaborate meanings (and other emotions) may be lost. Moreover, patients ultimately must develop the capacity to mentalize in the midst of emotion for the sake of being able to engage in resolving conflicts in re-lationships as they are unfolding. Striking while the iron is warm, for example, expressing annoyance while still feeling the annoyance, is more likely to influence another person than mentioning the annoyance after the fact in a detached way—or worse, building up resentment and eventually exploding in a rage.

As we have stated, emotions are evaluative responses to situations and relationships; as we mentioned earlier, modulating emotion in-volves *revaluing* affects in a continual process of reappraisal:

> This is a crucial moment within the process of affectivity, as it brings out that one does not necessarily adopt new affects as much as one reinter-prets the meaning of the same affects. So through revaluing affects one comes to have a greater sense of the complexity of one's affective expe-rience. (Fonagy et al. 2002a, p. 438)

In its broadest manifestation, the process of revaluing affects re-quires a mentalizing stance—that is, an exploratory attitude of inquisi-tiveness and curiosity about mental states and their basis as well as their influences on the self and relationships.

The third element of mentalized affectivity is *expressing* feelings. Plainly, identifying affect is a prerequisite to expressing it; feeling clearly is crucial to expressing feelings clearly. Similarly, modulating af-fect is also essential to expressing it effectively. Obviously, downward modulation of intense affects is essential to their effective expression; rage will not be well received. Yet upward modulation of affect also may be essential for effective expression; inhibited anger expressed as mild annoyance will not have the needed interpersonal force compared to direct expression of justified outrage.

Often it is not desirable or possible to express affects outwardly (e.g., when feeling put out by a boss's urgent demands). In these instances, Fonagy and colleagues point out that it is also possible to express affects *inwardly*, that is, to oneself, which requires mentalizing emotion in the sense of reflecting on affect while in the midst of emotional arousal:

> to express the affect, it can be sufficient to let one feel the affect anew without having it emerge in the world. For example, a patient realized how angry he was at his wife because she blamed him for her preg-nancy, although he believed at the time that his wife was feeling too vul-nerable to hear this from him. The point is that it was helpful for him to experience his anger at a deeper level than he had done, but it was equally important to confirm the choice not to convey his affect directly to his wife. We want to stress here how this account differs from one in which one recognizes one's anger from an intellectual standpoint. Men-

talized affectivity goes further in pushing us to own our affects; being able to express affects inwardly adds an option in situations where outward expression is not desirable. (Fonagy et al. 2002a, pp. 339–340)

We should not be misled into thinking that mentalized affectivity involves a lockstep sequence of identifying, modulating, and expressing affect (e.g., recognizing that you feel angry, calming yourself down somewhat, and then asserting yourself accordingly). Rather, an emotional episode in a relationship—whether it be a psychotherapeutic relationship, a love relationship, or a friendship—will entail a continual alternation among identification, modulation, and expression of emotions. Ideally, for example, in the context of a secure attachment relationship in which mentalizing is occurring reciprocally, expressing feelings is likely to contribute to clarifying them further, which is likely to contribute to modulating them downward or upward. In the course of expressing and clarifying feelings, additional layers and textures are likely to come to light. Indeed, we cannot overemphasize the importance of expressing feelings (at least to oneself if not to others) for the sake of further clarifying them. As we stated earlier in this chapter, this whole process of reciprocally expressing and clarifying emotion is self-constituting; mentalizing emotion entails making up one's mind. Solomon gives a fine example of what we would construe as self-constituting mentalizing in a continual flux of emotion:

In a tense situation, I suddenly realize (that is, recognize) that I am upset. I am agitated, sweating, edgy. But I was so before I noticed that I was so, and it is evident that my emotional disturbance did not begin just when I noticed it. Now that I notice my upset, however, I am not sure what I am upset about. Then I remember a brief confrontation I had with a colleague on the way out of the office and the way I slammed the door, and I realize that I must have been angry. But at what? I may or may not be able to pin this down, given the brevity and the seeming banality of that particular meeting. But then I remember earlier confrontations, a few of which were downright offensive. So now I understand my present anger not so much in terms of this one brief meeting but in terms of a whole history with this fellow. And I notice, as I have before, that the person's demeanor more than superficially resembled the behavior of my older brother: dismissive, disdainful, superior. (Solomon 2007, p. 229)

Solomon does not leave it at that; in his example, the emotions continue to course through different paths, with feelings of anger waxing and waning in the process. He reflects on being an angry person and notes his difficulty relaxing. The whole episode culminates in being angry about being angry, and the anger ultimately is diminished somewhat in amusement about this convoluted twist.

Agency in Mentalizing Emotion

As Solomon's example of reflection on a cascade of emotions evoked by an intense situation exemplifies, mentalizing emotion requires a sense of agency—owning emotion as a vital aspect of the self. Too often, emotion is seen as a passive response, as in "passion" (Solomon 2007). Doubtlessly, emotion sometimes can be fast and reactive, as when one is suddenly frightened or infuriated. Yet, the emotional experience is unlikely to come to an abrupt halt after the initial burst of intense feeling. At the very least, agency will be evident in the unfolding process of *working with* the emotions—understanding, regulating, and expressing them—as Solomon's example also attests. Mentalizing emotions is effortful mental work, especially when the emotions are intense and unwanted.

In the spirit of existentialism, Solomon extends agency in emotions beyond working with them as we have just summarized it here. Solomon proposes that we view emotions as *strategies*. Sometimes emotional strategies can be consciously intended and relatively deliberate, as when a person cultivates anger for the purpose of intimidating and bullying others to get his way. Sometimes the strategy can be relatively automatic, as when a person suddenly flees in fear. Sometimes the strategy can be unwitting, as when a resentful husband punishes his wife with depressive complaints and withdrawal. Earlier, we made the point that emotions are *potentially* adaptive. As these examples also illustrate, emotional strategies vary widely in their effectiveness. Most emotions, depending on their level of intelligence, vary in their effectiveness as strategies. Anger, for example, can be justifiably righteous, unreasonably petty, or inappropriately menacing. Solomon contends that, among the emotions, envy is unusual in being an invariably ineffective strategy:

> Its inclusion on the list of the "seven deadlies" is no mistake. Envy is not just wanting what someone else has. It is wanting *undeservedly* and usually *without recourse* what someone else has. That means that it is almost always a strategy for making oneself miserable, if not bitter, frustrated, and unhappy. It is, in short, a bad strategy. (Solomon 2007, p. 183, emphasis in original)

Viewing emotion as intentional strategies underscores the value of mentalizing not only with regard to what emotions are about but also what their purposes are, the appropriateness of these purposes, and the emotion's effectiveness in relation to the purposes. Agency implies responsibility, and mentalizing enhances responsibility. Solomon proposes heuristic inquiries into emotions that will be familiar to psychotherapists: "What am I doing this for? What am I getting out of this?" (p. 199).

Solomon's (2007) construal of emotions as being strategies manifesting agency and responsibility brings out the ethical dimension of emotions, namely, their prominent role in a life well (or badly) lived. This ethical dimension goes beyond "adaptation" in the Darwinian sense, and beyond "getting it right" in the intentional sense. Here we come back to the existential value of emotion: "The aim of our emotions, and the reason we have emotions in the first place, is to enhance our lives, to make them better, to help us get what we want out of life" (p. 182). Plainly, the life-enhancing potential of emotions requires mentalizing. And Solomon caps off this ethical view of emotion in advocating *emotional integrity*, by which he refers to achieving some degree of unity in a rich and complex emotional life. Consistent with Grayling's (2002) view, Solomon does not advocate a conflict-free life: "I would want to allow for a mixed, even conflicted, repertoire of feelings, emotions and reflections, including dissatisfaction, self-criticism, lack of contentment, and real ethical dilemmas, that is, impossible choices and engagements" (p. 267). He construes emotional integrity as integral to happiness, but he does not equate happiness with *feeling* happy; on the contrary, "A happy life with emotional integrity is not a life without conflict but a life in which one wisely manages emotional conflicts in conjunction with one's most heartfelt values" (p. 268). And, to take it one step farther, happiness is a kind of meta-emotion, involving an appraisal of our emotional life in toto: "Happiness depends on these moments (which may be plentiful or sparse) in which one gets a glimpse of our lives as a whole or, at least, of some substantial portion of our lives" (p. 266). Yet, as Solomon cautions: "This, perhaps more than any other emotional judgment, is liable to self-deception" (p. 266).

We have borrowed liberally from Solomon's work not just to bolster our point that mentalizing is and should be an emotional process but also to elucidate the sheer complexity in mentalizing emotion. Emotional integrity and happiness as Solomon construes it pose the greatest challenges for mentalizing. What better aspirations might we have for psychotherapy?

Recapitulation

Mentalizing is a fundamental human capacity that all but those in the autism spectrum generally take for granted: mentalizing is our capacity to relate to each other as persons—as minded beings. Albeit fundamental, mentalizing is anything but simple. The range of mental states we mentalize is vast (motives, feelings, beliefs, intentions, dreams, hallucinations, and much more); we mentalize not only consciously and deliberately by creating explicit narratives but also non-consciously and automatically in our implicit attunement and responsiveness; we mentalize states of mind in others and ourselves; and we attribute meaning to mental states on the basis of their wider context in the history of relationships.

Furthermore, although it comes naturally, mentalizing is by no means always easy. Skillful mentalizing entails accuracy, richness, and flexibility in perceiving and interpreting mental states and their meaning. We may fail to mentalize skillfully in many respects and in many contexts. When we are temporarily mindblind—inattentive or oblivious to mental states—mentalizing does not get off the ground. And, even when we are engaged in mentalizing, attentive to mental states, we are prone to distorted perceptions and interpretations, often as a result of projection (e.g., projecting self-criticism onto others) or defensiveness (e.g., failing to recognize anger for fear of aggression). Ironically, rich imagination— as in empathy— requires projection, which opens the door to defensive distortions. Above all, strong emotions in close relationships render mentalizing most difficult. We have emphasized the centrality of attention to mentalizing, and we have highlighted *effortful* attention because great effort is required to attend to and reflect on mental states, especially when striving to hold multiple perspectives in mind in the midst of strong emotions.

Given that our mentalizing capacity is ancient, we already have a rich language in folk psychology (Bruner 1990), most evident in our multiplicity of words for mental states. Our closest ordinary-language synonym for mentalizing is "empathy" (Baron-Cohen 2003, 2005), and we are inclined to endorse empathy for oneself as part and parcel of mentalizing. But we now have an array of more technical terms that overlap with mentalizing, such as theory of mind, metacognition, mindfulness, and psychological mindedness. Do we need yet another— "mentalizing"?

We advocate "mentalizing" as an inclusive term for the mental activity most central to our humanity, a term that focuses our clinical efforts to rectify the complex and multifaceted impediments to stable attachment relationships and self-regulation. Can there be any unity to this all-encompassing term that ranges over such diverse mental states, non-conscious and conscious processes, and pertains to self and others? Unity is the point: complexity notwithstanding, we relate to persons— ourselves among others—as constituted by a more or less unified self.

Moreover, rather than splitting non-conscious and conscious processes apart, we aspire to unify them, with implicit and explicit processes becoming mutually enhancing, as the implicit is increasingly available to explication and the explicit gradually becomes more procedural and automatic.

Perhaps the greatest divide we breach by mentalizing is the seeming gulf between self and other. Yet, as we will trace in the next chapter, this self-other boundary is a developmental achievement, not a given: the self is created through mentalizing in relation to mentalizing and mentalized others—attachment figures especially. Thus we believe that the concept of mentalizing is uniquely suited to encompass the unifying mental activity that is essential not only for creating selves in relationships but also for maintaining and enriching relationships suffused with emotions, imagination, and meaning.

Key Clinical Points

- *Mentalizing is multifaceted,* pertaining to a panoply of mental states in self and others, explicit and implicit processes, and time frames ranging from past to present and future; interventions must be tailored to what the individual experiences as the most relevant area of difficulty at any given time.

- *Two broad failures of mentalizing* are 1) not paying attention to mental states, for example, being indifferent or oblivious to others' mental states; and 2) mentalizing in a distorted and often intrusive fashion, as in paranoid interpretations of others' motives.

- *Egocentrism is the default mode of mentalizing,* and empathizing entails the effortful work of differentiating between oneself's and others' perspectives.

- *Although mentalizing is generally adaptive,* it can be painful (e.g., empathizing with suffering) and excessive (e.g., hypervigilant).

- *Much of psychotherapy enhances the mentalizing of emotion;* this entails 1) identifying emotional states and their context and causes, 2) modulating emotions downward and upward, and 3) expressing emotion while also thinking about its meaning, not only to others but also to oneself. Optimally, psychotherapy promotes mentalizing while remaining in the emotional state.

Chapter 3

Development

We articulated the multifaceted nature of mentalizing in the previous chapter, and we concluded by proposing that, of all the ordinary language and clinical concepts, *mentalizing* is uniquely suited to capture the essential unity of understanding oneself and others. As we elaborate in this chapter, the basis of that unity is the developmental process of coming to be a self in relation to others.

Of course, as a clinician, you need not know how mentalizing develops in order to engage your patients in mentalizing; you have been doing that all along. Yet we aim to promote more refined attention to mentalizing in clinical practice, and understanding the developmental conditions that enhance and inhibit mentalizing makes a crucial contribution to that refinement. Accordingly, we summarize current research on the development of mentalizing that we consider essential to understanding how to facilitate mentalizing in clinical practice.

Understanding the development of mentalizing requires counterintuitive thinking. Having acquired mentalizing capacities long ago, we adults are accustomed to taking a rich and private inner world for granted. We are naturally sympathetic with Descartes's dictum: I think, therefore I am. Moreover, we routinely employ our inner world to empathize with others through imagination and simulation (Goldman 2006; Stueber 2006). The use of inner experience to understand others creates a sense of the unity of minds and entails reasoning from the inside out: others are like me. Intuitively, we apply this line of reasoning to development: the child somehow comes to have a mind and then infers that others do too.

This natural Cartesian way of thinking obscures what Peter Hobson (2002) claims: "To put it bluntly, if an infant were not involved with other people, then she would not come to think" (p. xiv). As he elaborated, "The links that can join one person's mind with the mind of someone else—especially, to begin with, emotional links—are the very links that draw us into thought" (p. 2). Accordingly, he titled his marvelous book *The Cradle of Thought*. Thus Descartes was speaking accurately for the adult; speaking for the child in the making, we might put it differently: Mother thinks I am, therefore I am. Accordingly, counterintuitively, we embrace Vygotsky's (1978) view that mind develops from the outside in: "*An interpersonal process is transformed into an intrapersonal one*. Every function in the child's cultural development appears twice: first, on the social level, and later, on the individual level; first, *between* people (*interpsychological*), and then *inside* the child (*intrapsychological*)" (p. 57, emphasis in original).

In this chapter we first describe the developmental steps through which mentalizing emerges in relationships, and then we elaborate the complex interplay among parental mentalizing, attachment, and the development of mentalizing in the child. We also introduce what will be one of the primary concerns of this book, namely, how attachment trauma undermines the development of mentalizing and thereby contributes to developmental psychopathology.

Developmental Progression

The capacity to mentalize is a multistage developmental achievement that develops out of a host of capacities evident in early infancy that promote *social engagement* (Hobson 2002; Klin et al. 2000; Stern 1985). We begin this section by presenting a broad overview of the developing appreciation of the representational nature of mental states, which constitutes the ultimate sense of selfhood (Fonagy et al. 2002a). Then we elaborate four developmental processes that play major parts in the sense of self and others as having representational minds: emotion regulation, joint attention, language, and pedagogical interactions. To aid the reader in holding this developmental complexity in mind, we provide an overview of these main contributions in Table 3–1. All facets of development exemplify a central theme of this chapter: *contingently responsive mentalizing on the part of the caregiver promotes the development of mentalizing in the child.* We conclude this section with a discussion of three prementalizing modes of functioning that can become regressively activated in psychopathology: psychic equivalence, pretend mode, and teleological mode.

Mental Representation

The progressive development of mentalizing capacities is intertwined with agency, which, in turn, is intertwined with a sense of self and others. Fonagy and colleagues (2002a) have traced this development in five steps, outlined in Table 3–2. Here we focus on the emergence of mental representation, which we introduced in the context of a sense of representingness of mental states in Chapter 1 ("Introduction") and revisited briefly in the context of theory of mind in Chapter 2 ("Mentalizing").

As sketched in Table 3–2, infants soon learn that they (and others) are physical and social agents, capable of influencing—and being influenced by—external objects and other persons. Then, by around nine months of age, adopting a teleological framework, they expect agents' actions to be rational and goal directed (Csibra and Gergely 1998; Gergely and Csibra 2003). For example, at nine months, infants take it as a matter of course that one computer-animated agent takes a straight path as if to make contact with another, or jumps over an obstacle to do so if need be; yet these infants register surprise when one agent jumps needlessly to reach the other when there is no obstacle in its path. Nonetheless, notwithstanding their budding appreciation of rationality, nine-month-old infants do not yet comprehend the goal-directed actions of the agent as based on mental states; rather, expectations of agents' "rational" actions are based solely on observable physical realities (e.g., a straight or obstructed pathway).

During the second year of life, however, infants begin *mentalizing the teleological stance* (Gergely et al. 1995); they develop a mentalistic understanding of goal-directed agency. Infants develop a number of pertinent cognitive competencies, albeit rudimentary, during this period (Fonagy 2006): they interpret intentional agents' actions as stemming from desires, wants, and intentions (Wellman and Lagattuta 2000); they have an implicit understanding of true and false beliefs (Onishi and Baillargeon 2005); they engage in shared imaginative play that facilitates coopera-

TABLE 3–1.   OVERVIEW OF CORE PROCESSES IN THE DEVELOPMENT
OF MENTALIZING

Process	Description
Understanding of mental representation	A mentalistic understanding of goal-directed actions develops in which multiple mental models or perspectives can be contrasted (e.g., actual versus possible, past from present or future) and, ultimately, meta-representation becomes possible (e.g., reflecting on the accuracy of beliefs and awareness of thinking and feeling as such).
Emotion regulation	Understanding emotions plays a formative role in mentalizing and arises from a mirroring process in which infants' emotional expressions elicit a high but imperfect level of caregiver responsiveness that is "marked" by ostensive cues that show the infant that the caregiver is representing the infant's emotional state— not expressing the caregiver's own emotional state; this process enables the infant to develop self-representations of emotional states that promote emotion regulation and expression.
Joint attention	Awareness of attention directed to the self is evident in early infancy, and this awareness is succeeded by awareness of attending conjointly with another to a third object and by purposefully drawing others' attention to objects. Joint attention includes implicit emotional commentary on objects (as in social referencing) and, in this context, the other's attention to the self ushers in a special sense of self-awareness (and self-consciousness) as a person among persons.
Language	Language acquisition and mentalizing evolve in a bootstrapping process inasmuch as language acquisition requires joint attention and the appreciation of a communicative intention; in turn, linguistic capacities permit explicit mentalizing along with a refined conceptual framework for articulating mental states and reasoning about them (i.e., meta-representation).
Pedagogy	The caregiver's contingent responsiveness to the infant's emotional states can be construed as a process of implicit teaching, and the development of mentalizing is part and parcel of a human-specific adaptation for pedagogy, that is, an efficient means for teaching and learning cultural information—including knowledge about mental states. Like language, mentalizing and pedagogical learning develop in a bootstrapping process.

TABLE 3–2.   LEVELS IN THE DEVELOPMENT AND REFINEMENT OF
               MENTALIZING CAPACITY

Level	Description
Physical	Infants first develop a sense of self and others as physical *agents,* as distinct from physical *objects,* on the basis of being self-propelled and animated; physical agency contributes to the sense of self as author of actions (e.g., making one's limbs move) and as having influence over external objects (e.g., making the ball move), thus facilitating self-other differentiation.
Social	In tandem with physical agency, infants develop a sense of self and others as social agents; social agency encompasses awareness that communicative displays exert influence over other social agents (e.g., smiling prompts mother to smile).
Teleological	In the second half of the first year of life, infants develop a sense of self and others as teleological agents whose actions are purposeful and goal directed; at this level, infants expect actions to be rational, that is, efficiently directed toward goal attainment within the constraints of external reality (e.g., taking the straightest path to a goal).
Mentalizing	During the second year of life, infants begin mentalizing the teleological stance in the sense of interpreting rational, goal-directed actions as governed by intentional mental states, ultimately taking into account the possibility that the mental states governing actions may not correspond to reality (e.g., false beliefs).
Autobiographical	By the sixth year of life, children organize memories of their actions and experiences into a causal-temporal framework that permits the development of an autobiographical self and the understanding of self and others through coherent autobiographical narratives.

tive skills (Brown et al. 1996); and they begin acquiring a language to represent internal states (Repacholi and Gopnik 1997). Nonetheless, at this early stage infants are unable fully to separate mental states from external reality; the distinction between internal and external remains blurred (Fonagy 2006).

As we noted in discussing theory-of-mind research in Chapter 2 ("Mentalizing"), between three and four years of age, children develop a full-fledged explicit understanding of representational mental states, as exemplified by passing false-belief tasks that require linguistic articulation (i.e., anticipating that a child will look for something on the basis of where he wrongly *believes* it is located rather than on where it is *actually* located). In effect, in coming to develop an explicit understanding of mind as representational, children's thinking comes into alignment with cognitive science, which is predicated on the representational theory of mind (Fodor 2003). Perner (1991) has described the monumental developmental significance of this shift:

> representation is not just one aspect among others of the mind, but provides the basis for explaining what the mind is. In other words, by conceptualizing the mind as a system of representations, the child switches from a *mentalistic theory of behavior,* in which mental states serve as concepts for explaining action, to a *representational theory of mind,* in which mental states are understood as serving a representational function. One can think of the concept of "representation" as playing a catalytic role in children's reconceptualization of what the mind is. (p. 11; emphasis in original)

As Perner (1991) outlines it, the development of representational capacity frees the mind from reality. Going beyond perceptual representations, in the second year of life infants are able to construct and employ multiple models of the same situation, enabling them to formulate means-end relationships (e.g., contrasting an existing state with a desired state) and temporal relationships (i.e., contrasting past, present, and future). Then it becomes possible to have in mind something that is not present as well as to experience something that *is* present in different ways. The capacity for pretend play best exemplifies this decoupling of mental representations from reality (Leslie 1987); an object is represented as if it were something else, thereby acquiring a mental existence. Hobson (2002) gave the example of his son pretending that a spoon was a car: "The car-thought could be applied to the spoon-object, so that the spoon became a thought-car" (p. 77). Yet the full flowering of mind comes with the capacity for *meta-representation* (i.e., representing representations, as in "I think, therefore I am"); then the mind becomes aware of itself and its place in the world. The move to this meta-representational level permits cognitive and affective self-regulation through metacognition, as described in Chapter 2 ("Mentalizing"). While we might seem to be getting abstruse here in delving into meta-representation, this level of understanding is critical to our clinical work: patients in the throes of depressive rumination, paranoid projections, and posttraumatic flashbacks have lost a sense of their mind as mental—a sense of representingness. Accordingly, to mentalize, they need our help to keep in mind that their mental states are the work of their mind.

In fostering mentalizing in adults for the purpose of improving their functioning, we rest on solid developmental ground. In children, full-fledged mentalizing as marked by meta-representation is associated with a wide range of social-developmental capacities (Fonagy 2006): empathic behavior (Zahn-Waxler et al. 1992) and good relationships with peers (Dunn and Cutting 1999); elaborate pretend play (Taylor and Carlson 1997); more conversational fluency (Slomkowski and Dunn 1996); and greater social competence (Lalonde and Chandler 1995). Notably, there is also a downside to mentalizing: understanding of false beliefs also enables children to deceive and to play tricks and jokes (Sodian et al. 1992). Lastly, meta-representation includes the capacity to understand that behavior is influenced not only by transient mental states but also by enduring personality dispositions, providing the foundation for an emerging self-concept (Flavell 1999). As noted in Table 3–2, self-representations ultimately become organized into an autobiographical narrative. Correspondingly, mentalizing includes the capacity to understand others on the basis of their autobiographical selves—as we routinely do in conducting psychotherapy. And, as the practice of psychotherapy attests, mentalizing the self and others at increasing levels of refinement—in terms of accuracy, richness, and flexibility—is a lifelong endeavor.

Contingent Responsiveness and Emotion Regulation

Back to the beginning: Hobson (2002) asserted that "It is through emotional connectedness that a baby discovers the *kind* of thing a person is" (p. 59, emphasis in original). Similarly, Gergely and Watson (1996) proposed that, on the grounds that basic emotions are universal and innate, "emotions are among (if not the) earliest mental states that infants attribute to minds" (p. 1183). These latter researchers pinpointed a mechanism that sets the stage for mentalizing emotion, that is, going from the behavioristic stance of using emotional signals to predict behavior to recognizing emotions as mental states in others and oneself. This developmental progression is prompted by a shift in attentional preference. In the first few months of life, infants prefer perfectly contingent response→stimulus contingencies (Bahrick and Watson 1985), for example, watching as they move their limbs. By three months of age, infants know that anything which is not invariably and perfectly contingent on their own actions belongs to the external world (e.g., I move my arm and the ball beyond reach stays put).

Gergely (2001) identified a *switch in contingent responsiveness* around three months of age, at which point infants shift from a preference for perfect contingency to high-but-imperfect contingency, that is, *slightly* out of sync, novel, and unpredictable. This shift has monumental consequences for psychosocial development and for the development of mind in particular: infants switch their preference from attending to their own actions to attending to the emotionally responsive social environment. The mother's facial responses to her infant's emotional states are a perfect example of high-but-imperfectly contingent responses— just what her infant has come to prefer. Whereas infants' initial focus on perfect contingencies enables them to discover their bodily self in the physical world, their subsequent focus on highly but imperfectly contingent social responsiveness enables them to discover their mental self in the social world. This developmental step leads to a corresponding shift in the nature of affect regulation in the mother-infant relationship. Prior to the switch in contingency preference, comforting is provided by the mother's direct physical ministrations (e.g., comforting touch); subsequently, comforting can be provided by emotional communications that foster the development of affect representations in the infant.

More specifically, affect representations arise out of the early mirroring interactions of caregiver and infant aimed at soothing and downregulating the infant's arousal. Mirroring—resonating with, reflecting on, and expressing the internal state that the infant displays—is a universal, biologically prepared (instinctual) response on the part of all adults (Meltzoff and Moore 1997). For affect mirroring to support a representational framework, however, the mother must indicate that she is not showing the baby her own feelings, but rather her awareness of the baby's state. This form of mirroring is characterized by *markedness* (Fonagy et al. 2002a; Gergely and Watson 1996), that is, "marked" in the sense of being marked for sale or tagged. By intermingling an accurate reflection with an incompatible affect, or by exaggerating her display of the affect, the caregiver marks the expression as being as-if or pretend. For example, a mother might successfully soothe her infant by intermingling a reflection of the infant's distress with irony in her facial expression, or she might mimic the baby's frustration while showing concern. More generally, typical features of marked emotion include an exaggerated, slowed-down, or partial expression of the emotion; expressions of mixed emotions, combined simultaneously or sequentially; and behavioral cues such as raised eyebrows that frame the expression as intended for the infant's attention (Gergely 2007).

This process of mirroring emotion can go awry in two ways: either by failing to mark the affect or by lack of contingent responding. That is, expressions that correctly mirror the baby's state, but lack markedness, may overwhelm him. For example, rather than responding to the infant's frustration with a marked expression, the mother may feel angry and express her anger directly toward the infant. The infant feels such emotional expressions to be the parent's own real emotion, making the infant's experience seem contagious, thus experienced as even more dangerous, potentially leading to trauma rather than containment. On the other hand, the mother may respond to the baby with a marked but non-contingent (i.e., inaccurate) reflection. For example, the mother who mirrors the baby's excited biting of the breast as aggression might say, "Ouch! You are an angry little beastie today!" To the extent that it is internalized, mismatched mirroring generates alien internal experience that contributes to a fragmented sense of self (Fonagy et al. 2002a).

To summarize, the growth in understanding the self as a psychological (emotional) agent begins with infants' discovery of their own affects through their primary attachment relationships. Infants' budding capacities to experience their emotions as *feelings* are based on internalizing the caregiver's contingently responsive marked emotional expressions. The caregiver's mental representations of the infant's emotional states are exemplified in her behavior; intuitively, she *presents* these expressions to the infant. In turn, the infant begins to develop a mental representation of his or her own emotional state as a feeling—an emerging form of emotional self-awareness. These representations gradually form the basis for *mentalizing emotion* and thereby for affect regulation and impulse control: feelings become recognizable; they do not have to be acted out; and they can be shared.

Joint Attention

Attention not only plays a cardinal role in the ongoing activity of mentalizing but also in the development of mentalizing capacity. Research on joint attention in infancy, like that on emotional mirroring, illustrates the Vygotskian perspective that the sense of self develops from the outside in (Vygotsky 1978). Developmental research (Eilan 2005; Franco 2005; Reddy 2005) has elucidated the progression of joint-attention behaviors as enumerated in Table 3–3.

Reddy (2005) contends that "the self is the first target of others' attention that the infant experiences" (p. 106) and that "attention to the self may be the most direct and powerful experience of attention that is possible" (p. 86). Awareness of others' attention to the self is evident in the first few months of infancy. First, two-to-four-month-old infants *respond* to others' gaze at the self in varied ways. Illustrating how closely emotions are tied to attention, infants show responses ranging from pleasure and interest to ambivalence to distress and avoidance. Second,

TABLE 3–3.   MILESTONES IN THE DEVELOPMENT OF JOINT ATTENTION

- Responding emotionally to others' attention to the self
- Directing others' attention to the self as a whole and later to specific aspects and actions
- Following others' gaze toward objects
- Directing others' attention to objects in hand
- Directing others' attention to distant objects by pointing
- Ensuring that others' attention is engaged before pointing
- Checking others' emotional responses to objects or situations (social referencing)

infants also *direct* others' attention to the self, for example, by making utterances to bring about face-to-face engagement. At this time, infants also seek to reengage attention when it has been disrupted. In later months, infants' direction of others' attention becomes more refined; at seven to eight months, for example, infants go beyond soliciting attention to the self as a whole when they draw attention to specific aspects of the self (e.g., an exposed tummy) or specific actions (e.g., showing off and clowning). Later, infants direct others' attention to objects in hand (9–11 months) and then to distal objects (e.g., at 10–14 months, by pointing). Reddy maintains that the *objects and topics* of attention, not the participation in attentional engagements, become more complex over the course of development.

Engagement in mutual attention in early infancy provides the infant with the experience of being the object of another's attention. Of course, the early infant's engagement in attention contact does not require a concept of attention as an internal, unobservable state of mind (Gómez 2005); much less does the infant have the capacity to *represent the self as being represented* in the mind of the other. As Reddy (2005) noted, the objects of mutual attention become increasingly complex over the course of development. Whereas mutual attention in early infancy is dyadic, joint attention in the second half of the first year becomes triadic, involving the self, another person, and a third object. This triadic self-other-world relationship is fundamental; knowledge of any one requires knowledge of all three (Davidson 2001). Accordingly, Tomasello (1999) characterized the development of joint attention in relation to objects as the "nine-month social-cognitive revolution" (p. 11). Hobson articulated beautifully the significance of this triangulation for developing a sense of multiple mental perspectives, the essence of mentalizing:

What triangulation gives is a fixed point, a kind of pivot, around which different things are brought together. The pivot is the world. The two attitudes bear upon the same thing in the world. A single thing is experienced as having two meanings. It is this that prompts the infant to separate out her own attitude from that of the other. It is not just that the mother reacts and the infant feels new things—it is also that the mother and the infant are reacting to the very same object. Through this experience of having both her own and her mother's attitudes to the same things, the infant learns something about things on the one hand and attitudes on the other. In reading her mother's reaction to a toy, the infant learns something about the toy; but at the same time, the toy tells her something about her mother. What it tells her is that her mother is different from herself, in a particular way. It tells her that her mother has an attitude to the toy that is separate from her own attitude to the same toy. (Hobson 2002, p. 109)

Triangulation in joint attention reflects a complex developmental process (Eilan et al. 2005). Joint attention entails first having the infant's attention directed toward an object by someone else (e.g., looking where mother looks) and subsequently the infant's directing another's attention to an object (e.g., prompting mother to look where the infant looks). Joint attention is involved not just in following gaze but also in pointing and gesturing for others, holding up objects to show others, bringing others to specific locations to see an object, and offering objects to others by holding them out. Thus, as Hobson (2002) described, through joint attention, the infant develops an inchoate sense of sharing and comparing experience with another person.

A distinction between two forms of pointing illustrates the infant's incipient transition from a behavioristic to a more mentalistic stance. Infants first learn that pointing has the instrumental effect of inducing another person to do something (e.g., by pointing to the cup, the infant can induce mother to bring it). Subsequently, they learn to point to direct the other's *attention* to something (e.g., wanting mother to see the kitty)—that is, for the sake of sharing attention in the sense of generating some joint emotional engagement in relation to the object (Liszkowski et al. 2004). An important milestone in the development of joint attention, evident at about 18 months, is checking to ensure that the other's attention is engaged before pointing—what Franco (2005) called "the seed of mentalizing" (p. 142). We will be discussing the pedagogical nature of such interactions shortly; here we note that pointing in joint attention also can have an interrogative function, that is, as a request for relevant information about the object of attention (Fonagy et al. 2007).

Joint attention serves a crucial epistemic function in enabling the infant to learn about the world. Closely related to joint attention is social referencing, although the relative developmental timing of the two phenomena is unclear (Reddy 2005). In *social referencing,* the infant checks the mother's emotional reaction to a novel object, such as a noisy mechanical toy, to determine how the infant should regard it; for example, as interesting or dangerous (Moses et al. 2001). More generally, joint attention entails *implicit emotional commentary* on objects of mutual interest, and Eilan (2005) maintains that such expressions of emotion can be construed as primitive predications: "Reciprocated smiles are reciprocated comments on the world" (p. 28). We discussed the adaptive aspects of mentalizing emotion in Chapter 2 ("Mentalizing"); to a considerable degree, we rely on emotional knowledge of the world, and we begin acquiring that emotional knowledge through social referencing:

> there must be some sense in which this use of affective responses is imbued with some sense of *getting it right* in some respect. Things are scary or not, funny or not. The suggestion is that this primitive sense of right and wrong begins to be manifested as social referencing sets in, where the appropriateness or not of the response is precisely what the child is seeking reassurance about. One way of putting this is that affect regulation becomes, at this stage, regulation of the appropriateness of the response to the world. (Eilan 2005, p. 28, emphasis added)

Thus far, we have described joint attention in its triadic form as involving the infant's and mother's attention to a third object. Yet Tomasello (1999) also has described how, in this triadic context, *attention to the self* takes on new significance; self-awareness at a new level of complexity emerges:

> As infants begin to follow into and direct the attention of others to outside entities at nine to twelve months of age, it happens on occasion that the other person whose attention an infant is monitoring focuses on the infant herself. The infant then monitors that person's attention to *her* in a way that was not possible previously, that is, previous to the nine-month social-cognitive revolution. From this point on the infant's face-to-face interactions with others—which appear on the surface to be continuous with her face-to-face interactions from early infancy—are radically transformed. She now knows she is interacting with another intentional agent who perceives her and intends things toward her. When the infant did not understand that others perceive and intend things toward an outside world, there could be no question of how they perceived and intended things toward *me....* infants at this age also become able to monitor adults' emotional attitudes toward them as well—a kind of social referencing of others' attitudes to the self. This new understanding of how others *feel* about me opens up the possibility for the development of shyness, self-consciousness, and a sense of self-esteem. (pp. 89–90; emphasis in original)

In this passage, Tomasello has captured the dawning of the sense of self as a special sort of object: a person among persons. There is unity here, a sense of being like the other in being mentalized by the other. To reiterate, at this stage, self-awareness (as awareness of others' awareness) is far from being mentalized explicitly on the part of the infant; yet, along with emotional mirroring, it is part of the foundation on which mentalizing develops.

Language

Mentalizing and language develop in a bootstrapping fashion: incipient mentalizing capacities evident in joint attention are required for the acquisition of language; yet increasingly refined linguistic capacities are required for the development of a full-fledged representational theory of mind:

> young children's entry into the world of possibility is the crucial route into other minds. Moreover, it is a route that opens up only as their language abilities develop.... language mediates our experience of the world—how it can be used to *re*-present events so that what is communicated need not match what is (or was) in the world. As children acquire language, they acquire the ability to think about possible, re-presented scenarios, and they become able to imagine what other people might think, want, or feel. A new world opens up for them as they realize that people's minds are private from one another and separate from the real world. (Astington and Filippova 2005, p. 210, emphasis in original)

Here we summarize this bootstrapping developmental process and then note how compromised mentalizing capacities, as are glaringly evident in autism-spectrum disorders, result in compromised language use.

Tomasello (1999) argues that linguistic reference can be understood only in the context of *joint attentional scenes,* which he defines as "social interactions in which the child and the adult are jointly attending to some third thing, and to one another's attention to that third thing, for some reasonably extended length of time" (p. 97). Furthermore, these joint attentional scenes are defined intentionally: "they gain their identity and coherence from the child's and the adult's understandings of 'what we are doing' in terms of the goal-directed activities in which we are engaged" (p. 98). In addition, children must be able to engage in *role reversal* within these joint attentional scenes: they are spoken to, and they speak. Consistent with the dependency of language acquisition on joint attention, children develop a large vocabulary if their mother is adept at following into their attention (i.e., talking about objects they are already paying attention to), and children who spend more time engaged in joint attentional activities with their mother subsequently develop a larger vocabulary.

Not only are other minds the route to language but also, as Astington and Filippova (2005) contend, language is "a route into other minds," because it "serves two purposes: communication and representation" (p. 211). More specifically, "human language is used both as an intraindividual representational system and as an interindividual communication system" (p. 212). The link between communication and representation is evident empirically in relations between language and mentalizing: children begin developing the capacity to mentalize explicitly when they learn to employ words for mental states, and individual differences among children in their inclination to refer to mental states (e.g., in conversations with siblings and friends) are predictive of their subsequent performance in theory-of-mind tasks (Brown et al. 1996; Hughes and Dunn 1998).

Both semantic and syntactical aspects of linguistic competence have been implicated in explicitly comprehending false beliefs (Astington and Filippova 2005; de Villers 2000). Children must learn to distinguish between "the way things are in the world and the way things are represented in the mind" (Tager-Flusberg 2000, p. 131); to do so, they must comprehend the attitude of the person whose actions they are interpreting. Mental-state verbs, such as "think," "know," "guess," and "forget," serve to qualify the attitude of the person being interpreted (e.g., knows versus forgets) with respect to a given proposition (e.g., the cookies are in the cupboard). Thus, the semantics and syntax of language facilitate such reasoning about mental states—and the ability to juggle knowledge of mental states and reality when the two are in conflict, as they are in false-belief tasks (Astington and Filippova 2005).

Fully competent use of language requires mentalizing capacity, and persons with autism who have developed some capacity for language illustrate this connection (Hobson 2002). Tager-Flusberg (2000) has noted impairments in pragmatic use of language across the entire autism spectrum. Examples of characteristic impairments include pronoun reversals (e.g., "I" versus "you"), failure to attend to providing new information in conversation, difficulty maintaining an ongoing topic of discourse, difficulty interpreting figurative speech, and failure to appreciate jokes or sarcasm. Persons with autism also have difficulty with narrative discourse, being unable to organize a sequence of events that coheres with respect to the motives, beliefs, and emotions of the characters. As Tager-Flusberg (2000) summarized:

pragmatic impairments in autism are found across different discourse contexts. These impairments include: a narrower range of functions served by language; problems understanding that communication is about intended rather than surface meaning; failure to view conversations as a means of modifying and extending the cognitive environment of a conversational partner; and failure to view narratives as a means for communicating about both events and psychological states. What is striking about these impairments in communication is that they occur to some degree across the entire spectrum of autistic disorder. Across all ages, ability levels, and language levels, deficits are found in some or all of these aspects of pragmatics and communication. They are even considered to be one component of a broader autism phenotype, found among some proportion of first degree relatives with autism. (p. 127)

Yet mentalizing-related deficiencies in linguistic communication are by no means restricted to autism. On whatever basis, a failure to mentalize—for example, to hold the other person's mind in mind so as to provide needed contextual information—is likely to be associated with such pragmatic impairments of language (Sperber and Wilson 2002). Clinically, the thorough entanglement of mentalizing with language is evident in alexithymia (Krystal 1988; Taylor and Bagby 2004)—literally, not having words for feelings:

> It is hard to deny...that a shallow or impoverished vocabulary for emotional self-description makes for a shallow emotional life; and, conversely, that richer conceptual resources make for correspondingly enriched possibilities of emotional response. A person whose conceptual universe of the emotions is limited to the two possibilities of feeling good and feeling not-so-good will certainly fail to be subject to (and not just fail to notice) the range of responses possible for some other person with the emotional vocabulary of Henry James. (Moran 2001, pp. 40–41)

Henry James, we therapists are not; yet some of our best work will be helping our patients find the right words for their feelings and enriching their feelings in the process.

Pedagogical Interactions

From the point of view of the infant's development, we might construe contingently responsive mentalizing on the part of the caregiver as *implicit teaching* regarding the infant's state of mind—and emotional states in particular. This teaching and learning process is crucial for the development of the subjective sense of self and emotion regulation (Fonagy et al. 2007). More specifically, Gergely and colleagues (Csibra and Gergely 2005; Gergely 2007; Gergely and Csibra 2005) have explicated the development of mentalizing as one facet of a broader "human-specific adaptation for 'pedagogy,' a communicative system of mutual design specialized for the fast and efficient transfer of new and relevant cultural knowledge from knowledgeable to ignorant conspecifics" (Gergely and Csibra 2005, p. 463). Knowledge about minds is a major component of cultural knowledge and, central to our concerns, pedagogical interactions include teaching about minds, including the mind of the learner.

This uniquely human capacity to teach and to learn cultural information is extraordinarily efficient in comparison to trial-and-error or observational learning. Observational learning is relatively efficient for naturalistic purposes; for example, the infant can learn to get an object in a box by means of taking off the cover through first observing someone else do it (where the other person is not intending to provide instruction). Yet pedagogical learning is essential for acquiring *arbitrary* cultural knowledge (e.g., learning how a gadget like a spoon is to be used and, of critical importance, learning a language of arbitrary symbols). Paralleling the point we just made regarding the relation of joint attention and mentalizing to language acquisition, the capacity to relate on the basis of the *pedagogical stance* develops earlier than language and full-fledged mentalizing and, indeed, facilitates their development. Yet, in another bootstrapping process, once acquired, language and mentalizing enhance the capacity for pedagogical learning.

The infant's capacity to take the pedagogical stance does not emerge *de novo* but rather depends on a set of innate proclivities, including a preference for eye contact and the characteristic intonation of infant-directed speech ("motherese"). These innate behavioral tendencies prepare the infant to be receptive to *ostensive communication cues* that signal the teacher's intent to convey information to the infant; such cues include establishing eye contact, raising the eyebrows, widening the eyes, tilting the head forward, and addressing the infant by name. The ostensive cues trigger in the infant a receptive attentional and interpretive attitude, namely, the pedagogical stance (Gergely 2007)—as if the infant were to say, "I get it; you want to teach me something. OK, I'm ready, go ahead!"

Once the pedagogical stance is established, the communication must specify the *referent* of the knowledge to be transmitted (e.g., an object that is novel to the infant) as well as the *relevance* of the information to the infant (i.e., as comprising new knowledge for the infant). Thus, for the teacher, pedagogy entails mentalizing (knowing what the infant knows) and metacognition in particular (the capacity to represent her own knowledge in a form that is accessible to the infant). Concomitantly, the pedagogical stance presupposes *benevolent intent* on the part of the teacher, that is, a helpful intent to convey accurate and useful information. As Gergely observes, this pedagogical effort is costly to the teacher, who must mobilize the needed attentional resources, cognitive effort, and attachment motivation. In short, pedagogy requires a benevolent, *infant-minded caregiver* (Gergely 2007)—attributes that characterize a secure attachment relationship. In the course of secure attachment, infants develop a receptivity to teaching that Gergely and colleagues characterize as *epistemic trust,* namely, confidence in the caregiver as a reliable source of information. Insecure attachment, by contrast, carries the risk of inadequate or misleading pedagogical interactions along with faulty learning—including faulty learning about one's own state of mind (Fonagy et al. 2007). Then epistemic *mistrust* is liable to develop.

In Gergely's (2007) view, all the interactive phenomena we have been discussing as foundational for mentalizing exemplify pedagogical communication, including joint attention, pointing for the purpose of drawing the other's attention to an object, imitative learning, and—not least—language. Crucially for present purposes, emotional mirroring exemplifies all the features of pedagogy: emotionally attuned caregivers intuitively teach infants about the infants' subjective emotional states. This pedagogical process of teaching infants about their own emotional states, albeit intuitive, is extremely complex. Consider, for example, a mother interacting with her infant son. The mother must employ ostensive cues to gain her infant's attention, while making it clear to her infant that *he* is the referent of her communication. The "markedness" of the mother's expression, as we discussed it earlier in this chapter, is an essential cue that her emotional expression refers to him and not to her. The infant, then, employs her communication to derive information about himself—a mentalized representation of his emotional state that he can employ in the service of self-representation and can integrate with his own internal (e.g., somatic) cues. Thus he mentalizes his emotional state by connecting his bodily and muscular sensations with a mental representation derived from his mother's marked emotional response. This developmental process of beginning to mentalize emotion extends mentalizing to include internal states of the self; in effect, the infant is being socialized to pay attention to himself and to his internal world. Concomitantly, the infant develops an increasingly solid subjective sense of self along with the capacity for emotion regulation (Fonagy et al. 2007).

Gergely and colleagues (2007) also applied their pedagogical account to the phenomenon of social referencing, which we discussed in the context of joint attention. Infants employ social referencing, for example, to adopt attitudes toward unfamiliar objects (e.g., checking their mother's emotional expression to see if a novel toy is safe to play with). Gergely and colleagues presented experimental evidence that a communicator's (e.g., mother's) ostensive cues prompt the infant to interpret the interaction as a teaching event such that they are informed about the quality of the *object*, not the mental state of the teacher. This is a minimalist account of mentalizing activity in social referencing in the sense that the infant need not fathom the mother's mental state as such but rather must gather information about the nature of the object. Yet such pedagogical learning entails a default assumption that teachers are conveying accurate and universally shared knowledge about the world. Mentalizing comes into play when children come to learn that not all others are bearers of accurate or trustworthy information; this lesson requires understanding that all others are not entirely like-minded but rather have separate minds with different mental contents (e.g., knowledge). Thus, as Fonagy and colleagues (2007) put it, in coming to mentalize, children must learn not only that others *have* minds but also that they have *separate* minds.

Prementalizing Modes

Shedding further light on the development of mentalizing, Fonagy and Target (Fonagy 1995, 2006; Target and Fonagy 1996) distinguished two modes of experience that ultimately become integrated in the mentalizing mode, namely, psychic equivalence and pretend. When mentalizing collapses, individuals are liable to revert to these prementalizing modes, which also include the teleological mode. We will be referring to these four modes of experience throughout this book, and we summarize them in Table 3–4.

In the *psychic-equivalence mode*, the very young child equates the internal world with the external world: the world *is* how the mind represents it; alternative perspectives cannot be generated. Equating appearance and reality, children under four years of age do not know that a sponge shaped like a rock is a sponge despite looking like a rock (Flavell et al. 1987). Accordingly, very young children are potentially beset by fears associated with their imagination: if they *think* there is a monster in the closet, a monster *is* in the closet (world=mind). They cannot understand that mental phenomena such as thinking, knowing, imagining, and dreaming are generated by the brain and mind (Estes et al. 1989). Our second author gives an example of his son's distress in the psychic equivalence mode:

TABLE 3–4. MODES OF EXPERIENCE

Mode	Description
Psychic equivalence	World=mind; mental representations are not distinguished from the external reality that they represent, such that mental states are experienced as real, as in dreams, flashbacks, and paranoid delusions.
Pretend	Mental states are separated from reality but maintain a sense of unreality inasmuch as they are not linked to or anchored in reality.
Teleological	Mental states such as needs and emotions are expressed in action; only actions and their tangible effects—not words—count.
Mentalized	Actions are understood in conjunction with mental states (as contrasted to the teleological mode), and mental states have neither an exaggerated sense of reality nor unreality but rather are appreciated as representing multiple perspectives on reality (as contrasted with the psychic equivalence and pretend modes).

Some years ago, at about age four, the second author's son asked him to bring a Batman costume from one of his trips abroad. Wanting to please his son, and with considerable effort, the author found a Batman costume in a shop that sold theatrical costumes. On his return, his son tried it on, looked at himself in the mirror, cried, and demanded that it should be taken off and put away immediately. He proceeded to put on an old skirt of his mother's around his shoulders and ran around happily pretending to be Batman. In the expensive costume he *appeared* to be Batman and therefore *was* Batman. This is psychic equivalence.

The *pretend mode* liberates children from psychic equivalence (Fonagy 2006): in play, with the decoupling of internal and external reality (Leslie 1987), children retain awareness that their experience does not mirror the outer world (Dias and Harris 1990). Yet inner and outer must be kept separate:

The second author's son, aged two and a half years, was playing that an upside down chair was a tank and that the legs were shooting ammunition. He was asked: 'Is this a chair or a tank?' He stopped playing immediately, put the chair the right way up, and walked away. He knew that the object was a chair and not a tank. Yet, in the pretend mode, bringing external reality into contact with the play undercut imagination.

Neither the pretend mode nor the psychic-equivalence mode can create the optimal relation of the mind to external reality, albeit for opposite reasons: psychic equivalence is too real, whereas pretend is too unreal. In normal development the child integrates these two modes in coming to mentalize: mental states represent reality (unlike pretense) but are not equated with reality (unlike psychic equivalence). The essence of the representational mind is to be capable of adopting *multiple perspectives* on the same interpersonal situation, thus linking—but not binding—the mind to reality. As Perner (1991) described, the mind represents reality *as being* a certain way; father is seen as driving recklessly or as being in a hurry or as being frustrated. Moreover, full development of mentalizing skills includes an *awareness* of this representational relation of mind to reality—other perspectives are possible. Linking representational mind and world, mentalizing enables the recognition—implicitly or explicitly—that others' actions are understandable given their mental states, that is, their particular take on a situation. Concurrently, mentalizing entails awareness—implicit or explicit—that others interpret oneself in this way. This concurrent recognition affirms one's existence as a mental agent, representing the full flowering of the intersubjective experience of the self as the object in joint attention that Tomasello (1999) identified in the nine-month social-cognitive revolution.

As we will discuss later in this chapter in connection with attachment trauma, integrating psychic equivalence and pretend in the mentalizing mode does not render them obsolete; older children and adults are capable of regressing into these two modes. Moreover, we all regress into the psychic-equivalence mode—world=mind—on a daily basis when we dream. Furthermore, the *teleological* mode always remains a third prementalizing regressive possibility in which mental states like desires and affects must be expressed in action (Fonagy 2006): unable to mentalize his emotion, the patient with borderline personality disorder cuts himself and displays his bleeding arms to express in action what he cannot express in words.

Clinical Implications

To explicate the implicit: psychotherapy, a decidedly pedagogical endeavor, potentially replicates the developmental processes we have outlined in this section to help patients function more consistently in the mentalizing mode. Psychotherapists' empathy will entail highly but imperfectly contingent marked emotional responding. The psychotherapy process can go awry to the extent that the psychotherapist expresses intense and unmarked (real) emotion, abetting contagion, or expresses emotion incongruent with the patient's emotion, abetting internalization of alien experience. These emotional interactions take place in the context of joint attention, wherein the patient is the object of the therapist's attention (and vice versa); the implicit and explicit emotional commentary ideally promotes emotional knowing of the self in relationship. To be effective as an agent of change, however, this interchange must take place in the mentalizing mode: flexibly linked to reality without becoming too intensely real (psychic equivalence) or too detached (pretend, as in intellectualizing or using psychological jargon).

As we will continue to reiterate, psychotherapy is best construed as providing developmental help (Hurry 1998). Furthermore, as our emphasis on high-but-imperfect contingency implies, the psychotherapist's interventions should be only slightly discordant with the patient's experience. In the context of child education, Vygotsky (1978) provided a model for experience-near interventions in his concept of the *zone of proximal development*, namely, *"the distance between the actual developmental level as determined by independent problem solving and the level of potential development as determined through problem solving under adult guidance or in collaboration with more capable peers"* (p. 86; emphasis in original). In moving patients forward, we must be just slightly ahead of them, providing the necessary scaffolding through our own mentalizing.

Attachment and Mentalizing

If mentalizing capacity develops through relationships, the *quality* of those relationships will be pivotal. This section proceeds as follows: First, we describe the complex interplay between parental mentalizing, secure attachment in the child, and the child's mentalizing capacities. Next, we examine the relations between mentalizing and attachment in the context of intergenerational transmission processes. Then we consider the impact of attachment trauma on mentalizing capacity, and we also include some qualifications regarding our general thesis that the benevolent relationship climate of secure attachment is optimal for mentalizing. We conclude the section with comments regarding the clinical implications of all these findings.

Secure Attachment

Research has demonstrated a complex developmental interplay among parental mentalizing of the infant and child, child mentalizing capacity, and attachment security in infancy and childhood. Extensive research suggests that secure attachment is conducive to children's mentalizing capacities, but *contingently responsive parental mentalizing within the attachment relationship* plays the key role in facilitating the child's mentalizing.

Meins and colleagues' longitudinal studies have contributed substantially to understanding the developmental trajectories of mentalizing in the context of attachment relationships, and her research program will serve to anchor our review of the broader literature. Meins (1997) proposed the concept of maternal *mind-mindedness* to refer to the mother's "recognition of her child as a mental agent, and her proclivity to employ mental state terms in her speech" (p. 127). Meins and colleagues (2001) measured mind-mindedness in mothers' interactions with their six-month-old infants in a play situation, employing an index directly reflecting explicit mentalizing: *mind-related comments* on the infant's activities that were appropriate to the infant's behavior at that moment (i.e., contingently responsive); examples include, "Do you recognize that?" "Are you thinking?" "You're just teasing me!" Such mind-related comments reflect "the mother's proclivity to use language to frame the interaction in a mentalistic context" (p. 641) and thus indicate the mother's inclination to relate to the infant on the basis of her own mental representations of the infant's mental states. In this groundbreaking study, the assessment of maternal mind-mindedness in the interaction at six months predicted the infant's security of attachment measured subsequently at 12 months. This finding makes intuitive sense: secure attachment is measured by the extent to which the infant confidently reaches out to the mother for comforting after a period of separation in a laboratory separation-reunion paradigm (Ainsworth et al. 1978); when distressed, an infant is more likely to reach out for comfort to a mind-minded caregiver.

Lundy (2003) extended Meins and colleagues' findings by assessing mind-minded comments in mothers and fathers in relation to interactional *synchrony* as well as subsequent security of attachment. Synchronous parent-infant interactions are conceptualized as reciprocal and mutually rewarding, and exchanges were considered synchronous in this study if they involved at least three contingent steps between parents and infants. Replicating Meins and colleagues' results, Lundy found that both maternal and paternal mind-mindedness predicted attachment security; moreover, she found that mind-mindedness was associated with interactional synchrony for both parents and that synchrony mediated the relationship between mind-mindedness and subsequent attachment.

In earlier research, Meins and colleagues (Meins 1997; Meins et al. 1998) had found that security of attachment at 12 months, in turn, predicted subsequent theory-of-mind performance on a range of tasks. For example, whereas 83% of children with previous secure attachment passed a false-belief test at age four, only 33% of those with insecure attachment did so. A subsequent longitudinal study (Meins et al. 2002), however, failed to replicate this earlier finding, showing instead that maternal mind-mindedness at six months of age but *not* attachment security per se at one year predicted theory-of-mind performance at four years. The authors concluded that "the relation between attachment and ToM [theory of mind] can be explained best in terms of individual differences in mothers' mind-mindedness" (p. 1723).

An extension of this research program (Meins et al. 2003) showed that maternal mind-mindedness at six months also predicted children's performance on a stream-of-consciousness task at 55 months, a task that assessed their inclination to attribute active thought processes to an experimenter in various states of activity (i.e., sitting quietly and waiting, looking at posters on a wall, and solving a puzzle). Children were asked: "What about her mind right now? Is she having *some* thoughts or ideas, or is her mind empty of thoughts or ideas?" Thus children who had mind-minded mothers at six months were more inclined to attribute thinking to another person at 55 months. Notably, these researchers also assessed mothers' mentalizing at the child's age of 48 months by asking mothers to describe their child and determining the extent to which their descriptions referred to aspects of the child's mental life (i.e., as opposed to behavioral, physical, or very general descriptions). Mothers' six-month mind-mindedness regarding the interactions related strongly to their mentalistic descriptions at 48 months, showing continuity in maternal mentalizing. Yet only the six-month measure and not the more concurrent 48-month measure related to children's performance on the theory-of-mind and stream-of-consciousness tasks, suggesting that general *descriptions* of the child are less predictive of the child's development than contingently responsive mentalizing *interactions*.

Meins and colleagues (2003) concluded that "mothers' appropriate comments on their infants' mental states might provide a linguistic and conceptual scaffold within which infants can begin to understand how mental states determine behavior" (p. 1208). Plainly, these interactions are occurring before the infant has developed the capacity to use language, much less the capacity to mentalize; hence the findings suggest that the mothers' proclivity to mentalize and to draw the infant into contingent interactions provides an interactive foundation for the *later* development of mentalizing:

> Appropriate mind-related comments at 6 months index the beginnings
> of mothers' and infants' joint attention to mind, in which mothers' ap-

propriate labeling of their infants' current mental states helps draw infants' attention to the existence (and perhaps functional significance) of mental states and processes. In due course, and perhaps at a slightly later stage in development, this kind of interaction presents infants with opportunities to integrate subjective information on their mental states with an external linguistic comment on the behavior that results from these states. (Meins et al. 2003, p. 1208)

As Meins and colleagues' research attests, there is nothing magical about the relation between secure attachment and mentalizing: secure attachment constitutes a relationship climate conducive to mentalizing *interactions*; conversely, as described earlier in this chapter, contingent mentalizing responsiveness is conductive to affect regulation that cements the secure emotional bond, as Meins and colleagues' (2001) findings also suggest.

Additional research is noteworthy in part for illustrating the range of assessments of parental mentalizing conducive to secure attachment and child mentalizing. Oppenheim and colleagues (Koren-Karie et al. 2002; Oppenheim and Koren-Karie 2002), for example, videotaped parents and children interacting in various contexts and then interviewed the parents regarding their perceptions of their children's thoughts and feelings as well as their own. This assessment can be done for infants (e.g., in free play) as well as for preschool children (e.g., when building a house together). These researchers focused on maternal *insightfulness* regarding the motives underlying their child's behavior in the interaction. Insightfulness encompasses understanding and acceptance of the child's motives; an emotionally complex and undistorted view of the child, including positive and negative features; and openness to unexpected behavior that leads to continual updating of her view of the child. This research showed that mothers who were classified as positively insightful regarding their interactions with their child were most likely to have securely attached children. Notably, insightfulness accounted for variability in attachment above and beyond maternal sensitivity, that is, appropriateness of responsiveness to the child in the interaction (Koren-Karie et al. 2002).

As we have indicated, there is a complex interplay between parental mentalizing of the child, secure attachment, and the child's subsequent development of mentalizing capacity. Although Meins and colleagues' research showed inconsistent relationships between security of attachment per se and the child's mentalizing capacities, Fonagy and colleagues (1997a, 1997b) found both concurrent and predictive relationships between attachment security and mentalizing capacities. Their research program assessed security of attachment in three- to six-year-old children with projective test stimuli depicting various separation scenarios to which the children told stories in response to specific prompts. The children also were administered a belief-desire reasoning task that required appreciation of false beliefs and disappointment. Not only did concurrent attachment security as measured by the projective test correlate with successful performance on the belief-desire reasoning task but also this successful child mentalizing was predicted by mother-infant and father-infant attachment security.

Sharp, Fonagy, and colleagues have carried the study of parent-child correspondence in mentalizing forward into later childhood (Sharp et al. 2006). As they point out, it is advantageous to study older children inasmuch as they can talk about what is on their mind. Employing 7- to 11-year-old children, the study used cartoon scenarios involving distressing peer-related scenarios (e.g., a child sitting alone on a playground). Children were asked to mentalize by imagining what the cartoon subject's peers were thinking, and their mothers were asked to mentalize by guessing their child's responses—mentalizing their child's mentalizing. Inaccurate maternal mentalizing was associated with inaccurate mentalizing in children, namely, children's unrealistically positive views of what other children might be thinking, an attributional bias that has been shown to relate to disturbances in peer relationships (Sharp et al. 2007). Moreover, inaccurate maternal mentalizing was associated with high levels of psychopathology in children, as measured by self-report and parent report.

Gottman and colleagues (1996) have studied what we would call optimal mentalizing of emotion in parents of older children. Specifically, they studied what they call parental "meta-emotion philosophy" and its relation to child functioning. By meta-emotion, they refer to attitudes toward emotion—what we would call a mentalizing stance toward emotions. Specifically, meta-emotion philosophy bears on "parents' feelings and thoughts about their own and their children's emotions, their responses to their child's emotions, and their reasoning about these responses" (p. 245). In researching parental meta-emotion, they observed that some parents adopted an emotion-coaching strategy with five components:

> parents (a) said that they were aware of low intensity emotions in themselves and in their children; (b) viewed the child's negative emotion as an opportunity for intimacy or teaching; (c) validated their child's emotion; (d) assisted the child in verbally labeling the child's emotions; and (e) problem solved with the child, setting behavioral limits, and discussing goals and strategies for dealing with the situation that led to the negative emotion. (p. 244)

As we would construe it, parents with an emotion-coaching philoso-phy are mentalizing emotion in themselves and their children as well as actively promoting mentalizing emotion in their children, although the researchers did not specifically assess children's mentalizing. In a longi-tudinal study of children beginning at age five and ending at age eight, Gottman and colleagues (1996) found that parental meta-emotion and emotion coaching were associated with children's lowered physiological arousal and greater emotion-regulation capacities as well as with better functional outcomes as measured by academic achievement and peer re-lations. Moreover, a subsequent study (Katz and Gottman 1997) showed that parents' meta-emotion philosophy contributed to resilience in their children, specifically, being one factor that buffered children against the adverse effects of marital discord, separation, and divorce.

We have reviewed research on parent-child interactions in detail be-cause this research provides a straightforward model for clinical inter-ventions. In closing this section, however, we mention some additional studies to underscore the sheer breadth of empirical support for the re-lation between attachment and mentalizing. Precocious mentalizing in childhood as reflected in theory-of-mind task performance has been as-sociated with more reflective parenting practices (Ruffman et al. 1999), the quality of parental control (Cutting and Dunn 1999; Vinden 2001), parental discourse about emotions (Denham et al. 1994; Meins et al. 2002), the depth of parental discussion involving affect (Dunn et al. 1991), and parents' beliefs about parenting (Baumrind 1991; Vinden 2001). We have argued that such effective parenting is likely to promote the child's acquisition of a coherent conceptual apparatus for under-standing behavior in mentalistic terms. It is not surprising, for example, that parents whose disciplinary strategies focus on mental states (e.g., a victim's feelings or the non-deliberate nature of transgressions) have children who learn quickly to appreciate the importance of mental states (Sabbagh and Callanan 1998). Furthermore, we would expect tol-erance for negative affect to be characteristic of secure attachment and, concomitantly, a family environment that facilitates mentalizing. Ac-cordingly, family-wide talk about negative emotions, often precipitated by the child's own emotions, has been shown to predict later success on tests of emotion understanding (Dunn and Brown 2001); this finding is consistent with the fact that reflecting on intense emotion without being overwhelmed is a marker of secure attachment (Sroufe 1996). Similarly, the number of references to thoughts and beliefs and the relationship specificity of children's real-life accounts of negative emotions relates to precocious mentalizing (Hughes and Dunn 2002).

Intergenerational Transmission of Attachment

To take a step back: What are the origins of parental mind-mindedness? Fonagy and colleagues' research program on the means by which attachment security is mediated by mentalizing (Fonagy et al. 1991a, 1991b, 1994; Steele et al. 1996) extended a productive line of investigation of the intergenerational transmission of attachment (Fraiberg et al. 1975; Main 1991; Main et al. 1985). While they were pregnant with their first child, mothers were interviewed about their own attachment history with the Adult Attachment Interview (Main and Goldwyn 1994). Fonagy and colleagues' initial study of 96 mother-infant pairs revealed that the mother's security of attachment in relation to her parents assessed *prior to the birth* of her infant predicted her infant's security of attachment with her at 12 months (Fonagy et al. 1991a). Fonagy and colleagues subsequently found the same pattern for father-infant pairs (Steele et al. 1996), and these findings have been replicated consistently by other research teams (Benoit and Parker 1994; van IJzendoorn 1995; Ward and Carlson 1995).

Fonagy and colleagues proposed that attachment security is transmitted in part by the securely attached parent's mentalizing capacity:

> we assume that the quality of the infant's attachment to the parent is intrinsically linked to two factors both present and measurable before the birth of the child: (1) the parent's internal working model; and (2) the parent's capacity to reflect on the current mental state of the child and to reflect on, and exert control over, his or her own expectations of relationships as these influence his or her behavior toward the child.... The child is likely to be securely attached if *either* the parent's internal model of relationships is benign, dominated by favorable experiences, *or*...the parent's reflective function [mentalizing] is of sufficient quality to forestall the activation of working models based on adverse experiences inappropriate to the current state of the relationship of child and caregiver. (Fonagy et al. 1995, p. 258)

Slade and colleagues (Slade 2005; Slade et al. 2005) further validated Fonagy and colleagues' (1995) model of intergenerational transmission by assessing not only mothers' security of attachment and mentalizing capacity with respect to their own attachment history but also the mothers' ability to mentalize in relation to their infant (at 10 months); they too assessed the infants' subsequent security of attachment (at 14 months). These researchers assessed mothers' mentalizing of their infant with a 90-minute Parental Development Interview. The interview covers such matters as the mother's perception of her infant and the infant's feelings; her thoughts and feelings about separations from her infant; and her view of herself as a parent as well as her view of the way her experiences with her own parents influenced her parenting. Mentalizing was assessed on the basis of the mother's awareness of mental states, her recognition of developmental aspects of mental states, and her awareness of mental states in relation to the interviewer.

As previous research had done, Slade and colleagues' study confirmed a strong relationship between the mother's security of attachment and her mentalizing capacity in relation to that attachment. In addition, the mother's security of attachment in relation to her parents predicted her ability to mentalize in relation to her child. Moreover, maternal mentalizing capacity in relation to the child was predictive of the child's attachment security. Finally, the researchers found suggestive evidence that the link between the security of the mother's adult attachment measured in pregnancy and her infant's security of attachment at 14 months was mediated by the mother's mentalizing capacity. As Slade (2005) asserted, "the centrality of the parent as mediator, reflector, interpreter, and moderator of the child's mind cannot be overemphasized" (p. 273). More specifically:

> A mother's capacity to hold in her own mind a representation of her child as having feelings, desires, and intentions allows the child to discover his own internal experience via his mother's representation of it; this re-presentation takes place in different ways at different stages of the child's development and of the mother-child interaction. It is the mother's observations of the moment to moment changes in the child's mental state, and her representation of these first in gesture and action, and later in words and play, that is at the heart of sensitive caregiving, and is crucial to the child's ultimately developing mentalizing capacities of his own. (p. 271)

Importantly, Slade and colleagues' research demonstrated that the mother's predominantly mentalizing stance toward her infant, consistent with her ability to mentalize in relation to her own attachment history, promoted attachment security in her infant. Yet attachment develops in relation to behavioral interactions with the infant. Thus Arnott and Meins (2007) took this line of investigation yet another step. As others had done, they assessed (prenatally) the mother's and father's security of attachment in relation to their own parents as well as their capacity to mentalize about their early attachment experience. In addition, as Meins and colleagues had done in their previous research, they independently assessed each parent's mind-minded comments to their six-month-old infant in a free play situation, and then they did a follow-up assessment of their 12-month-old infant's security of attachment to each of them. Thus they were able to put all the components of the developmental pathway together.

Although there were some differences between mothers and fathers, the following general pattern held for both parents: security of parental attachment (to their parents) was positively related to mentalizing capacity (regarding those attachments); both security of attachment and mentalizing capacity were related to mind-minded comments to the infant at six months; and mind-minded comments were predictive of the infant's security of attachment at 12 months. Two general developmental pathways for both parents were identified: parental secure attachment was linked to infant secure attachment through high parental mind-mindedness, and parental insecure attachment was linked to infant insecure attachment through low parental mind-mindedness. Thus the combination of parental secure attachment and mind-mindedness was a powerful predictor of infant attachment for both parents.

To summarize this line of research we have reviewed, the capacity to mentalize in the attachment relationship is part and parcel of secure attachment. As Slade and colleagues' work demonstrates, parents who demonstrate mentalizing capacity in relation to their own childhood attachments are thereby more likely to develop rich, accurate, and flexible mental representations of their infant; as Meins and colleagues' work shows, this mentalizing capacity is manifested in mind-minded, contingently responsive interactions with their infants. In turn, paralleling their parents, the infants develop secure attachment as well as mentalizing capacities. This broad intergenerational trajectory is summarized in Figure 3–1. Fonagy (2006) has articulated the import of this developmental process:

> As we currently formulate it, the mother's secure attachment history permits and enhances her capacity to explore her own mind and promotes a similar enquiring stance towards the mental state of the new human being who has just joined her social world. This stance of open, respectful exploration makes use of her awareness of her own mental state to understand her infant—but not to a point where her understanding would obscure a genuine awareness of her child as an autonomous being. The awareness of the infant, in turn, reduces the frequency of behaviours that would undermine the infant's natural progression towards evolving its own sense of mental self through the dialectic of interactions with the mother. (p. 70)

Attachment Trauma

Just as secure attachment relationships are the crucible for optimal mentalizing, trauma in attachment relationships is inimical to mentalizing (Fonagy et al. 2007). *Attachment trauma* carries a double meaning, refer-

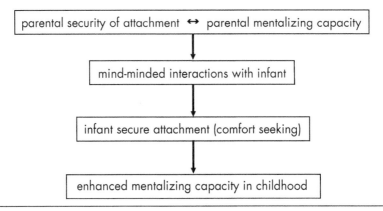

FIGURE 3-1.   INTERGENERATIONAL TRANSMISSION OF SECURE
ATTACHMENT AND MENTALIZING.

ring to trauma inflicted in an attachment relationship as well as to the
concomitant undermining of the capacity for secure attachment (Allen
2001). Abusive and emotionally neglectful behavior plainly reflects an
absence of empathizing in the caregiver; inflicting trauma exemplifies
mindblindness (Allen 2007). Consequently, whereas parental mentalizing is conducive to secure attachment, childhood maltreatment engen-
ders the most profound form of attachment insecurity, namely, disorganized attachment (Main and Solomon 1990; van IJzendoorn et al. 1999).
The disorganized infant is not able to develop any consistent strategy
for relating to the attachment figure; accordingly, Main (1999) characterized disorganized attachment as *fright without solution.*

As Fonagy and Target (1997a, 2002) have proposed, childhood maltreatment undermines the development of mentalizing capacity and
thus poses a dual liability: the maltreatment evokes distress and simultaneously undermines the *development* of capacities for affect regulation. More specifically, attachment trauma promotes a defensive
withdrawal from the mental world—at worst, a phobic avoidance of
mentalizing (Fonagy et al. 2007). Awareness of the mind of the abuser
is terrifying to the child, because "he will be confronted with attitudes
toward himself which are extremely painful to recognize: hatred, cruelty,
indifference" (Fonagy and Target 1997a, p. 693). This self-protective retreat from the mental world undermines the child's reflective capacities,
for example, as shown by poor performance on theory-of-mind tasks,
diminished capacity for pretend play, and the relative absence of language referring to internal states. Impaired mentalizing, in turn, undermines coping with an abusive relationship in a vicious circle:

Poor comprehension of mental states associated with maltreatment amplifies distress, activating the attachment system. The need for proximity persists and perhaps even increases as a consequence of the distress caused by abuse. Mental proximity becomes unbearably painful, and the need for closeness is expressed at a physical level. Thus, the child may paradoxically be driven physically closer to the abuser. The child's ability to adapt to, modify, or avoid the perpetrator's behavior is likely to be constrained by limited mentalizing skills, and exposure to further abuse is likely to occur. The paradox of proximity seeking at the physical level concurrent with psychological avoidance lies at the root of the disorganized attachment consistently seen in abused children. (Fonagy et al. 2000, p. 111)

Main and Hesse (1990) proposed that *frightening* or *frightened* behavior on the part of the parent is the key contributor to disorganized attachment; such behavior might include looming or invading the child's space, playing frightening games, timidity, or parental dissociative states. Lyons-Ruth and colleague (Lyons-Ruth and Jacobvitz 1999) identified two patterns of maternal behavior associated with attachment disorganization: *hostile intrusiveness* and *helpless withdrawal*, both of which reflect misattunement and aversion to the child's attachment behavior along with an inability to empathize with the child—a failure to mentalize in the context of attachment-related interactions.

Building on Lyons-Ruth's approach, Slade and colleagues' (Grienenberger et al. 2005; Slade 2005; Slade et al. 2005) research program also considered the adverse side of attachment. These researchers were especially interested in "a mother's capacity to regulate her child's affect at times of heightened arousal," and they hypothesized that "her behavior at times of distress and negative affect (rather than global sensitivity, per se) will be most crucial in determining the child's attachment security" (Grienenberger et al. 2005, p. 300). Non-mentalizing maternal behavior included affective communication errors (e.g., laughing when the infant is crying), role or boundary confusions (e.g., demanding a show of affection), fearful behavior (e.g., as evident in a squeaky voice), intrusive behavior (e.g., pulling the infant by the wrist), and withdrawal (e.g., not acknowledging the infant after a separation). The research showed that these non-mentalizing interactions were associated with high levels of infant insecurity, especially as manifested in disorganized attachment. Notably, paralleling secure attachment, an intergenerational transmission process also has been demonstrated for disorganized attachment. Parental disorganized attachment is associated with atypical maternal behavior and with disorganized infant attachment (Goldberg et al. 2003). Moreover, preliminary evidence that the capacity for change in attachment organization decreases over development underscores the danger that persistent trauma will lead to long-term disorganization of attachment, with attendant poor development of social cognition and substantially raised risks of psychopathology (Kobak et al. 2006).

Slade and colleagues' research buttresses the conceptual links between trauma and impaired mentalizing (Fonagy and Target 1997a). On the one hand, as these researchers proposed, "mothers who were able to openly reflect on their children's affect and intentions would be better equipped to handle infant vulnerability without becoming overwhelmed by their own unintegrated fear or hostility." On the other hand, "Parents who are lacking in RF [reflective functioning] may become easily dysregulated or disorganized by their infant's distress as they fail to distinguish between their own feelings and those of their children" (Grienenberger et al. 2005, p. 308). If we take egocentrism—attributing one's own mental states to others—to be the default non-mentalizing mode (Decety 2005), we can see how attachment trauma exemplifies its worst instantiations. Owing to their own trauma history, parents are liable to relate to their distressed child, in effect, in the psychic-equivalence mode. As Slade (2005) summarized:

> Disturbed and abusive parents obliterate their children's experience with their own rage, hatred, fear, and malevolence. The child (and his mental states) is not seen for who he is, but in light of the parents' projections and distortions. The infant then takes on the parent's hatred and aggression, a primitive form of identification with the aggressor. (p. 273)

Consistent with the foregoing review, a wealth of research links maltreatment to developmental deficits that we would anticipate to be associated with impaired mentalizing. Maltreated children's narratives show disturbances in parental representations as well as self-representations (Macfie et al. 2001). Specifically, abused children's capacity to generate complex representations of the parent in conflict-imbued settings decreases with development; similarly, their self-representations become increasingly simplified and exaggerated (Toth et al. 2000). Maltreated children are impaired not only in cognitive aspects of mentalizing, such as theory-of-mind tasks (Cicchetti et al. 2003; Pears and Fishler 2005) but also in emotion-focused mentalizing (Pears and Fishler 2005; Rogosch et al. 1995; Smith and Walden 1999). For example, as Fonagy and colleagues' (2007) review of research indicates, maltreated children are less likely to respond empathically to other children's distress; they show more emotionally dysregulated behavior; they talk about internal and emotional states less often; and they have difficulty understanding emotional expressions. Hence, in construing emotionally modulated conversations as the royal road to mentalizing, Fonagy and colleagues draw an analogy from the effects of maltreatment to those of sensory deficits: the learning environment is not only frightening but also impoverished, lacking the open and reflective communication about mental states that most nourishes mentalizing.

In sum, given all we now know about the adverse effects of maltreatment on the development of mentalizing, we might view the extensive empirical evidence linking secure attachment to mentalizing from two perspectives: secure attachment not only entails the *presence* of mentalizing-promoting behaviors (e.g., mind-mindedness) but also the *absence* of mentalizing-undermining behaviors (e.g., hostile intrusiveness and neglect). In short, mentalizing begets mentalizing and, conversely, non-mentalizing begets non-mentalizing. Hence the intergenerational transmission process for secure attachment (as depicted in Figure 3–1) is mirrored by an adverse intergenerational transmission process for insecure attachment as depicted in Figure 3–2.

Qualifications

In the preceding review, we have documented a well-researched global correspondence between accurate mentalizing and secure attachment, on the one hand, and mentalizing failures and insecure attachment, on the other hand. Yet we also have noted that mentalizing is highly context-dependent, fluctuating within a given attachment relationship depending on the nature of the interaction at the moment. As we will dis-

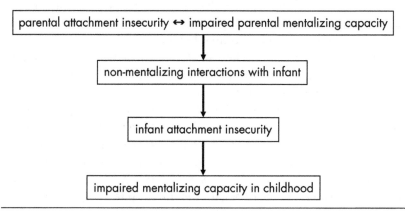

FIGURE 3–2.   INTERGENERATIONAL TRANSMISSION OF INSECURE ATTACHMENT AND IMPAIRED MENTALIZING.

cuss further in Chapter 4 ("Neurobiology"), recent neuroimaging findings have led to some refinements in our understanding of the relationship of attachment to mentalizing. Quite obviously, dynamic fluctuations in the emotional quality of the secure attachment relationship will determine the extent to which mentalizing is active at any given point in time (Fonagy 2006; Fonagy et al. 2007). There are three conditions under which mentalizing will be inhibited or inactive in the overall context of a secure attachment relationship. First, activating loving feelings, be they those of a mother for her baby or those in a romantic relationship, sometimes inhibits mentalizing—as will be unsurprising to readers whose passion occasionally has overridden their judgment of romantic partners. Second, threat-related activation of attachment, such as might occur at times of separation, can undermine mentalizing by virtue of evoking overwhelming affect that is uncharacteristic of the relationship generally. Third, a stable secure attachment relationship can obviate the need to mentalize, for example, insofar as there is no need to contend with threatening or stressful interactions or to make judgments of trustworthiness.

On the other hand, there are three broad reasons for secure attachment being conducive to mentalizing. First, inevitable challenges, conflicts, and fears in the relationship will prompt mentalizing, and the emotional containment the relationship provides will modulate the emotional arousal to a level conducive to mentalizing. Second, while not necessitating mentalizing, a secure attachment relationship promotes positive emotional arousal conducive to an interest in mentalizing. Third and most crucial: as we have been emphasizing, in a secure attachment relationship the attachment figure is frequently mentalizing the child, and mentalizing is conducive to further mentalizing. In effect, as the "pedagogical stance" implies, the secure attachment relationship is the ideal practice ground for mentalizing.

While we generally associate mentalizing with benevolence, and the link between secure attachment and mentalizing is consistent with this association, there are important exceptions. As we have just implied, one reason to mentalize is social threat: when relationships are potentially exploitative or injurious, mentalizing serves not only to detect the threat but also to facilitate self-protective interactions and negotiations. Thus we learn to mentalize in a competitive-threatened mode as well as in a securely attached, exploratory mode. Hence *in*secure attachment can promote mentalizing of negative emotions (Harris 1999). Of course, mentalizing in the competitive-threatened mode can be compromised when affect escalates; then we see distortions characteristic of mentalizing in a downright paranoid mode. Thus we have a double-edged sword: social competition and threat, which likely fueled the evolution of mentalizing capacities and associated brain structures (see Chapter 4, "Neurobiology"), can either enhance or undermine mentalizing. On the other hand, partly by alleviating competitive pressures, secure attachment can promote the fullest flowering of mentalizing capacities (Fonagy et al. 2007).

The flip side of this competitive-threatened-paranoid relationship paradigm is also noteworthy: mentalizing skills can be employed to threaten, exploit, or harm others (Fonagy 2006; Fonagy et al. 2007; Sharp 2006). Thus, developmentally, mentalizing skills can be associated with malicious teasing, bullying, deception, and relational aggression (e.g., in girls who elicit intimacy and disclosure and then manipulate the relationship by threatening to expose secrets). Notoriously, psychopathy can be associated with exceptional mindreading skill employed for manipulative, exploitative, and malevolent purposes.

All these instances of antagonistic social behavior reflect skillful but *partial* mentalizing; something is missing, namely, empathy (Sharp 2006). In Baron-Cohen's (2003, 2005) terms, for example, psychopathy entails mindreading without empathy, that is, mentalizing without an appropriate emotional response to the mental states being mentalized accurately (see Chapter 4, "Neurobiology"). We consider mindreading without empathy to be impoverished mentalizing in the sense of a *failure of emotional knowing* (or knowing through emotion). Thus the lack of appropriate emotional responsiveness reflects a profoundly significant lacuna in otherwise intact mentalizing.

Finally, while we have argued that mentalizing is the developmental wellspring of secure attachment and vice versa, mentalizing is employed, practiced, and refined in the full range of interpersonal relationships throughout life. As Dunn's (1996) research attests, the practice of mentalizing beyond relationships with caregivers begins in childhood in interactions with siblings and peers. Nonetheless, the parallels with secure attachment are noteworthy:

> The *quality* of the child-child relationship was important here: it was during playful cooperative interactions that the children discussed mental processes, and the length of their friendship and frequency of their interaction were positively related to explicit reference to mental processes. (Dunn 1996, p. 512; emphasis added)

Notably, despite mothers' frequent use of mental state language with their children, four-year-old children use mental state terms more often in conversing with siblings and friends than with their mother, often in the context of pretend play (Brown et al. 1996). Moreover, children's performance on theory-of-mind tasks and emotion understanding is correlated with the extent of their conversations about mental states in dyadic play (Hughes and Dunn 1998). Thus discourse about emotional states plays a central role in the development of mentalizing capacities (Harris 1999), and such discourse occurs in a wide range of relationships. We hardly strain common sense in extrapolating: what is characteristic of childhood holds throughout life, namely, that positive relationships of all sorts promote mentalizing and vice versa. Of course, antagonistic, competitive, and insecure relationships also can prompt mentalizing when they are short of overwhelmingly threatening.

Clinical Implications

As we described in Chapter 1 ("Introduction"), Bowlby (1988) recognized that the secure base of attachment not only promotes exploration of the outer world but also enables the exploration of the world of the mind. Research reviewed in this chapter has begun to clarify the means by which psychotherapists provide this much needed secure base.

Ideally, *mind-minded* therapists keep up a mind-related commentary appropriate to the patient's current state (Meins et al. 2001), engaging in contingently responsive mentalizing interactions. Ideally, therapists are *insightful* in the sense of understanding and accepting patients' motivation, developing an emotionally complex view of patients that subsumes positive and negative features, while remaining open to continually updating their views on the basis of new information without introducing distortions based on preconceptions (Oppenheim and Koren-Karie 2002). Similarly, therapists construct autobiographical narratives of their interactions with patients that predominantly reflect their patients' intentional nature (Slade et al. 2005). Conversely, hostile intrusiveness and helpless withdrawal on the part of therapists will undermine their patients' mentalizing capacities (Lyons-Ruth and Jacobvitz 1999). Yet we must not convey that a continuously warm and benevolent climate will best promote mentalizing in psychotherapy, any more than it would have done in childhood development. Developing greater ability to mentalize in the context of challenge and threats to attachment security requires that these emotional states be evoked—and mentalized—in the psychotherapy process.

Two aspects of these clinical implications bear underscoring. First we focus primarily on the patient's current mental state rather than exploring past mental states. Such a focus on the present might appear to be non-contingent when the patients are considering how they "were" rather than how they "are," but the mentalizing therapist moves fluidly between these states, considering the current motivation for exploring the past as well as the impact of exploring past states on the current mental state. Second, the "insightful" therapist promoting mentalizing is not seeking causal *explanations* (i.e., explaining the present on the basis of the past) but rather is continually striving to stimulate a coherent and emotionally *meaningful narrative* for both patient and therapist. Moreover, as we just noted, this narrative is best developed in the midst of emotional states, positive and negative.

Naturally, a therapist's ability to hew to these ideals will vary from patient to patient and from time to time with any given patient (Diamond et al. 2003)—just as is true of mothering, fathering, or any other relationship. Moreover, we have focused relatively exclusively on the impact of the attachment figure's mentalizing on the child's mentalizing, just as we emphasize the impact of the psychotherapist's mentalizing on the patient's mentalizing. But we should keep in mind that mentalizing is always a two-way street. Fonagy and colleagues (2007) refer to the often neglected child-to-parent effect; for example, that non-mentalizing behavior in children can evoke controlling behavior in parents. The same applies to patient-to-therapist effects. Of course, as the ideal parent would do, we psychotherapists should aspire to mentalize in the face of non-mentalizing behavior.

Recapitulation

We introduced this chapter by proposing that, in contrast to concepts such as empathy, mindfulness, metacognition, psychological mindedness, and the like, mentalizing is uniquely grounded in developmental research. We recognize that all clinicians necessarily mentalize and aspire to promote mentalizing in their psychotherapeutic work, whether or not they have heard the word and whether or not they are privy to mentalizing's developmental foundations and trajectory. But we have argued that owing to this developmental grounding, knowledge of mentalizing promises to refine our clinical work: understanding development clarifies the relationship conditions that promote and undermine mentalizing and enables us to provide needed developmental help—ideally, sooner rather than later.

Recall the extensive developmental ground we have covered in this chapter. We have characterized the development of the self in terms of increasingly sophisticated agency: infants begin life as *physical* and *social* agents, exerting influence over their body, physical objects, and other persons; they develop *teleological* understanding when they perceive agents as being engaged in rational goal-directed actions. During the second year of life, when infants begin *mentalizing* the teleological stance, they become able to interpret goal-directed actions as based on mental states such as desires and intentions. By the close of their third year of life, having passed the litmus test of passing false-belief tasks, children fall into line with modern cognitive scientists in employing a representational theory of mind. The representational view of the self continues developing throughout life into a rich inner world associated with an increasingly complex autobiographical narrative, ideally accompanied by a correspondingly rich understanding of other persons. As we have contended, all this mental development goes from the outside in: caregivers' contingently responsive mentalizing in the form of emotional mirroring, joint attention, and pedagogical interactions instigate and scaffold this development of the self. But the mentalizing mode of functioning, once achieved, is not consistently maintained; psychopathology associated with attachment trauma, for example, entails regression to prementalizing modes: psychic equivalence, pretend, and the action-oriented teleological mode.

Following in Bowlby's footsteps, we have conveyed one overriding message: to promote mentalizing, psychotherapy must recapitulate optimal development by creating a climate of secure attachment. Yet this message would be relatively uninstructive without all the developmental research we have described. Decades ago, Bowlby's collaborator, Mary Ainsworth (Ainsworth et al. 1978), rightly linked secure attachment to *sensitive responsiveness*. But we have learned since that the core of sensitively responsive caregiving is mentalizing—and mentalizing emotion in particular. Hobson characterized variations in this process well:

> Suppose an infant is in a particular state of mind and is needing an appropriate response from a caregiver. She might be excited and joyful, deeply upset, or screaming with rage. The contrast is between an adult who has the mental space to pick up and be sensitive to the infant's state, so that the infant feels responded-to and somehow encompassed within the adult's attentive care, and an adult who either cannot perceive or cannot take on board what the baby is feeling. (Hobson 2002, p. 125)

Owing to extensive clinical observations and research, we now know a great deal more about how the development of mentalizing flourishes and, sadly, with research on attachment trauma, we also know how it founders. Thus we are in an increasingly strong position to provide—however belatedly—needed developmental help that will foster a stronger sense of self-agency, greater capacities for emotion regulation and impulse control, and an enhanced sense of connection with others.

Bowlby (1982) maintained that secure attachment is essential for us all throughout life—"from the cradle to the grave" (p. 208). Many of our patients struggle to attain or maintain secure attachment relationships, and an important function of psychotherapy is to assist them in those efforts. As the research reviewed in this chapter attests, we psychotherapists assist them in the ways that infant-minded parents do: by mentalizing and promoting mentalizing in a benevolent yet challenging relationship. Employing attention and imagination, we must develop accurate and rich mental representations, always open to novel elaborations while remaining mindful of skewing preconceptions and countertransference distortions. Psychotherapy is indeed a pedagogical relationship insofar as it is characterized by contingently responsive, implicit and explicit mentalizing interactions in which our patients can make use of our representational capacity to enhance their sense of self; inherent in this process is enhanced agency stemming from the process of knowing oneself and making oneself known.

Key Clinical Points

- *Conditions that promote and undermine mentalizing:* Attachment research illuminates the relationship conditions that promote and undermine the development of mentalizing. Contingent, mind-oriented responding promotes mentalizing in psychotherapy as well as in development; the mind-minded mother is a model. Conversely, non-mentalizing interactions (e.g., intrusiveness and withdrawal) are as inimical to psychotherapy as they are to development.

- *Role of contingent emotional responsiveness:* As it does in development, contingent emotional responsiveness in psychotherapy provides an external representation of emotional states; this process can go wrong in two ways. First, if the therapist's emotional responses are too intensely real (unmarked), the patient's emotional state will escalate. Second, if the therapist's responses are out of sync with the patient's emotions (non-contingent), a number of things can happen: at best, patients who are unable to correct the misunderstanding will ignore the intervention; at worst, they will internalize the therapist's misrepresentation. In the face of persistently non-contingent responses, patients may cease to look to the therapist as someone who is able accurately to re-present their experience.

- *Prementalizing modes:* When mentalizing is lost, three prementalizing modes of subjectivity can come to the fore: psychic equivalence (equating reality with the current mental state, as in concrete thinking), pretend (not relating mental states to reality, as in dissociation), and teleological (expressing mental states through action or somatic reactions). Evidence of prementalizing modes of functioning in therapy is an indication that the therapist's primary task is not to explore, elaborate, explain, or correct the patient's productions but rather to work with the patient to recover mentalizing.

Chapter 4

Neurobiology

If mentalizing required understanding the neurocognitive basis of this activity, none of us would have learned to do it. Yet we clinicians have ample reason to become familiar with the general direction of neurobiological research on mentalizing. First, neuroscience is putting some steel reinforcement in the scientific foundation of the developmental research we reviewed in the last chapter. Second, we have delineated both heterogeneity and unity in the concept of mentalizing, and neurobiological research is putting our conceptualization to the test; the brain, through its responses to our neuroimaging probes, can inform our ways of mentalizing it. Third, appreciating how neurobiological deficits contribute to impaired mentalizing can point our attention to strategies for clinical intervention. Finally, the neurocognitive perspective underscores the potential therapeutic value of psychopharmacological treatment in tandem with psychosocial interventions.

Taking Bowlby's (1982) lead, we begin this chapter by considering the pivotal role of mentalizing in the evolution of attachment. Then, relying largely on recent neuroimaging research, we devote the bulk of the chapter to delineating brain regions that contribute to various components of mentalizing. More concerned with mind than brain, we organize this review around emotional, cognitive, and interpersonal processes to reinforce our understanding of mentalizing. A word of caution to the uninitiated: with the advent of neuroimaging, the research literature pertinent to mentalizing is mushrooming; the complexity of the findings is staggering, and we aim merely to highlight some general trends. Finally, we conclude the chapter with a consideration of two neurodevelopmental mentalizing disorders with genetic bases: autism and psychopathy. Both disorders exemplify mentalizing failures associated with impaired functioning in brain regions that contribute to mentalizing.

Evolution

As we have already noted, Premack and Woodruff (1978) introduced "theory of mind" into the literature in their study of chimpanzee social intelligence. Individuals were construed as having a theory of mind if they were capable of predicting behavior on the basis of imputing unobservable mental states to conspecifics. Although Premack and Woodruff presented evidence that a chimpanzee imputed unobservable intentions to an actor who was engaging in solving various problems, subsequent researchers have varied in their inclination to attribute mentalizing to nonhuman primates; hence among researchers themselves, some are more willing than others to mentalize in imputing mentalizing to chimpanzees and other animals (Macedo and Ober 2006). Tomasello and Call (1997) reviewed evidence for primates' sophisticated social skills: they can recognize familiar individuals and their relationships to one another; interpret behavioral cues so as to predict others' actions; formulate social strategies and communicate to influence others' actions; and learn from observing the behavior of others. Yet Tomasello and Call argued that Premack and Woodruff's initial results have not held up to further scrutiny, concluding that "there is no solid evidence that nonhuman primates understand the intentionality or mental states of others" (p. 340), notwithstanding their ability to make sophisticated behavioral predictions.

While not disagreeing about the lack of evidence that primates can impute hidden mental states, Gómez (2004) argued for a broader and more pluralistic conception of theory of mind that would encompass *overt* mental states, that is, mental states observable in behavior, such as expressing emotion, paying attention to something, or intending to do something—an example being "who is trying to do what to whom and with what final goal" (p. 236). Gómez concluded that "Chimpanzees and other primates may have some rudimentary version of these basic mentalistic schemas for making sense of the social world" (p. 236) and, further, that "primates perceive other primates' behaviors as intentional, in the sense that they may see each other as being connected with particular targets in particular ways" (pp. 236–237). Notably, the comparative literature parallels the developmental literature here: *investigators* differ from one another not only in the breadth of their concepts of mentalizing but also in their inclination to mentalize, that is, to entertain mentalistic interpretations of infants' and young children's behavior (Hobson 2002).

Without splitting hairs, we might conclude that nonhuman primates demonstrate incipient mentalizing and that we humans have taken a quantum leap forward in our capacity to develop a fully representational theory of mind that enables us to impute covert as well as overt mental states and to reason in sophisticated ways about them, not only in regard to others but also in relation to ourselves. Accordingly, the traditional view that practical problem solving—foraging and tool making—drove the evolution of the neocortex has been supplanted by the view that, in evolution, an escalating demand for social intelligence has fueled the cognitive equivalent of an arms race (Bogdan 1997; Humphrey 1988). Alexander, for example, proposed that our superior intelligence evolved not for the sake of dealing with the hostile forces of nature but rather for the sake of competition with each other; we became our own "principal hostile forces of nature" (Alexander 1989, p. 469).

Thus, while we also master folk physics and folk biology (Carey 1985), the sheer cognitive complexity of folk psychology (Godfrey-Smith 2004) has provided the greatest impetus to neocortical development. Group (and inter-group) living requires highly complex social skills not only for the purpose of competition (e.g., for resources or mates) but also for cooperation; indeed, we often *cooperate for the purpose of competing*; for example, in forming alliances to strengthen a competitive advantage. We need dedicated brain apparatus to keep track of our own and others' alliances as well as the social hierarchies within which these alliances are embedded (Byrne and Whiten 1988; de Waal 1989). Such social cognition required increasingly sophisticated problem-solving skills of a unique sort. Bogdan (1997) characterized these relationships skills in terms of the capacity for *interpretation*—yet another term for mentalizing—defined as "a competence that allows primates to make sense spontaneously and effectively of each other in terms of behavioral dispositions and psychological attributes, such as character traits, emotions, feelings, and attitudes" (p. 1).

Tomasello (1999) proposed that our mentalizing capacity solves an otherwise inexplicable evolutionary puzzle: given the near-total overlap in genetic makeup between chimpanzees and humans, the mere six million years since the splitting of the genetic lines is insufficient time for genetic variation and natural selection to account for the evolution of the diverse cognitive skills evident in our technology, communication, and social organizations. The genus, *homo*, evolved a mere two million years ago, and species-specific cognitive skills emerged only a quarter of a million years ago with *Homo sapiens*. Tomasello (1999) proposes that our extraordinarily rapid cognitive development required social and cultural transmission of knowledge, gradually ratcheting forward with new creative inventions continually building upon prior accumulated knowledge. He identified three types of social learning: imitative learning, instructed learning, and collaborative learning, all founded on mentalizing:

> These three types of cultural learning are made possible by a single very special form of social cognition, namely, the ability of individual organisms to understand conspecifics as beings like themselves who have intentional and mental lives like their own. This understanding enables individuals to imagine themselves "in the mental shoes" of some other person, so that they can learn not just *from* the other but *through* the other. (pp. 5–6)

As we described in Chapter 3 ("Development"), Gergely and Csibra (2005) have developed this line of thinking further in characterizing our species-specific capacity for *pedagogy* as adaptive in permitting rapid and efficient cultural learning. Mentalizing capacity is the common denominator in this evolutionary leap.

Fonagy (2006) proposed that "Evolution has charged attachment relationships with ensuring the full development of the social brain" (p. 60). In this sense, the evolutionary function of attachment goes far beyond providing protection of the offspring by assuring physical proximity, as Bowlby (1982) originally proposed. As Fonagy (2006) notes, attachment is associated with the exceptional dependence of the human infant on caregivers for a prolonged period of time, coupled with the emergence of intensive parenting. Accordingly, attachment, in synergy with mentalizing, organizes physiological regulation (Hofer 2003) and promotes brain development (Fonagy et al. 2007; Schore 2001; Siegel 1999). We should not lose sight of the enormous plasticity of the brain during this formative period: brain volume quadruples between birth and age six, and traumatic experience during this period can have a significant adverse effect on brain development (Giedd 2003).

Through genetic variation, individual differences are the engine of evolution; to date, short of autism, the evidence for genetic contrIbutions to individual differences in mentalizing capacity remains equivocal. An initial study with a relatively small sample found that theory-of-mind scores of 120 40-month-old twins were powerfully influenced by genetic factors (Hughes and Cutting 1999). Specifically, the study estimated heritability at 67%, with the remaining 33% of variance accounted for by non-shared environmental factors. Yet a longitudinal study employing a substantially larger sample of 1,116 60-month-old twin pairs who completed a comprehensive battery of theory-of-mind tasks (Hughes et al. 2005) found environmental contributions to be predominant. Behavioral-genetic models of the data showed that environmental factors explained the largest portion of the variance in theory-of-mind task performance and that environmental influences affecting both twins and non-shared environmental influences (i.e., parental and other non-genetic influences that are specific to each child) on theory-of-mind performance were substantial. To the extent that genetic factors contributed to theory-of-mind performance, they overlapped with the genetic contribution to verbal ability. Shared environmental influences also contributed to overlapping variability in verbal ability and theory of mind. Yet, based on the substantial environmental influence that appeared to be specific to theory of mind, the authors speculated that a number of social influences such as we have already reviewed (Chapter 2, "Development") come into play.

No doubt, we have much to learn about the phylogeny of mentalizing capacities (Tomasello and Call 1997) as well as the early cultural evolution in which the uniquely human capacities for symbolization and language came into being (Corballis 2002; Mithen 1996). We have introduced the evolutionary perspective in part to expand our purview beyond ontogeny to phylogeny and thereby to underscore the centrality of mentalizing to our humanity: attachment is a mammalian adaptation (MacLean 1990), but we human primates catapulted ourselves forward in evolution on the basis of whatever subtle neurobiological tweaks gave us the capacity to learn to mentalize in our attachment relationships, which yielded our unique capacity for rapid cultural learning and the expansion of culture.

Neurobiological Basis of Mentalizing

Consistent with the evolutionary perspective, mentalizing can be construed as innate in the broad sense of "developmental outcomes that are more or less inevitable for a given species" (Elman et al. 1996, p. 22).

Evidence for innateness of mentalizing includes a culturally invariant developmental sequence, relative independence from level of intelligence, little individual variation, and a narrow time window for development (Fletcher et al. 1995). Accordingly, mentalizing is one function of what we loosely call the "social brain" (Brothers 1997). In using this terminology, however, we should not imply that brain regions active in mentalizing are exclusively devoted to processing social stimuli (Fernandez-Duque and Baird 2005). This caveat accepted, converging evidence from human and nonhuman primate studies with a wide range of methodologies (e.g., effects of brain lesions, neuroimaging, and single-cell recording) implicates several brain areas in the processes of social engagement and mentalizing. Indeed, the sheer diversity of brain structures that are active in mentalizing tasks is consistent with the multifaceted nature of mentalizing (Fonagy et al. 2007); to highlight this diversity, Table 4–1 provides a rough sketch of the functions of key brain structures implicated in mentalizing, which we discuss in more detail in the text.

Recognizing that many clinicians are less interested in neuroanatomy than in the psychology of mentalizing, we organize this review around key mental activities: we begin with the neurobiological basis of perceiving social cues and resonating emotionally, as a prelude to dis-

TABLE 4–1. FUNCTIONS OF KEY BRAIN STRUCTURES IMPLICATED IN MENTALIZING

Structures	Functions
Fusiform gyrus	Identification of individuals
Superior temporal sulcus	Perceiving agency and intentionality in behavior
Amygdala	Assigning emotional significance to behavior
Temporal poles	Generating semantic contexts for behavior
Mirror neurons	Resonating with observed actions and emotions
Anterior insula	Experiencing and observing pain and disgust
Anterior cingulate	Effortful control of attention, cognition, and emotion
Orbitofrontal cortex	Monitoring changing reinforcement contingencies
Medial prefrontal cortex	Mentalizing region proper (overlapping anterior cingulate)

cussing brain areas implicated in mentalizing emotion and interpersonal interactions. Then we discuss seemingly paradoxical findings suggesting that attachment can *de*-activate brain areas associated with mentalizing, and we conclude with a discussion of mentalizing impairments associated with excessive emotional arousal.

Perceiving Social Cues

We start with two temporal lobe structures implicated in the input side to mentalizing: the *fusiform gyrus* (sometimes called the fusiform face area) is activated by static figures (animals or faces) and thus plays a role in perception of appearances and identification of individuals, whereas the *superior temporal sulcus* is activated in response to biological motion and the active behavior of living things (Adolphs 2003; Frith and Frith 2003). The superior temporal sulcus integrates complex visual-perceptual information and is strongly interconnected to the full range of cerebral structures involved in social cognition: it is involved in perceiving animacy, agency, and intentionality as manifested in overt behavior; it is responsive to changeable aspects of behavior (e.g., facial expressions as well as eye and mouth movements); and it thus plays a key role in facilitating prediction of the next move in a behavioral sequence. Notably, these perceptual processes are extremely rapid: global categorization of faces occurs within 100 milliseconds, and specific discrimination of individual identity occurs within 170 milliseconds (Adolphs 2003).

The *amygdala* can be construed as the sensory gateway to the limbic system (Schore 2001), and it plays a significant role in assigning emotional significance to highly processed input from the superior temporal sulcus (Aggleton and Young 2000; Rolls 1999). Hence the amygdala is highly responsive to social cues, including facial expressions, gaze (e.g., someone looking at you), and body movements (e.g., someone approaching you). Brothers (1997) assigned the amygdala a pivotal role in social cognition inasmuch as the amygdala is highly sensitive to facial cues, and the face plays such a prominent role in social communication. In her view, the amygdala functions as an "editor" in the social brain by biasing information processing such that faces receive preferential attention. More specifically, the amygdala directs the visual system to attend to the eye region to make use of information pertinent to identifying emotions such as fear (Adolphs et al. 2005). Consistent with this view, Stone (2000) concluded that the amygdala "forms an important *input system* to the theory of mind circuit" (p. 265, emphasis added). In assigning social significance to stimuli, for example, the amygdala contributes to judgments of trustworthiness (Adolphs 2003).

Researchers have debated the extent to which the amygdala is responsive only to fear, to emotion with a negative valence, or to a broader range of emotion (Davidson et al. 2000). Clearly, the amygdala plays a central role in fear conditioning (Armony and LeDoux 1997; LeDoux 1996), and it is especially responsive to stimuli signifying threat and danger (Aggleton and Young 2000; Davidson 2000). Illustratively, PET scans of subjects looking at photographs of faces expressing varying intensities of happiness and fear revealed monotonic increases in amygdala activity from the most happy to the most fearful face (Morris et al. 1996), and an fMRI study of responses to facial expressions showed amygdala activation in relation to expressions of fear but not disgust (Phillips et al. 1997). Yet Rolls (1999) presented evidence for amygdala activation in both rewarding and punishing contexts and concluded that it is "most unlikely that the amygdala is specialized for decoding of *only* certain classes of emotional stimulus, such as fear" (p. 110, emphasis added). Instead, Rolls views the amygdala as involved in stimulus-reinforcement associative learning and as coding the social significance of faces generally. Consistent with this view, Bonda and colleagues (1996) employed neuroimaging to study perception of biological motion using point-light displays by which movement can be depicted by means of isolated points of light attached to the body's main joints. This research showed that, in contrast to the superior temporal sulcus, which was generally active in the perception of biological motion, the amygdala was activated by *emotionally* expressive movements (i.e., in dancing).

Neuroimaging studies demonstrate that the amygdala response to emotional stimuli can be extremely rapid and non-conscious. Whalen and colleagues (1998) showed participants pictures of human faces expressing fear or happiness; the pictures were presented for 33 milliseconds and followed by a neutral face that served to mask the emotional stimulus such that participants only reported seeing the neutral face. Nonetheless, fMRI showed increased amygdala activity to the fearful faces and decreased amygdala activity to the happy faces, suggesting that the amygdala is involved in non-conscious monitoring of emotional stimuli. Notably, the amygdala deactivation suggests that a happy face might be construed as a safety signal. An additional study of amygdala activation in response to fear-conditioned stimuli (Morris et al. 1998) showed that the right amygdala was activated by the masked stimulus, whereas the left amygdala was activated by the unmasked (consciously perceived) stimulus; these results are consistent with other findings suggesting that the left cerebral hemisphere is more involved in conscious processing and the right hemisphere is more involved in non-conscious processing. Of course, the amygdala does not stop functioning after an immediate appraisal but rather contributes to processing at several stages: rapid non-conscious appraisals of stimuli can influence the course of further conscious reappraisal, in the course of which the prefrontal cortex serves to modulate amygdala activity and thus to regulate emotional responses (Adolphs 2003; Hariri et al. 2003).

The *temporal poles* also are active in interpreting social cues and situations and thus are active in mentalizing tasks. The anterior temporal lobe integrates information from all sensory modalities as well as the limbic system, and the left temporal pole is especially active when linguistic processing is involved in social cognition. Thus Frith and Frith (2003) proposed that "this region is concerned with generating, on the basis of past experience, a wider semantic and emotional context for the material currently being processed" (p. 465). They note, for example, that behavior is often interpreted in terms of normative scripts (e.g., a restaurant script); that the left temporal pole might be engaged in the retrieval of social scripts; and that unexpected deviations from social scripts call for mentalizing.

Domes and colleagues' (2007) research provides a noteworthy addendum to findings regarding the input side to mentalizing. Consistent with evidence that the peptide oxytocin mediates social affiliation and attachment, these authors found that an intranasal administration of oxytocin improved performance on the Reading the Mind in the Eyes Test (Baron-Cohen et al. 2001), a measure of participants' ability to infer mental states from photographs of the eye region. The authors speculated that oxytocin might influence activity in the fusiform gyrus, superior temporal sulcus, and amygdala, among other brain regions pertinent to mentalizing.

Resonating Emotionally

Nowhere is the self-other unity in mentalizing more concretely evident than in the burgeoning research on *mirror neurons* (Rizzolatti and Craighero 2004). This research has begun to provide clues about the neurobiological basis of empathy, although research on mirroring emotions (i.e., feelings evoked by observing another person in an emotional state) has lagged behind research on mirroring actions. We begin with the latter.

Mirror neurons were first observed in the ventral premotor cortex of monkeys; the same neurons are activated by *performing* an action and by *observing* conspecifics performing the same action, suggesting an overlapping neural representation (Jeannerod 1997). Thus, in the midst of observing others' action, mirror neurons encode the self's *potential* action as part and parcel of the perception (Rizzolatti and Luppino 2001). Rizzolatti and colleagues thus proposed a direct matching hypothesis:

> we understand actions when we map the visual representation of the observed action onto our motor representation of the same action. According to this view, an action is understood when its observation causes the motor system of the observer to "resonate".... we understand others through an "internal act" that recaptures the sense of their acting. (Rizzolatti et al. 2001, p. 661)

Mirror neurons are active not only in the spontaneous execution and observation of a given action but also in imitation-based learning (Buccino et al. 2004). Thus the motor system creates multipurpose internal representations, which may be employed variously in action generation, action understanding, and imitation (Rizzolatti and Luppino 2001). Moreover, mirror neuron activity does not depend on the action's actually being observed; mirror neurons are also active when the final part of an action is hidden from sight and thus must be *inferred* (Umilta et al. 2001).

Mirror neurons have been found not only in the prefrontal cortex but also in the superior temporal sulcus and parietal cortex; Iacoboni and colleagues (2001) hypothesize the following cascade: the superior temporal sulcus neurons provide an initial description of the action to the parietal mirror neurons; the parietal neurons add somatosensory information for the prefrontal cortex; and the prefrontal cortex encodes the action. Of course, the nature of the action will determine the location of the neural activation. Listening to speech, for example, activates areas of the ventral premotor cortex involved in speech production (Wilson et al. 2004).

Mirror neuron activity also is evident in conjunction with the perception of sensation. An fMRI study (Keysers et al. 2004) showed activation in the somatosensory cortex of participants who either observed someone else's leg being touched or experienced their own leg being touched; more specifically, the overlapping activation was evident in the secondary somatosensory cortex (an area that shows rough somatotopic organization but also integrates information across body parts). Owing to this shared neural representation, the authors concluded that "we do not just *see* touch but also *understand* touch through an automatic link with our own experience of touch" (p. 343)—a phenomenon evident in a creepy sensation when we observe the tarantula crawling over James Bond's chest in a movie scene or when we flinch while watching a fighter being punched in the jaw in a boxing match.

The discovery of mirror neurons provides an intriguing avenue to understanding the neurobiological basis of empathy (Gallese 2001). Research on empathy for others' physical pain is on solid footing, given relatively extensive research delineating patterns of brain activation associated with both somatosensory and affective components of pain experience. Jackson and colleagues (2005) used fMRI to scan participants who were shown numerous photographs depicting hands and feet in painful and non-painful situations. They found significant activation in the *anterior cingulate cortex* and *anterior insula* during the perception of others' pain; these areas are known to be activated in conjunction with the affective experience of pain. Singer and colleagues (2004) went one step farther, employing fMRI to scan participants' brain activity while either experiencing pain or observing their romantic partner undergoing the same painful stimulus. Consistent with prior research, pain in the self was associated with a widespread pattern of activation, including the anterior cingulate cortex and anterior insula; yet observing pain in the partner was associated only with activation in these latter structures. Moreover, participants who scored higher on an individual-differences measure of empathy showed greater activation of the anterior cingulate cortex as well as the anterior insula. Importantly, the affective and not the somatosensory component of pain is the basis of empathy:

> the understanding of someone else's emotional reaction to pain does not necessitate such a detailed sensory-discriminative representation of the noxious stimulus but rather a representation of the subjective relevance of the stimulus as reflected in the subjective unpleasantness that the other person feels. Such decoupled representations—which are independent of the sensory inputs of the outside world—have been postulated to be necessary for our ability to mentalize. (Singer et al. 2004, p. 1161)

A subsequent study on empathy for pain provides an intriguing qualification to these findings (Singer et al. 2006). Prior to having their empathy for pain assessed, male and female participants interacted with an experimenter's confederate in a trust-and-reciprocity game in which the confederate either behaved cooperatively and fairly or selfishly and unfairly. When observing the cooperative confederate in pain, both male and female participants showed a neurobiologically empathic response (i.e., evident in activation in the anterior insula / fronto-insular cortex and the anterior cingulate cortices). Moreover, as in the previous study, both male and female participants with more empathic general dispositions showed relatively high cortical activation. Striking gender differences emerged, however, in relation to empathy for the selfish confederate's pain. Whereas females showed no significant difference in empathy (as manifested by cortical activation) between the cooperative and selfish confederate, males showed enhanced empathy for the cooperative but not the selfish confederate. Moreover, not only did men report a higher desire for revenge against the selfish confederate but also men (but not women) who experienced a desire for revenge showed greater activity in reward-sensitive brain regions (striatum/nucleus accumbens) when observing the selfish confederate in pain.

Research on the experience and observation of disgust also shows overlapping neural substrates (Wicker et al. 2003). Participants viewed movies of others smelling the contents of a glass and showing facial expressions of disgust, and the participants themselves also inhaled disgusting odorants. Observing and directly experiencing disgust was associated with activation of the anterior insula and, to a lesser extent, the anterior cingulate cortex. The anterior insula is an olfactory and gustatory center that regulates visceral sensations and associated autonomic responses; in addition, the anterior insula receives input from the superior temporal sulcus, which is responsive to facial expressions. The authors note that the insula activation during observations of disgust reflects an automatic sharing of the emotion. Like the automatic activation of pain-related affect when observing others in pain, this automatic capacity to share feelings while observing others serves the evolutionary function of promoting avoidance (e.g., of painful situations or toxic foods) on the basis of observational learning.

We noted earlier that a single mental representation flexibly supports spontaneous experience, observation, or imitation. Carr and colleagues (2003) employed fMRI to compare participants' brain activity while observing facial expressions of several emotions (happiness, sadness, anger, surprise, disgust, and fear) with activity when they imitated the various expressions while aspiring to feel the emotions internally as well. They found that generally overlapping areas were activated by observing and imitating emotions, although a number of areas were more active during imitation than observation, including temporal areas, the anterior insula, and the amygdala. These findings of increased activation with imitation (e.g., in the amygdala) are interpreted as consistent with the long-held idea that emotions can be evoked by voluntary facial expressions (Ekman and Davidson 1993).

Gallese and colleagues (2004) summarize the research on action and emotion understanding by proposing that "Social cognition is not only thinking about the contents of someone else's mind" but rather employs a "mirror mechanism" that "gives us an experiential insight into other minds" (p. 401). They describe how "a bridge is created between others and ourselves" (p. 400) as follows:

With this mechanism we do not just "see" or "hear" an action or an emotion. Side by side with the sensory description of the observed social stimuli, internal representations of the state associated with these actions are evoked in the observer, "as if" they were performing a similar action or experiencing a similar emotion.... crucial for both first- and third-person comprehension of social behavior is the activation of the cortical motor or viscero-motor centers, the outcome of which, when activating downstream centers, determines a specific "behavior," be it an action or an emotional state. When only the cortical centers, decoupled from the peripheral effects, are active, the observed actions or emotions are "simulated" and thereby *understood*. (Gallese et al. 2004, p. 400, emphasis added)

Yet it is not clear how much is "understood" from mirror neuron activity alone. Empathy involves more than automatic resonance; the resonance must be mentalized, that is, mentally elaborated. As we indicated in Chapter 2 ("Mentalizing"), Preston and de Waal's Perception-Action Model of empathy (Preston and de Waal 2002; Preston et al. 2007) includes subject-object state matching, as reflected in mirror neuron activity. Yet true empathy also requires subject-object differentiation, emotion regulation, and imagination; empathy thus includes at least implicit awareness of multiple perspectives, for example, my take on your take on your situation. Thus, as we emphasized in Chapter 2 ("Mentalizing"), mentalizing entails mental *work*; empathy goes beyond affective resonance (Decety 2005) and includes the need to "quarantine" one's own perspective at times. As we noted in our earlier discussion of empathy, however, the need to quarantine one's own perspective for the sake of accurate empathy will depend on the similarity of one's own experience to the experience of the other (Preston et al., in press). We now turn to the more elaborate levels of mentalizing.

Mentalizing Emotion

On the basis of their systematic review of neuroimaging research on patterns of brain activation associated with mentalizing tasks, Frith and Frith (2003) identified the *mentalizing region:* a broad area in the medial prefrontal cortex that also includes a portion of the anterior cingulate cortex. As we noted in Chapter 2 ("Mentalizing"), contrasting internally and externally focused aspects of social cognition, Lieberman reviewed evidence that processes that focus on the "mental interior (thoughts, feelings, experiences)"—whether directed toward self or others—are associated with medial prefrontal (as well as parietal) activation (Lieberman 2007, p. 3).

The functional overlap between the medial prefrontal and anterior cingulate cortices in the mentalizing region that Frith and Frith (2003) identified is not surprising inasmuch as the prefrontal and anterior cingulate cortices not only are co-activated (Kringelbach 2005) but also overlap anatomically: some investigators refer to the medial prefrontal area as the "paracingulate," and one specialist colloquially dubbed the anterior cingulate cortex the "metropolitan frontal lobes" (Goldberg 2001, p. 142). Indeed, terminological variation abounds in this literature. The *medial prefrontal cortex* is part of the *orbitofrontal cortex,* which includes distinct medial and lateral areas as well as more dorsal and ventral areas (Elliott et al. 2000; Kringelbach 2005); the ventral portion of the medial orbitofrontal area, known as the ventromedial prefrontal cortex, has been the focus of clinical observation and extensive research pertinent to mentalizing (Damasio et al. 2003). Admittedly, identifying a mentalizing region in this large prefrontal area with fuzzy boundaries is a bit like pinpointing a location to "greater Los Angeles."

The complementary functions of the two overlapping cortical areas in the mentalizing region, the anterior cingulate and the medial prefrontal cortex, have been investigated apart from mentalizing. Extensive evidence supports distinguishing affective (rostral and ventral) and cognitive (dorsal) regions in the anterior cingulate (Bush et al. 2000). The affective region registers emotional salience of situations and regulates emotion, whereas the cognitive region modulates attention and executive functions in cognitively demanding situations. Thus the anterior cingulate bridges emotion and attention (Davidson et al. 2003)—for example, playing an active role in monitoring conflict (Botvinick et al. 1999) and detecting conditions under which errors are likely (Carter et al. 1998). Registering affect, the anterior cingulate can influence the allocation of attention and the marshalling of cognitive resources in other cortical areas, including the prefrontal cortex. In short, anterior cingulate activation as a whole is associated with effortful control of attention, cognition, and emotion in situations that involve selecting among potentially competing responses (Davidson et al. 2003). Intriguing recent neuroimaging research involving simultaneous scanning of interacting participants also suggests that the differentiation of self-other agency (i.e., me versus not-me) is registered in different regions of the medial bank of the cingulate gyrus (Tomlin et al. 2006).

In conjunction with the anterior cingulate, the medial prefrontal cortex also plays a central role in flexible responding to changing circumstances that call for self-regulation. The medial prefrontal cortex is active in ambiguous and potentially conflict-laden situations, being particularly responsive to changing reinforcement contingencies (Rolls 1999). That is, the medial prefrontal cortex keeps track of situations and actions that are potentially rewarding or punishing, continually updating this information on a moment-to-moment basis. Damasio and colleagues (2003), for example, described how somatic states ("gut feelings") registered in the ventromedial region "steer the decision-making process toward those outcomes that are advantageous for the subject, based on the subject's past experience with similar situations" (p. 83). Similarly, Elliott and colleagues (2000) propose that the orbitofrontal cortex is active "when there is insufficient information to determine the appropriate course of action" and when "the problem of what to do next is best solved by taking into account the likely reward value of stimuli and responses" (p. 308). Thus the orbitofrontal cortex is involved in acquiring and monitoring changing stimulus-reinforcement relations—holding reward values in mind and flexibly updating them. Moreover, the *medial* orbitofrontal cortex is active in monitoring associations between stimuli, responses, and outcomes under changing circumstances; whereas the *lateral* orbitofrontal cortex is active in inhibiting previously rewarded actions that are no longer likely to be rewarded owing to changed conditions (Elliott et al. 2000; Kringelbach 2005). Consistent with the view that the lateral orbitofrontal cortex is involved in response reversal, this region is activated by exposure to angry faces, which serve as a cue to inhibit unacceptable behavior (Blair 2003, 2004).

In sum, the anterior cingulate and medial prefrontal cortices make use of internal cues (emotions and incentives) to regulate attention and action in changing circumstances that call for continual decision making and self-regulation. Hence it is not surprising that these areas are central to *social cognition:* social interactions require coordinated awareness and understanding of others' emotional states and one's own as well as continually adapting interactive behavior to changing reinforcement contingencies in accordance with this awareness. Accordingly, Damasio and colleagues (2003) propose that activity in the ventromedial region "permits cognitive processes to incorporate certain types of emotional knowledge" (p. 83) and that such knowledge is "indispensable when making decisions about social matters" (p. 85).

Lane (2000) reviewed research indicating that representations of emotional states are established in the mentalizing region. Notably, emotional arousal per se activates more caudal regions of the anterior cingulate, whereas the conscious *awareness* of emotion activates more rostral areas of the cingulate along with the medial prefrontal cortex. The same is true of pain (Singer et al. 2004): painful stimulation activates the more caudal region of the anterior cingulate, whereas the affective awareness of pain and empathy for others' pain is associated with activation of the rostral anterior cingulate and paracingulate cortex.

Thus the mentalizing region is active in conscious awareness of the emotions of oneself and others as well as in the mental elaboration of emotion. This process of mental elaboration is consistent with Lane's (2000) proposal of multiple levels of emotional awareness (ranging from the experience of physical sensations to appreciating complex blends of emotion in oneself and others), which he links to the mentalizing region as follows:

> The interaction between representations of emotional experience and the phenomenal experience of emotion may at least in part be mediated by the tight anatomical linkage…between the rostral and dorsal anterior cingulate cortices. The dynamic interaction between phenomenal experience, establishing a representation of it, elaborating that representation (e.g., identifying the source of the emotional response), and integrating it with other cognitive processes are the fundamental processes involved in the cognitive elaboration of emotion addressed by the levels of emotional awareness model. (p. 360)

To reiterate, the distinction between *being* in an emotional state (or in pain) and *awareness* of emotion (or pain) is crucial to mentalizing emotion (or pain): as Frith and Frith (2003) explained, the mentalizing region is involved in creating *representations* that are decoupled (or one step removed) from sensation and perception, and this decoupled representation can be employed in further cognitive processing. As we described in Chapter 2 ("Mentalizing"), mentalizing emotion entails *working with feelings:* identifying, modulating, and expressing them. The research we have just highlighted suggests that the mentalizing region of the anterior cingulate and medial prefrontal cortexes is crucially active in this work. Buttressing this view, Lieberman and colleagues (2007) reported an elegant demonstration of the emotion-regulating role of the medial prefrontal cortex in conjunction with what we call mentalizing. These researchers showed that, compared to a range of experimental control conditions, affect labeling (choosing a word to match facial expressions of emotion) increased activation in the right ventrolateral prefrontal cortex and, correspondingly, diminished activity in the amygdala and related limbic regions. Moreover, of particular interest here, activity in the medial prefrontal cortex mediated the relation between right ventrolateral prefrontal activation and reduced amygdala activity. As Lieberman and colleagues note, their findings are consistent with previous neuroimaging research relating more complex cognitive reappraisal processes to decreased negative affect; yet it is noteworthy that the mere labeling of emotions can have this effect and that the medial prefrontal cortex plays a mediating role in it.

Mentalizing Interpersonal Interactions

Phineas Gage was a 25-year-old railroad worker in 1848 when an explosion shot a metal rod through his head, and he gained posthumous fame as exemplifying the frontal lobe syndrome (Damasio 1994). Damasio and colleagues' (2003) description of Gage's personality change is typical of lesions to the ventromedial prefrontal cortex: "Whereas Gage had been a diligent, reliable, polite, and socially adept person before his accident, he subsequently became uncaring, profane, and socially inappropriate in his conduct" (p. 82)—a change that was especially remarkable in light of his generally preserved intellectual functioning. More precisely, Stone (2000) reviewed a host of deficits in real-time social interactions associated with orbitofrontal damage: impairment in the pragmatics of conversation, inability to take into account the listener's point of view or interest, insensitivity to the partner's signs, inability to judge one's impact on others, and inability to model others' mental states. Hence orbitofrontal damage is associated with difficulty maintaining friendships and with vulnerability to being exploited interpersonally.

With recent neuroimaging research, we can now more specifically link deficits in social cognition associated with frontal lobe lesions to mentalizing. In conjunction with its role in emotion, the mentalizing region of the medial prefrontal cortex (Frith and Frith 2003) is distinctly active in the performance of a wide variety of theory-of-mind tasks. Notwithstanding the overlap we continually emphasize, we can make some distinction between mentalizing emotion (i.e., perceiving one's own and others' emotional states as such) and mentalizing cognition (i.e., thinking about others' thinking, as in theory-of-mind tasks); paralleling our psychological thinking, neuroimaging findings show that overlapping yet somewhat distinct neural networks are involved in mentalizing emotion and cognition (Fonagy et al. 2007). For example, there is some evidence that within the medial prefrontal cortex, mentalizing emotion activates the more ventral areas, whereas mentalizing cognition activates the more dorsal areas (Mundy 2003; Volkmar et al. 2004). Yet research to date has been more successful in pinpointing activity associated with attributing true and false beliefs (in the dorsal area of the medial-prefrontal cortex) than with attributing emotional states (Saxe et al. 2004); moreover, contrasts between attention to thoughts and attention to emotions show activity in contiguous areas of the medial prefrontal cortex (Frith and Frith 2003). Employing inferences about mental states of cartoon-sequence characters, Vollm and colleagues (2006) conducted a direct comparison between mentalizing emotion and cognition in contrasting patterns of brain activity associated with empathy ("What will make the main character feel better?") and theory of mind ("What will the main character do next?"). Exemplifying the overlap, both mentalizing tasks activated the medial prefrontal cortex, superior temporal lobe, and temporal pole. Yet there were also a number of differences between tasks; most notably, the empathizing task also recruited networks involved in emotion processing (i.e., amygdala).

We should note that although we focus on the prefrontal region here, well-controlled studies also show activation of the temporoparietal junction in theory-of-mind tasks (Saxe and Kanwisher 2003; Vollm et al. 2006); moreover, the inferior parietal cortex (with its extensive reciprocal connections with prefrontal cortex) has been shown to be active when research participants adopt the perspective of another person (Decety 2005) and has been implicated in maintaining the distinction between self and other when one is in the midst of empathizing (Lawrence et al. 2006). Nonetheless, extensive reviews of neuroimaging research consistently highlight medial prefrontal activation in conjunction with a wide range of mentalizing tasks (Adolphs 2003; Frith and Frith 2003; Gallagher and Frith 2003; Lieberman 2007; Saxe et al. 2004), and we merely describe one relatively dramatic study for illustrative purposes.

Gallagher and colleagues (2002) conducted an elegantly controlled demonstration of the selective activation of the medial prefrontal cortex in a mentalizing interaction. They engaged normal volunteers in a computerized version of the children's game "rock, paper, scissors," under different mindsets. The critical contrast compared patterns of brain activity when participants believed that they were playing against another person versus believing that they were playing against a computer; otherwise, the task demands were equivalent (i.e., programmed). The experimental conditions were highly effective:

> In discussing the mentalizing condition, volunteers unanimously depicted the opponent as an intentional agent. They all described guessing and second guessing their opponent's responses, and attempting to identify characteristic patterns of behavior in the opponent. To a lesser extent, they described their opponent as reading their own patterns of behavior. Volunteers spoke of strategies for response, which they related to imagined mental states of their opponent. (Gallagher et al. 2002, p. 817)

As the researchers hypothesized, the mentalizing condition was associated with selective activation of the paracingulate cortex, that is, "just anterior to the most anterior part of the anterior cingulate proper between the putative cognitive and emotional divisions" (p. 819). In conjunction with comparable results from a host of related neuroimaging studies, the authors propose that "the paracingulate cortex has a special role in the ability to use information to make attributions about mental states" (p. 820), and they contend more specifically that this brain region might enable the critical process of mentalizing, that is, the decoupling of mental representations from reality:

> When explaining a person's behavior in terms of a belief we have to recognize that this belief might not correspond to reality. Even when it conflicts with reality it is the belief not the reality that determines behavior. We also have to distinguish the representation of the reality by the other person from our representation of reality. Perhaps activity in the paracingulate cortex is necessary to maintain these decoupled representations in the face of competition from representations of the actual state of the world. This function is analogous to the function of the adjacent, more posterior part of the ACC [anterior cingulate cortex]. This region is active in tasks which elicit response conflict.... We speculate that paracingulate cortex has a similar role in handling possible conflict between actual and virtual representations, but in the more abstract domain of mental states rather than motor responses. This ability to handle different representations of the world is an essential requirement for adopting an intentional stance. (Gallagher et al. 2002, p. 820)

Notably, a similar fMRI study employing a trust-and-reciprocity game also found greater activation in medial-prefrontal cortex when participants played a person compared to when they played a computer (McCabe et al. 2001). Yet this difference held only for those participants who engaged in cooperative strategies (to maximize financial gain for both participants). For those (selfish) participants who adopted a competitive strategy, there were no differences in medial-prefrontal cortical activation associated with playing a person versus a computer—a rather disquieting finding from the standpoint of mentalizing. Plausibly, the authors inferred that the non-cooperators were playing on the basis of game-based rules rather than employing theory-of-mind related inferences and strategies.

Attachment Paradoxes

We have emphasized repeatedly that secure attachment relationships are conducive to mentalizing and vice versa (see Chapter 3, "Development"). Yet some neuroimaging findings also reveal a seemingly paradoxical finding, namely, that loving feelings in attachment relationships can *deac*tivate the cortical areas associated with mentalizing (Fonagy 2006).

It is hardly surprising that seeing a photograph of one's partner when one is in the throes of the very early stages of intense romantic love would increase activity in dopamine-rich brain areas associated with reward, including the ventral tegmental area and the caudate nucleus. Nor is it surprising that seeing the photograph would decrease activity in an area associated with fearful responsiveness, the amygdala (Aron 2005). Yet, in light of the attachment-mentalizing link, it might seem surprising that evoking attachment feelings would deactivate areas associated with mentalizing. Bartles and Zeki conducted two studies of attachment relationships, one in which participants saw photographs of their romantic partners (Bartles and Zeki 2000), the other in which mothers saw photographs of their infants (Bartles and Zeki 2004). Both studies included careful controls, such as photographs of friends as contrasted with romantic partners and photographs of other children with whom the mothers were acquainted as contrasted with their own infants. These researchers found considerable overlap between romantic and maternal love in reward-related areas of activation (e.g., in the striatum as well as the middle insula and dorsal anterior cingulate cortex) as well as some differences. Most notably, for both romantic and maternal love, they found overlapping patterns of deactivation, and this deactivation included the medial prefrontal/paracingulate cortex (i.e., the mentalizing region) as well as the amygdala.

Bartles and Zeki (2004) interpreted the patterns of deactivation as reflecting a *decreased* need for mentalizing in love relationships:

> both romantic and maternal love activate specific regions in the reward system and lead to suppression of activity in the neural machineries associated with the critical social assessment of other people and with negative emotions.... once one is closely familiar with a person (in a positive or negative way), the need to assess the social validity of that person is reduced. This correlates with a reduction of activity in the systems necessary for doing so; these findings therefore bring us closer to explaining in neurological terms why "love makes [us] blind." (p. 1164)

These interesting findings point to some complexity in the relation between attachment and mentalizing and underscore the dynamic and context-dependent nature of mentalizing in attachment relationships. As these findings attest, under many circumstances, secure attachments might *obviate the need* for mentalizing. The findings also mesh well with an all too common conjunction between passionate love and mind-blindness. Yet we do not believe that these recent neuroimaging findings contradict the extensive literature we have reviewed in Chapter 3 ("Development") that supports a robust relationship between secure attachment and mentalizing. We must consider the nature of the task involved in these studies showing deactivation of mentalizing regions: gazing lovingly at photographs. We might infer that a state of admiring love precludes mentalizing, especially in the early, infatuated stage of a love relationship; but that observation hardly precludes the possibility of mentalizing effectively when engaged in an *interaction* with a loved one (as in the mother-infant research) or when *reflecting on relationships* with loved ones (as in the Adult Attachment Interview). Indeed, this latter point about mentalizing when reflecting on relationships was employed in the interpretation of the findings of a similar study that were in the opposite direction to those of Bartles and Zeki. Liebenluft and colleagues (2004) showed increased activity in mentalizing regions (anterior paracingulate cortex and posterior superior temporal sulcus) when mothers viewed pictures of their own children as contrasted to familiar and unfamiliar children. The authors interpret these findings as follows: "familiarity with a face is related not only to the face's appearance, but also to the representation of that person's mental state and personality, and...this information is spontaneously retrieved when viewing a familiar individual" (p. 230).

Such conflicting findings regarding the conjunction of loving feelings and mentalizing underscore the dynamic and complex relations between attachment and mentalizing. For example, when the child feels securely attached to the parent, the child can relax mentalizing, in the sense of not needing to monitor the parent's state of mind (e.g., by being vigilant regarding the parent's trustworthiness); at the same time, this security allows the child to mentalize in the exploratory sense of finding his or her own mind in the mirroring response of the parent. In short, one facet of mentalizing is relaxed while another facet is activated.

No doubt, love can be blind. But we must temper our generalizations by distinguishing love from preoccupied infatuation:

> Love is not, as such, irrational. Like any emotion, it can be on target or off, warranted or unwarranted, based on the facts or wrong about the facts, wise or foolish, life-enhancing or self-destructive. Thus falling in love with a conman or a liar, if one can see the truth but refuses to, is irrational. It is in such cases that "love is blind." But this is not usually the case. Usually, love sees more clearly and deeply, with much more attention to and appreciation of details, than ordinary perception. (Solomon 2007, p. 56)

The consistent relations between secure maternal attachment and mentalizing exemplify mature love "seeing more clearly and deeply," and we will reiterate this point in the context of psychotherapy in Chapter 5 ("The Art of Mentalizing").

Frazzled Mentalizing

A useful tip in helping patients navigate conflicts in attachment relationships: mentalizing goes offline in the context of intense emotional arousal as the fight-or-flight response comes online. Arnsten (1998) neatly captured this process in the title of her article "The Biology of Being Frazzled."

In understanding the relation between emotional arousal and mentalizing, it is essential to go beyond a unitary concept of arousal (Robbins 1997). Key neuromodulators, for example, contribute to different forms of arousal: norepinephrine contributes to alerting, vigilance, and controlled attentional processing in the face of stress; dopamine energizes approach behavior in response to potentially rewarding incentives; and serotonin modulates arousal in the norepinephrine and dopamine systems (Pliszka 2003). Furthermore, the effects of arousal in any of these systems vary not only with the extent of transmitter secretion but also with the receptor subtype activated (Arnsten and Goldman-Rakic 1998; Arnsten et al. 1999; Mayes 2000). Through dynamic changes in patterns of excitation and inhibition, these intertwined arousal systems modulate the relative balance of activity in various cortical and subcortical areas.

Two points are critical for understanding impairments in mentalizing. First, owing to what can be construed as a *neurochemical switch* associated with escalating levels of emotional stress (Arnsten 1998; Mayes 2000), patterns of brain functioning can shift from flexibility to automaticity, that is, from relatively slow executive functions mediated by the prefrontal cortex to faster habitual and instinctual behaviors mediated by posterior cortical (e.g., parietal) and subcortical structures (e.g., amygdala, hippocampus, and striatum). Concomitantly, mentalizing goes offline as defensive responses (fight-flight-freeze) come online. This capacity for rapid switching in modes of functioning in response to threat has the presumed evolutionary value of promoting immediate and adaptive behavioral responses to danger. Yet this automatic responding is typically maladaptive in less dire situations of interpersonal stress, where complex cognitive-emotional functioning (i.e., mentalizing) is most adaptive.

Second, there are intra-individual variations as well as enduring individual differences in the threshold for switching from executive (mentalizing) to automatic (fight-or-flight) responding. Moreover, the threshold for switching can be lowered as a result of exposure to early stress and trauma. As Mayes (2000) summarized,

> This threshold for overactivation is individually variable based on time of day (circadian rhythms), immediate and past contexts and experiences, developmental age, and genetic endowment…. the balance between facilitative and inhibitory effects on PFC [prefrontal cortex] and

attentional functions may also be *permanently altered* and more apparent under stressful or arousing conditions. (p. 276, emphasis added)

These neurobiological perspectives on shifting patterns of brain activity in relation to escalating stressful arousal underscore our contention that mentalizing is a context-dependent dynamic skill (Fonagy and Target 1997a). Clinicians have developed a wide range of emotion-regulation strategies for patients with a history of attachment trauma who have become exquisitely sensitized to stress and thus have acquired a lower threshold for switching into the fight-or-flight mode. In addition to preventing destructive and self-injurious defensive behavior, these emotion-regulation strategies are intended to promote adaptive interpersonal and intrapersonal functioning by keeping mentalizing online in the face of stress (Allen 2001, 2005; Lewis 2006).

Mentalizing Disorders

As we have just noted, this book emphasizes dynamic variations in mentalizing, largely those associated with challenges in attachment relationships. These dynamic impairments of mentalizing are responsive to clinical interventions that foster emotion-regulation skills and secure attachment. Yet clinicians also are confronted with more enduring mentalizing impairments associated with neurobiological disorders, and we will consider two of these here: autism and psychopathy. Research on these conditions promises to refine our understanding of mentalizing impairments as well as the related neurocognitive deficits. We anticipate that, as research on mentalizing progresses, we will appreciate the neurobiological contributions to mentalizing impairments in a wider range of disorders; for example, Fonagy and colleagues are in the process of employing neuroimaging in interpersonal interactions to investigate neurobiological contributions to impaired mentalizing in persons with borderline personality disorder.

Autism

As we noted at the outset of this book, "mentalizing" (Frith et al. 1991; Morton 1989) and "mindblindness" (Baron-Cohen 1995) were introduced in the context of developing a theory of the core deficit in autism. Autistic disorder is a complex syndrome composed of impairment in social interaction and communication (including language delays and deficits) along with repetitive and stereotyped patterns of behavior; the diagnosis requires an onset prior to three years of age (American Psychiatric Association 2000). Much pertinent neurobiological research encompasses a spectrum of conditions, including pervasive developmental disorder as well as high-functioning autism and Asperger syndrome, notwithstanding that these diagnostic distinctions are fraught with controversy (Volkmar et al. 2004).

Autism exemplifies impaired mentalizing most starkly; the core deficits in mentalizing associated with autism are listed in Table 4–2. Most distinctive to autism is a profound lack of *social engagement* such that, in effect, mentalizing does not get off the ground (Hobson 2002, 2005). Parents of children subsequently diagnosed with autism retrospectively report atypical social interactions as early as three to six months (Berger 2006). Mundy (2003) proposes a fundamental disturbance in *social orienting* in infants with autism, and Volkmar and colleagues (2004) regard the lack of a preferential orientation to social stimuli and the corresponding lack of motivation for social engagement as the root problem that eventuates in a cascade of deficits in emotion and social cognition. Hence parental disengagement is now seen as a consequence rather than a cause of autism; that is, parents disengage *in response* to their infant's inability to engage.

Berger (2006) has focused on deficits in *face expression processing* as a critical facet of the lack of social engagement. He notes that normal infants smile in response to another's smile at one month and actively seek eye contact by nine weeks. Infants with autism, however, fixate less on eyes, focus more on the mouth region and, more generally, focus on specific features rather than the gestalt of the face—as well as showing less preferential interest in faces on the whole. Berger proposes that the key dysfunction in autism resides in "the system that initiates positive hedonic states to social stimuli in the main sensory domains" (p. 360); although he focuses on the face, he also notes that infants with autism fail to find pleasure not only in eye contact and smiles but also in touch and the sound of the voice.

Given their lack of orientation to social stimuli, children with autism fail to engage in *joint attention* (Hobson 2005). Mundy (2003) notes, however, that children with autism are somewhat inclined to capture others' attention for instrumental purposes (e.g., pointing to some object they want) and that their relative unresponsiveness to others' bids for attention diminishes with age. Most crucially, however, their inclination to *spontaneously initiate* coordinated attention with a social partner remains profoundly deficient, and this deficiency affects their capacity to establish relationships with peers on into adolescence. In sum, as Hobson (2005) put it, children with autism "do not seem to share the world with other people, and they do not relate to the world-according-to-the-other" (p. 197).

TABLE 4–2. KEY MENTALIZING DEFICITS IN AUTISM

- Lack of preferential orientation to social stimuli

- Low levels of emotional engagement and responsiveness

- Failure to engage in and initiate joint activities

- Impaired language learning

- Poor performance in theory-of-mind tasks

- Lack of engagement in pretend play and imaginative activities

- Deficient self-awareness and misuse of personal pronouns ("I" vs. "You")

Extensive research on autism has focused on mentalizing deficits under the rubric of theory of mind (Baron-Cohen 2000; Volkmar et al. 2004), the development of which is founded on social engagement and joint attention (see Chapter 3, "Development"). Children with autism spectrum disorders notoriously show deficits in the theory-of-mind litmus test, the false-belief task. Yet they also perform relatively poorly on a host of related tasks and abilities: inferring desires from gaze direction; appreciating that seeing leads to knowing; distinguishing between physical and mental entities; distinguishing between appearance and reality; understanding that the brain provides for a set of mental functions, including thinking; recognizing mental-state words and using them spontaneously in speech; tailoring speech to the perspective and knowledge of the listener; detecting deception; and spontaneously engaging in pretend play and imaginative activity (Baron-Cohen 2000).

We have noted in Chapter 3 ("Development") that mentalizing originates in the context of emotional responsiveness (Gergely and Watson 1996), and we can construe the lack of social engagement in autism as largely due to the lack of *emotional engagement:* an inability to become engaged with others' emotional states and to be moved by them (Hobson 2002, 2005). Hence children with autism find social interactions to be unrewarding (Berger 2006). Consistent with this initial lack of emotional engagement, persons with autism-spectrum disorders are deficient in their capacity to mentalize emotion: they are relatively inattentive to facial expressions of emotion, unresponsive to others' distress, and unmoved by others' emotions (Hobson 2002). Like typical children, children with autism can identify what an actor is *doing* from observing point-light displays, but they cannot identify what the actor is *feeling* (Hobson 2005). As Hobson (2002) put it, "the child with autism may not perceive a smile *as a smile* but as a contorted face; he may not perceive a gasp of fear as a fearful expression but as an unusual sound" (p. 14, emphasis in original).

As Hobson (2002) reviewed, persons with autism-spectrum disorders not only have difficulty mentalizing in relation to others but also in relation to *the self*. Deficient self-awareness is reflected in lack of self-consciousness: "they may not conceive of themselves as selves in the minds of others. In this sense, many children with autism are not self-conscious" (p. 89). Hence, for example, a person with autism might unthinkingly walk around in the nude with guests in the house. Reflecting a core deficit in the sense of self, children with autism have difficulty with personal pronouns (e.g., "I" and "you") and are liable to refer to themselves by name. In Hobson's terms, there is a *thin* quality to their self-concepts, which lack subtle emotional qualities and do not include the significance of their relationships with other persons. This deficient sense of self originates in the lack of relatedness with others, as Hobson (2002) summarizes:

> In the case of self-awareness, then, we have a variation on a familiar theme: what happens between people is intimately connected with what happens within the individual. If the child with autism is not engaged with other people, and especially with the attitudes of others, then he is not going to be very concerned with other people's attitudes towards himself. More than this, he does not identify with others, so in the extreme case (and this is not true of all people with autism) he may not even move to the position of taking *any* attitude towards himself. (p. 225; emphasis in original)

As we have stated, autism has been identified as a disorder of mentalizing, distinguished by its prominent neurobiological etiology as well as its high heritability; the genetic predisposition is doubtlessly complex, perhaps involving interactions among anywhere from three to ten loci (Volkmar et al. 2004). The search for affected brain regions has been broad; as Volkmar and colleagues state, "At one point or another, malfunction of nearly every neural system in the brain has been proposed as central to the pathobiology of autism" (Volkmar et al. 2004, p. 145). Broad impairment, for example, is suggested by accelerated overgrowth of the brain coupled with reduced connectivity in the first two years of life; brain volume in toddlers with autism may be enlarged by as much as 10 percent. Considerable interest has focused on structural abnormalities in the cerebellum, which plays a significant role not only in motor coordination but also in attention and orienting.

The wide search for regions of brain impairment associated with autism is narrowing somewhat: Volkmar and colleagues (2004) noted "the discovery of generalized hypoactivation of an entire social processing brain network in individuals with autism" (p. 144) which they construed as "indicative of a pervasive lack of social interest, engagement, motivation, or reactivity" (p. 145). Hence hypoactivation has been observed in what now have become the usual suspects: the fusiform face area, superior temporal sulcus, amygdala, anterior cingulate, and prefrontal cortex (Berger 2006; Mundy 2003; Volkmar et al. 2004). In addition, mirror neuron dysfunction that compromises capacities for imitation has been implicated in autism-spectrum disorders (Dapretto et al. 2005; Nishitani et al. 2004; Williams et al. 2001). For example, Dapretto and colleagues (2005) found that, compared to controls, when they were imitating and observing emotional expressions, children with autism showed no mirror neuron activity in the inferior frontal gyrus and, moreover, preserved activity in this region was inversely related to social symptom severity.

Mundy (2003) has reviewed extensive evidence of impairment associated with autism in the mentalizing region of the prefrontal cortex, namely, in the anterior cingulate and dorsal medial-frontal cortex. Moreover, impairment in this region is associated with deficits in joint attention as well as theory-of-mind tasks, suggesting developmental continuity insofar as theory of mind builds upon joint attention. Moreover, Mundy proposes that the anterior cingulate and dorsal medial-frontal cortex play a key role in intersubjectivity, supporting the comparison of self-representations with representations of others' mental states. Mundy (2003) summarizes this cascade of mentalizing deficits as follows:

> impairment in the early tendency to initiate and organize social behaviors, such as social orienting and joint attention bids, may be especially pernicious to the development of the child with autism because it disrupts his/her capacity for social action, which ultimately contributes to the foundation of social self-knowledge requisite to social-cognitive development. (p. 805)

To reiterate, this developmental cascade in autism begins with a lack of *orientation* to social stimuli—faces, for example. As described earlier, Berger (2006) pinpoints the lack of reward associated with social interaction as the core problem, and he points out that this problem might have multiple neurobiological origins:

> it is hypothesized that the social features of autism arise when sensory access to the affect system through a final common pathway such as a sensory convergence area of the amygdala is dysfunctional. This can

occur either because the networks leading to the affect system, or the affect generating system itself, or both, are dysfunctional. Hence, if for any of a number of reasons, the system that initiates positive hedonic states to social stimuli in the main sensory domains is dysfunctional, the social features characterizing autism will occur. (p. 360).

Gergely's (2001) intriguing hypothesis regarding the early origins of autism falls squarely within our account of the development of mentalizing in focusing on impairments of contingent responsiveness (see Chapter 3, "Development"). To recap, Gergely has noted how in the first few months of life, infants shift from a preference for perfectly contingent response→stimulus associations (e.g., watching their limbs move) to high-but-imperfect response→stimulus associations (e.g., watching mother smile in response to their own smile). Gergely and Watson (1999) have proposed that this shift in preferences is based on an innate contingency-detection perceptual mechanism with a *contingency switch* that takes place around three months. Gergely (2001) presented evidence that infants with autism fail to make this switch, resulting in a lack of orientation to contingently responsive caregivers and a cascade of social deficits, including aversion to social objects, inattention to faces, lack of social responsivity and, consequently, lack of social understanding. This model also has the advantage of encompassing the intolerance children with autism show for variation in routines and their preference for stereotypic motor activities, which generate extremely high response-stimulus contingencies.

While autism cannot be diagnosed reliably until two years of age by current criteria (Volkmar et al. 2004), the developmental failure begins early in infancy with the lack of orientation to social stimuli and the lack of social-emotional engagement; these are the foundations of mentalizing through the developmental route of joint attention, perspective taking, self-awareness, symbolizing, and representational theory of mind. Pathological conditions often have a way of illuminating normal development, and autism has brought mentalizing into bold relief by highlighting the devastating personal and social consequences of its absence. As we have just described, autism also provides compelling converging evidence for the contribution of key brain regions to various facets of mentalizing-related functions—again, by the absence of normal activation.

Psychopathy

Psychopathy exemplifies a *partial* but fundamental impairment of mentalizing—as Baron-Cohen (2003, 2005) construes it, mindreading without empathizing. Cleckley's (1976) astute clinical observations are fascinating in delineating the seemingly anomalous intermingling of preserved and deficient mentalizing capacities; thus we begin with some of his lucid descriptions.

Commenting on the psychopath's superficial charm, Cleckley observed, "There is nothing at all odd or queer about him, and in every respect he tends to embody the concept of a well-adjusted, happy person" (p. 338). Yet he noted extraordinary immunity from anxiety: "Even under concrete circumstances that would for the ordinary person cause embarrassment, confusion, acute insecurity, or visible agitation, his relative serenity is likely to be noteworthy" (p. 340). Moreover, in the context of chronic and damaging unreliability, untruthfulness, and insincerity, he highlighted the total lack of remorse or shame: "If Santayana is correct in saying that 'perhaps the true dignity of man is his ability to despise himself,' the psychopath is without a means to acquire true dignity" (p. 343). Moving to the core domain of impairment, he proposed the criteria of pathologic egocentricity and incapacity to love as well as general poverty in affective reactions. With great wisdom, he pondered,

> In considering the general shallowness of affect…in connection with their incapacity for object love, there is temptation to wonder about the possible interdependence of these faculties. Is it possible for tragic or transforming emotion to arise in any person without that peculiar and indescribable personal commitment to another? (p. 350)

Finally, although the psychopath's shallow emotional ties to others generate the most alarming interpersonal consequences, Cleckley captured with great acumen the associated failures in mentalizing the self:

> He has absolutely no capacity to see himself as others see him…no ability to know how others feel when they see him or to experience subjectively anything comparable about the situation. All of the values, all of the major affect concerning his status, are unappreciated by him…. Some of these patients…spoke fluently of the psychopathic personality, quoted the literature, and suggested this diagnosis for themselves. Soon this apparent insight was seen to be…a consistent and thorough artifact. Perhaps it was less a voluntary deception than a simulation in which the simulator himself fails to realize his lack of emotional grasp or that he is simulating or *what* he is simulating. The patient seems to have little or no ability to feel the significance of his situation, to experience the real emotions of regret or shame or determination to improve, or to realize that this is lacking…. Here is the spectacle of a person who uses all the words that would be used by someone who understands, and who could define all the words but who is still blind to the meaning. (pp 350–351, emphasis in original)

Psychopathy as Cleckley identified it instructively parallels autism in reflecting stable impairment of mentalizing rooted in neurobiology. As Blair and colleagues (2005, 2006) state, psychopathy is a neurodevelopmental disorder of genetic origin. Neither the neurobiological insults (e.g., as associated with physical anomalies or birth complications) nor the molecular genetics have been characterized definitively, but psychopathy is highly heritable, and no shared environmental influence has been identified in twin studies. Most pertinent for present purposes, dysfunction has been identified in brain regions associated with mentalizing (Blair et al. 2006).

In the diagnostic classification system (American Psychiatric Association 2000), psychopathy has not been distinguished from either antisocial personality disorder in adults or conduct disorder in children. Nonetheless, building on Cleckley's (1976) clinical observations, Hare and colleagues (Hare 1980; Hare et al. 1991) have developed reliable criteria for teasing out psychopathy within the heterogeneous spectrum of antisocial behavior. Two clusters of characteristics can be distinguished: an interpersonal-affective cluster, characterized, for example, by callousness and lack of remorse; and a pattern of antisocial behavior, for example, characterized by impulsivity and an unstable lifestyle. The emotional deficits can be viewed as fundamental to psychopathy, and the antisocial pattern of behavior is "best viewed as a secondary symptom or consequence of psychopathy" (Cooke et al. 2004, p. 337)—and not an invariable consequence. Blair and colleagues (2005, 2006) reported that the *callous-unemotional* mode of relating intrinsic to psychopathy characterizes about 25% of individuals in the otherwise heterogeneous diagnostic categories of antisocial personality and conduct disorder. Thus, short of creating a separate diagnosis, it is important for clinical purposes to identify the severity of psychopathy within the existing diagnostic categories (Meloy 2001)—not least because psychopathy is associated with higher rates of recidivism and violent re-offending in particular as well as with a paradoxical *increase* in antisocial behavior following treatment and rehabilitative interventions (Blair et al. 2005).

Building on Hare's conceptualization, Blair and his colleagues (Blair 2004; Blair et al. 2005, 2006) have developed a comprehensive understanding of the intertwining psychosocial and neurobiological facets of psychopathy, predicated on their conviction that emotional deficits are the crucial component. The callous-unemotional facet of psychopathy reflects a general under-responsiveness to emotional cues (Herpertz et al. 2001b) and especially to the aversive consequences of behavior, most particularly as reflected in the lack of concern for the distress of others (Blair et al. 1997). The lack of an aversive response to others' emotional distress has significant consequences for moral socialization; the psychopathic child will not be deterred, for example, by parental disapproval, disappointment, or concern:

> Due to their impairment in the response to the sadness and fear of other individuals and in the formation of aversive stimulus-reinforcement associations, individuals with psychopathy are less able to take advantage of…"moral" social referencing. They should be, and are…more difficult to socialize through standard parenting techniques. They will not learn to avoid using instrumental antisocial behavior to achieve their goals. This is because of relative indifference to the "punishment" of the victim's distress and impairment in learning the association between this "punishment" and the representation of the action that caused the victim's distress. (Blair et al. 2006, p. 268)

Blair (2004) ties the emotional deficit in psychopathy to different forms of aggression; namely, instrumental and reactive aggression. A proclivity for *instrumental aggression* best distinguishes psychopaths from their non-psychopathic antisocial and conduct-disordered counterparts. In contrast to reactive (affective) aggression, which typically is impulsive in stemming from frustration and anger, instrumental aggression is deliberate, calculated, goal-directed behavior. The lack of responsiveness to socialization plays a major role in the etiology of such behavior—nothing deters it. In contrast, trauma plays a greater role in *reactive aggression*, inasmuch as trauma sensitizes individuals to stress, lowering the threshold for emotional reactivity (Allen 2001). Blair and colleagues propose that psychopaths are *less* vulnerable to potentially traumatic stressors by virtue of their emotional under-reactivity.

As Blair and colleagues (2006) summarized, the neurobiological impairments in psychopathy evidenced by neuroimaging studies are consistent with the literature we have reviewed on mentalizing deficits. The callous-unemotional pattern of responding reflects not only a relative fearlessness but also a failure to empathize as Baron-Cohen defines it: "Empathizing occurs when we feel an appropriate emotional reaction, an emotion *triggered by* the other person's emotion, and it is done in order to understand another person, to predict their behavior, and to connect or resonate with them emotionally" (Baron-Cohen 2003, p. 2, emphasis in original). In short, empathizing entails being moved by others' emotions. Consistent with this clinical picture, psychopaths show both reduced amygdaloid volume and reduced amygdala activation when they are exposed to emotional cues as well as when they participate in aversive conditioning tasks (Blair 2003, 2004); accordingly, they are emotionally unresponsive to others' expressions of fearful and sad emotions. Thus, without the amygdalar contribution to perception, their mindreading lacks emotional coloring and responsiveness; they are unmoved by the emotional pain they evoke in others. Accordingly, psychopaths lack the normal violence inhibition mechanism (Blair et al. 2005): they fail to mentalize in the sense that an impulse to do harm does not evoke an inhibiting aversive mental representation of the other person's potential emotional distress. In short:

> psychopathic individuals represent the developmental case where sad and fearful expressions are not aversive unconditioned stimuli. As a consequence of this, the individual does not learn to avoid committing behaviours that cause harm to others and will commit them if, by doing them, he receives reward. (Blair 2003, p. 566)

Although psychopathic individuals are distinctive in their instrumental aggression, they are not immune to reactive aggression. Yet their reactive aggression has a different basis from that of non-psychopaths (e.g., traumatized persons). Blair and colleagues (2005, 2006) review evidence for impaired orbital/ventrolateral functioning in psychopathy and, as described earlier in this chapter, these prefrontal areas also have been implicated in mentalizing. The orbital/ventrolateral impairment contributes to reactive aggression insofar as the ventrolateral cortex plays a significant role in inhibiting responses to stimuli that have been rewarded previously but are no longer rewarded currently. Thus this prefrontal area plays a critical role in response reversal, for example, in adapting behavior to changing reinforcement contingencies (e.g., when teasing no longer is experienced as amusing but rather becomes hurtful). Blair and colleagues propose that, owing to impaired orbital/ventrolateral functioning, psychopaths are more likely to perseverate in unrewarding behavior; then, being unable to shift gears, they are more liable to frustration and thereby more vulnerable to reactive aggression in that context.

Recapitulation

Mentalizing in psychotherapy—for example, responding empathically to a patient's distress—involves attending, seeing, hearing, feeling, thinking, moving, and talking; thus mentalizing will be associated with activity in the entire brain—a multiplicity of regions interacting in concert. Nonetheless, the territory of mentalizing is narrower than perceiving and thinking writ large, and there is some justification for narrowing our focus (slightly) to the "social brain."

To summarize, on the social orienting and input side, the fusiform face area contributes to identifying individuals, and the superior temporal sulcus interprets patterns of actions such as emotional expressions; the amygdala adds emotional coloring to the perception, especially when threat looms. The overlapping regions of the anterior cingulate and medial prefrontal cortex have been identified as the mentalizing region proper, contributing not only to the awareness of emotions in self and others (and in emotional self-regulation) but also to interpreting impersonal situations as in theory-of-mind tasks. To reiterate, this medial prefrontal region covers a large and heterogeneous territory, and linking the more specific facets of mentalizing to more narrowly defined brain regions will be the next frontier of neuroimaging research in mentalizing.

As we stated at the beginning of this chapter, the combination of developmental and neurobiological research is establishing a firm scientific foundation for our concept of mentalizing. Both domains of research underscore the multiplicity of emotional and cognitive processes that we are subsuming under this broad rubric. Developmental and neurobiological research will continue to refine our understanding of the many facets of mentalizing and their interactions. Yet, multifaceted as it may be, we highlight the unity in mentalizing for clinical purposes, and nowhere is this unity more apparent than in the like-mindedness ensured by our shared social brain and culture, which enables the mind of each individual to come into being through the minds of other individuals.

Yet we have seen that optimal development of mentalizing capacities is by no means assured—even short of neurodevelopmental disorders such as autism and psychopathy. Most conspicuously, attachment trauma undermines the development of mentalizing capacity. But various degrees of impaired mentalizing associated with a wide range of psychopathologies also merit clinical attention. Moreover, whether focusing on mentalizing impairments or a host of other problems, all interventions require mentalizing on the part of the patient and clinician. Hence, in the spirit of Frank (1961), we proposed at the outset of this book that mentalizing is the most fundamental common factor in psychotherapies. As we have reviewed in the first part of this book, the past several decades of attachment research, recently abetted by neuroimaging, have enabled us greatly to refine our understanding of the common core of therapeutic relationships. Part II of this book ("Practicing Mentalizing") considers a range of potential applications.

Key Clinical Points

- *Trauma and arousal thresholds:* Neurobiological research illuminates the challenges of mentalizing while remaining in the emotional state: beyond a certain threshold of emotional arousal, patterns of brain activity switch from being conducive to mentalizing to promoting reflexive fight-or-flight responding; thresholds for switching out of mentalizing can be lowered by early trauma.

- *Autism:* Autism is the prototype of impaired mentalizing; genetically based neurobiological deficits impede the initial process of social-emotional engagement, which is the wellspring of mentalizing. Hypoactivation in diverse brain regions that support mentalizing has been identified in autism-spectrum disorders.

- *Psychopathy:* Like autism, psychopathy is associated with genetically based neurobiological deficits. Yet psychopathy entails a *partial failure of mentalizing,* namely, a callous-unemotional manner of relating that can be construed as mindreading without empathy. Impaired emotional responsiveness associated with amygdala hypoactivation, coupled with impaired inhibition associated with orbital/ventrolateral hypoactivation, contribute to failures in socialization and a proclivity for instrumental aggression.

PART II

Practicing Mentalizing

Chapter 5

The Art of Mentalizing

We assume that, having diligently reviewed the theory and research on mentalizing in the first part of this book, readers are eager to find out how to translate theory into practice, and the second part of this book aspires to do just that. Yet, banking on readers' frustration tolerance, we begin discussing practice in this chapter by spelling out the limits as to how prescriptive we can be. These exist because the activity of mentalizing—*doing it* at any given moment—is an art, not a science. Within these limits, we will be discussing mentalizing interventions in the next chapter. But first we are giving thorough consideration to the spirit of our approach, because the essence of mentalizing-focused therapy is reflected in the clinician's *attitude* toward the process—what we have been calling the mentalizing stance—rather than in technique. Moreover, in addition to giving our science-weary readers a non-technical interlude, this chapter continues our effort to humanize "mentalizing" in light of its technical and intellectual connotations.

We construe the skillful conduct of psychotherapy as the artful use of science (Allen, in press). To elaborate this point, in this chapter we present some exceptionally fine work done by others whom we regard as super-mentalizers. Table 5–1, for example, lists characteristics of discourse characterizing secure attachment relationships as viewed by Main and Goldwyn (1994).

TABLE 5–1. CHARACTERISTICS OF DISCOURSE INDICATIVE OF SECURE ATTACHMENT

- Reflectiveness
- Lively consciousness
- Freshness of speech
- Capacity for humor
- Little self-deception
- Ease and openness with the ability to alter one's views
- Ease with imperfections in self and others
- Compassion

All these criteria are consistent with what we have called the mentalizing stance, and we should highlight the fact that Main was focusing on research participants, not clinicians, in the Adult Attachment Interview. No special training is required to be a fine mentalizer—or a super-mentalizer, for that matter. We would expect to find some super-mentalizers among Meins's mind-minded mothers (Meins et al. 2002). But the ideal characteristics Main identified in her research participants apply equally to the functioning of clinicians conducting psychotherapy. These criteria exemplify the subjective emotional engagement, spontaneity, and sheer creativity characteristic of mentalizing as contrasted with the objective, detached, rule-oriented approach we associate with scientific procedures.

To elaborate our view of mentalizing activity as an art, we begin by distinguishing mentalizing from scientific thinking, employing Simon Baron-Cohen's cardinal distinction between empathizing and systemizing. Next, explicating the implicit, we underscore the point that our basic therapeutic leverage is our humanity. Then we highlight the artful nature of what we construe as exemplary mentalizing by quoting liberally from the writings of two psychoanalysts and one ethicist. We conclude with some comments about integrating science and art in practicing mentalizing-focused interventions.

Empathizing Versus Systemizing

In Chapter 2 ("Mentalizing"), we described the "theory-theory" of the acquisition of theory of mind, wherein the prospective mentalizer is likened to a scientist who develops mentalistic constructs to interpret behavior. We are in accord with philosopher Jane Heal (2003) in believing that the analogy to science is misguided:

> Our relations with other people do not have the same structure as our relations with inanimate objects, plants or machines. We do not deal with our family members, friends, colleagues or fellow citizens as we do with volcanoes, fields of wheat or kitchen mixers, namely, by trying to figure out the nature and layout of their innards so that we can predict and perhaps control them…. What we hope of another with whom we interact is not that he or she will go through some gyrations which we have already planned in detail, but that he or she will make some contributions to *moving forward the joint and co-operative enterprise* in which we are both, more or less explicitly, engaged. (pp. 42–43; emphasis added)

"Moving forward the joint and cooperative enterprise" is precisely what mentalizing accomplishes. Paralleling Heal's protest against equating persons with kitchen mixers, Baron-Cohen (2003, 2005) proposed a fundamental distinction between empathizing—the territory of mentalizing—and systemizing, of which scientific thinking is representative. Baron-Cohen defines systematizing as the "drive to analyze, explore, and construct a system. The systemizer intuitively figures out how things work, or extracts the underlying rules that govern the behavior of a system. This is done in order to understand and predict the behavior of a system" (Baron-Cohen 2003, p. 3). He defines a system as an entity that takes inputs and delivers outputs according to rules; here is the kind of thinking that goes into systemizing: "If I do x, a changes to b. If z occurs, p changes to q" (Baron-Cohen 2005, p. 475, emphasis in original). Baron-Cohen proposed that the human brain can analyze six kinds of systems: technical (e.g., computers), natural (e.g., tides), abstract (e.g., mathematics), social (e.g., elections), organizable (e.g., libraries), and motoric (e.g., musical techniques). In short, working with a system entails developing and utilizing an *algorithm*, defined in the *Shorter Oxford English Dictionary* as a procedure or set of rules for calculating or problem solving. If we aspired to manualize psychotherapy to the hilt, we would arrive at a set of algorithms.

Having distinguished empathizing from systemizing, Baron-Cohen (2005) makes a strong claim:

Systemizing works for phenomena that are indeed ultimately lawful, fi-
nite, and deterministic…. *Systemizing is of almost no use when it comes to
predicting the moment by moment changes in a person's behavior.* To predict
human behavior, empathizing is required. Systemizing and empathizing are wholly different kinds of processes. (p. 476, emphasis added)

Baron-Cohen (2005) goes on to characterize systematizing and empathizing as not only fundamentally different but also *opposite* to each
other, and he adds, "Empathizing involves an imaginative leap in the
dark, in the absence of much data" (p. 476). Moreover, he contends that
the two kinds of thought processes depend on independent brain regions. The dissociation between empathizing and systemizing is most
stark in autism, which is characterized by markedly impaired empathizing, often in conjunction with superior systemizing (Baron-Cohen
et al. 2005). To a lesser degree, the dissociation is evident in gender differences: extensive overlap notwithstanding, male brains are better designed for systemizing, whereas female brains are better designed for
empathizing; notably, incipient gender differences in these activities are
evident in newborns (Baron-Cohen 2003).

To conclude, we have no doubt that systemizing plays a role in conducting psychotherapy; without knowledge, principles, and strategies,
the process would founder for lack of direction—nor could we improve
our effectiveness through research. But the moment-to-moment interactive process requires empathizing.

Our Humanity

In the context of trauma therapy, Pearlman and Saakvitne (1995) proposed,
"We are the tools of our trade" (p. 185). To take Baron-Cohen's (2005)
point, it is only through our fundamental humanity—our empathizing capacity—that we can make any clinical use of all our scientific and professional knowledge. And our professional training can be beneficial only to
the extent that it refines—and does not undermine—our natural mentalizing ability. Taking our natural mentalizing capacity for granted, we believe
that professional training—as we are aspiring to do here—is helpful primarily by virtue of reorienting and sharpening attention.

In writing about the abilities of psychoanalysts, Strenger (1991)
made the same point about our humanity in proposing the continuum
principle:

Appeal to special abilities of analysts must not violate the following
principle: *It must be possible to show that the claimed capacities are refinements of ordinary human capacities, and it must be made plausible why under*

specified circumstances such refinement can actually occur. This can be called
the *continuum principle*, because it postulates that the abilities claimed
for analysts must be on a continuum with ordinary human abilities.
(p. 95; emphasis in original)

We agree with Strenger's view that the "picture of the natural scientist does not apply to the psychoanalyst" and his opinion that other
forms of expertise might also serve as models: "the historian, the art
dealer, the professor of literature, and the financial counselor" (p. 130).
These are practical arts. And, as we are also stating, Strenger proposes,
"The psychoanalytic therapist's competence does not reside in the mastery of a formal, well-established theory;" rather, the crucial qualities
that pertain to competence are personality characteristics such as "ma-
turity, objectivity, flexibility, and empathy" (p. 131). Nor does identifying countertransference require any "mysterious faculties" but rather
awareness of the "ordinary human reactions to a person who seduces,
attacks, admires, or devalues" (p. 93).

While we are single-mindedly focusing on empathizing and mentalizing capacity, we must not lose sight of the fact that the structure of the
treatment situation is critical to the optimal employment of this capacity. The boundaries of the treatment afford an exceptional opportunity
to mentalize—as Strenger construes it, *freedom from the pressure to act*.
Expanding on his point that the analyst acquires knowledge about the
patient by employing "abilities every sane human being possesses and
uses effortlessly in everyday life," Strenger states,

> The analyst can refine these capacities and use them with greater sensi-
> tivity than we (including the analyst himself) generally do in everyday
> life. This is possible because the analyst is, as a therapist, exempt from
> the pressure of reacting directly to the patient's promptings and can
> thus concentrate on his perception of, and emotional reaction to, the pa-
> tient. (p. 85)

We often use the metaphor of pushing the pause button in mentalizing, and the treatment situation affords the luxury of doing so—for
both the patient and the therapist. Accordingly, in the design of the psychotherapy situation, we have stacked the odds of mentalizing in our
favor, to the benefit of the patient. Mentalizing in everyday life is not so
easy; therapy is preparation.

Exceptionally Artful Mentalizing

Learning psychotherapy is not different from other crafts; we learn best
by observing masters. We have chosen a few writers whom we regard

as exceptional mentalizers: Hans Loewald, Daniel Stern, and Iris Murdoch. Only one of them, Daniel Stern, used the word (in passing).

Hans Loewald

Loewald (1960) contended that therapeutic neutrality "should not be confused with the 'neutral' attitude of the pure scientist" (p. 18) and that the identification of the analyst with the patient (and vice versa) "has nothing to do with scientific detachment and the neutrality of a mirror" (p. 19). Noting that Freud considered scientific man to be the most advanced form of human development, Loewald emphasized instead the need to question the assumption that psychoanalytic therapy is a purely scientific activity. On the contrary, he asserted that therapeutic activity "requires an objectivity and neutrality the essence of which is *love and respect* for the individual and for individual development" (p. 20, emphasis added). Of course, Freud was as far from narrow-minded as one could be, and Loewald (1960) made good use of Freud's analogy between the psychoanalyst and the artist:

> In sculpturing, the figure to be created comes into being by taking away from the material.... In analysis, we bring out the true form by taking away the neurotic distortions. However, as in sculpture, we must have, if only in rudiments, an image of that which needs to be brought into its own. (p. 18)

For this therapeutic process of bringing the imagined into being, Loewald used the parent-child relationship as a model: "The parent ideally is in an empathic relationship of understanding the child's particular stage in development, yet ahead in his vision of the child's future and mediating this vision to the child in his dealing with him" (p. 20). He went on to note that the child then internalizes the parent's image of the child—a process we have detailed in the development of mentalizing in attachment relationships (see Chapter 3, "Development").

Yet, no more narrow-minded than Freud, Loewald (1970) was too wise to place a rigid boundary between the practice of psychoanalysis and scientific inquiry; he questioned not only the view of psychoanalysis as purely scientific activity but also the practice of science as detached and dispassionate, motivated solely by seeking objective truth:

> It also needs to be said that the love of truth is no less a passion because it desires truth rather than some less elevated end. In our field the love of truth cannot be isolated from the passion for truth to ourselves and truth in human relationships. In other fields, too, the scientist is filled with love for his object precisely in his most creative and "dispassionate" moments. Scientific detachment in its genuine form, far from ex-

cluding love, is based on it. In our work it can be truly said that in our best moments of dispassionate and objective analyzing we love our object, the patient, more than at any other time and are compassionate with his whole being. (p. 65)

Daniel Stern

In writing about love and compassion, Loewald brought out the essential role of emotion in therapeutic understanding. Love and compassion are not derived from scientific procedures; they flow from empathizing, not systemizing. In the same vein, Stern and colleagues' work (Stern 2004; Stern et al. 1998) attests to the role of spontaneity and creativity in the therapeutic process; these, too, cannot be predicated on algorithms.

In his emphasis on "present moments" and "moments of meeting," Stern (2004) has, in effect, articulated the phenomenology of mentalizing in the therapeutic process. Stern's present-centered focus on the here and now contrasts with most psychodynamic treatments in which he believes "there is a rush toward meaning, leaving the present moment behind" (p. 140). Consistent with our emphasis on art, he articulates the "creative virtues of 'sloppiness' in the psychotherapeutic process" (p. 156) in which the task for the patient and therapist is to continue *moving along* in a therapeutic way—much in the spirit that Heal articulated. In describing this process, Stern (2004) alludes to what we would call the non-mentalizing alternative (in parentheses):

> Moving along, while it is happening, is largely a spontaneous, locally unpredictable process. The therapist cannot know exactly what the patient is going to say next, let alone what he is going to say next, until he says it or does it. And the same applies for the patient.... (If the therapist thinks she knows, she is treating a theory and not a person). (p. 156)

Consistent with the mentalizing stance, Stern advocates "holding theory at a further distance during the session so that the immediate relationship can be lived more fully" (p. 224).

Stern highlights *present moments*, typically spanning several seconds, as warranting special attention: these moments have special therapeutic value in being novel, engaging, unpredictable, and also potentially problematic so as to require some sort of mental action and psychological work. The potentially most mutative present moments are *moments of meeting*, which he refers to as mindreading; we would call this mentalizing interactively in the transference:

> The present moments that interest us most are those that arise when two people make a special kind of mental contact—namely, an intersubjec-

tive contact. This involves the mutual interpenetration of minds that permits us to say, "I know that you know that I know" or "I feel that you feel that I feel." There is a reading of the contents of the other's mind. Such readings can be mutual. Two people see and feel roughly the same mental landscape for a moment at least. These meetings are what psychotherapy is largely about. (p. 75)

Stern is describing mentalizing at its best in characterizing psychotherapy as having the main implicit task of regulating the immediate intersubjective field, carrying out the regulation by "probing, testing, and correcting the reading of the other's mental state in light of your own" (p. 120). As the following example illustrates, exemplary mentalizing is truly artful:

The nature of a now moment usually demands something beyond a technically acceptable response: It demands a moment of meeting.... It requires an authentic response finely matched to the momentary local situation. It must be spontaneous and must carry the therapist's personal signature.... Take, for example, the patient who suddenly sat up to look at her therapist. Right after the patient also sat up, the two found themselves looking at each other intently. A silence prevailed. The therapist, without knowing exactly what she was going to do, softened her face slowly and let the suggestion of a smile form around her mouth. She then leaned her head forward slightly and said, "Hello." The patient continued to look at her. They remained locked in a mutual gaze for several seconds. After a moment, the patient laid down again and continued her work on the couch, but more profoundly and in a new key, which opened up new material. The change was dramatic in their work together. (pp. 168–169)

Stern notes that such nodal moments of meeting are the exception rather than the rule; none might occur over a span of several sessions. Yet these poignant moments are merely a peak form of what the parent-infant interactions characteristic of secure attachments exemplify on a more mundane basis, for example, in Meins and colleagues' (2002) description of mind-minded mothering (see Chapter 3, "Development"). Stern does not underplay the importance of meaning making and narrative, but he makes it clear that the meeting of minds is the foundation on which explicit narrative understanding must develop.

Iris Murdoch

Although she might have balked at the word, the ethicist and novelist Iris Murdoch brought what we call mentalizing to a high art and, like Loewald, she drew an intimate connection between love and the capacity to understand other individuals in their own right (Antonaccio 2000;

Murdoch 1971, 1992). Simply put, "Love is knowledge of the individual" (Murdoch 1971, p. 27).

Now with ample scientific backing, we have followed in Murdoch's footsteps in placing considerable burden on *attention* as the basis of mentalizing: "I have used the word 'attention'...to express the idea of a just and loving gaze directed upon an individual reality" (Murdoch 1971, p. 33). As we also have done, Murdoch gave great weight to *imagination* as "an ability to picture what is quite other; especially of course to picture and realise, make real to oneself, the existence of other people" (Murdoch 1992, p. 322). Furthermore, in line with the pervasive distorting influence of egocentrism on mentalizing that we have emphasized, Murdoch construed surmounting egoism—what she called *unselfing*—as the core challenge in perceiving human reality for what it is. Thus Murdoch made a point of distinguishing egoistic fantasy from truth-seeking creative imagination; she viewed fantasy as "mechanically generating narrowly banal false pictures" and imagination as "freely and creatively exploring the world, moving toward the expression and elucidation (and in art celebration) of what is true and deep" (Murdoch 1992, p. 321).

No stranger to what we might loosely construe as the distorting effects of neurosis, Murdoch (1992) proposed that "Egoistic anxiety veils the world" (p. 175), and she viewed the role of attention and imagination as removing "the usual egoistic fuzz of self-protective anxiety" (p. 244). Indeed, she construed "extreme nervous self-consciousness" as the "most selfish of all states to be in" (Conradi 2001, p. 153). As she recognized, employing attention and imagination to overcome egoism is no mean feat: "our ordinary consciousness is full of illusions. Our 'grasp' is superficial. Anxiety, malice, envy, greed, all sorts of selfish preoccupations and instinctive attachments may deform or hide what confronts us.... At every moment we are 'attending' or failing to attend" (pp. 295–296)

Murdoch (1971) construed "reality" as "that which is revealed to the patient eye of love" (p. 39) and, as we have just described, she believed that keen attention and imagination are required to overcome the distorting influences of egocentrism and fantasy. She appreciated the sheer amount of mental effort required to do this; hence she rightly construed aspiring to see the reality of another person as a loving act. Murdoch illustrated her view with what has become a celebrated example of a mother, M, who initially feels hostility toward her daughter-in-law, D (pp. 16–17). Perceiving D as "pert and familiar, insufficiently ceremonious, brusque, sometimes positively rude, always tiresomely juvenile," M feels that her son has married beneath him. Murdoch proposes that

M, being a very "correct" person, consistently behaves with impeccable manners toward D; Murdoch is concerned solely with what happens in M's mind, not with her overt behavior. She notes that M could settle into a "hardened sense of grievance" exemplified by the conviction that "my poor son has married a silly vulgar girl." But "the M of the example is an intelligent and well-intentioned person, capable of self-criticism, capable of giving careful and just *attention* to an object which confronts her." Being reflective, M begins to see herself as being snobbish, and she is aware of her jealousy. She persuades herself to look again. The mental process unfolds:

> Here I assume that M observes D or at least reflects deliberately about D, until gradually her vision of D alters. If we take D to be now absent or dead this can make it clear that the change is not in D's behaviour but in M's mind. D is discovered to be not vulgar but refreshingly simple, not undignified but spontaneous, not noisy but gay, not tiresomely juvenile but delightfully youthful, and so on. (p. 17)

Murdoch points out that, in principle, neither view is inherently more accurate than the other, but she takes the revised view to be more appropriate for the sake of her argument: "When M is just and loving she sees D as she really is" (p. 36); to reiterate, the work of effortful attention was necessary to counteract egoistic states of illusion.

In the course of her argument, Murdoch brought to light the *ethical texture* of what we call mentalizing. She put this point starkly: "consciousness is a form of moral activity: what we attend to, how we attend, whether we attend" (Murdoch 1992, p. 167). More elaborately,

> it is perfectly obvious that goodness is connected with knowledge: not with impersonal quasi-scientific knowledge of the ordinary world, whatever that may be, but with a refined and honest perception of what is really the case, a patient and just discernment and exploration of what confronts one, which is the result not simply of opening one's eyes but of a certainly perfectly familiar kind of moral discipline. (Murdoch 1971, p. 37)

Accordingly, Murdoch (1992) argued that we practitioners of psychotherapy "cannot avoid being involved in moral judgment, in moral reflection and insight in the widest sense" inasmuch as "It is the soul that is being treated" (p. 307). No doubt, embracing this ethical dimension of moralizing puts us on an unavoidable slippery slope: we must find a way to engage in this inescapably moral activity without moralizing (Allen, in press).

We psychotherapists could hardly do better in aspiring to mentalize—to see the reality of self and others—than to follow Murdoch's

lead. When feeling persistent animosity or disdain for a patient, for example, one might think of M's attentive work to develop an alternate
view of D. As Murdoch articulated it, making this shift in perspectives
is a high aspiration:

> The love which brings the right answer is an exercise of justice and real-
> ism and really looking. The difficulty is to keep the attention fixed upon
> the real situation and to prevent it from returning surreptitiously to the
> self with consolations of self-pity, resentment, fantasy and despair…. It
> is a *task* to come to see the world as it is…. We act rightly "when the time
> comes" not out of strength of will but out of the quality of our usual at-
> tachments and with the kind of energy and discernment which we have
> available. And to this the whole activity of our consciousness is relevant.
> (Murdoch 1971, p. 89; emphasis in original)

With these glimpses of Murdoch's mind in mind, and with the ethical texture of mentalizing in view, we can construe mentalizing at its
fullest not only as a skill but also as a virtue. Murdoch set the bar high,
hewing to an ideal standard of perfection. Yet she acknowledged that
the distance from potentially fantasy-laden subjectivity to truly loving
objectivity is considerable: "it's terribly distant, farther than any star"
(Murdoch 1999, p. 518). The "not-knowing" stance we advocate in the
next chapter is a good place to start: "We have…a natural impulse to de-
realise our world and surround ourselves with fantasy. Simply stopping this, refraining from filling voids with lies and falsity, is progress"
(Murdoch 1992, p. 503).

When aspiring to attain virtue, the only reasonable attitude is one of
humility. Here is consolation for the aspirant mentalizing psychotherapist: "To think about the virtues is to take measure of the distance separating us from them. To think about their excellence is to think about
our own inadequacies or wretchedness" (Comte-Sponville 2001, p. 5).
In this light, we all can be grateful for the idea of the good-enough
mother as we aspire to become good-enough therapists; as mothers and
therapists all know, that is no mean aspiration.

Help From Science

Having given science its due in the first part of this book, we have given
it short shrift here, where we are focusing not on the importance of our
knowledge about mentalizing but rather on actually *doing it*. But knowing and doing are conjoined; the art is in the *application* of the science.
Through the developmental research we have reviewed, we have solid
knowledge about the relationship conditions that facilitate and impair

mentalizing. Meins (1997) and Murdoch (1971) are not far apart. We are more likely to do something effectively if we have a clear idea about what we are trying to do, and developmental research has provided that much.

Yet, beyond the developmental research, there is another domain of scientific knowledge that we find extremely helpful in aspiring to mentalize in the sense of seeing reality aright and less fettered by our egocentric perspective: our knowledge of psychopathology. We are likely to find it most difficult to *mentalize non-mentalizing*. The challenge of working with children with autism—adapting to their limited mentalizing—is the most glaring example of needing to mentalize non-mentalizing. But the same point applies to our scientific knowledge of many other psychiatric conditions in which mentalizing is compromised, ranging from psychopathy and borderline personality disorder to severe depression or acute anxiety states. Failing to appreciate the nature of the psychopathology will be associated with inadequate mentalizing and ineffective or downright harmful interventions.

Finally, we must rely on scientific methods for gauging the effectiveness of our interventions in relation to treatment outcomes; over the past half-century, these methods have become highly refined. The effectiveness of mentalizing interventions has been researched most systematically in the treatment of patients with borderline personality disorder (see Chapter 9, "Borderline Personality Disorder"), but as the rest of the present book attests, some inroads have been made in other areas, and opportunities for further scientific investigation of the practical value of the mentalizing stance abound.

Recapitulation

In winding our way from Mary Main to Iris Murdoch, we have set the bar high for mentalizing. But we must acknowledge the distance between the ideal and the real. Owing to good-enough mentalizing, most children are adequately raised and most psychotherapy patients are adequately treated. Of course, we are obligated professionally to use accumulated scientific knowledge, training, supervision, and consultation to continue improving our practice; we have presented this chapter in that spirit.

Our emphasis on the art of mentalizing in psychotherapy is fitting inasmuch as we have given more weight to ways of thinking and relating—emphasizing the mentalizing stance and considering content as secondary to process—than to specific techniques and procedures. We are a long way from algorithms and, as Baron-Cohen's (2005) work makes plain, algorithms are antithetical to mentalizing. Thus we face a paradox: in the present mental healthcare climate, one needs manuals to be practicing evidence-based treatment; yet developing a manual to an extremely high level of specificity would undermine precisely what we are striving to cultivate: mentalizing. To reiterate, the art is in the application. As Roth and Fonagy imply, there is no substitute for practical wisdom, especially in helping patients who are seriously disturbed or treatment resistant:

> manuals have much to contribute to the training of psychotherapists, and…models of good training practice would include formally assessing their capacity to adhere to these. However…while good knowledge of the key components of a technique is an important foundation for effective practice, expert practitioners may be those who are able to use technical recommendations flexibly, and deviate and go beyond them at times, when the clinical situation seems to require this. (Roth and Fonagy 2005, p. 476)

Moreover, continuing on the theme of the crucial role of clinical judgment, Roth and Fonagy point out: "There is irony in the fact that although there is an increasing requirement for practice to be based on evidence, we are not aware of systematic evidence demonstrating the benefit of this process" (p. 502).

Given the limits of scientific procedures, there is an advantage in refining a therapeutic approach in relation to a basic human capacity. Indeed, as we have stated, a significant part of what we do in training moves clinicians away from technical theories and back toward common sense. This last point sets the stage for considering mentalizing interventions a bit more concretely—but only a bit, for reasons we have just strived to make clear.

Key Clinical Points

- *Modes of thinking:* The art of psychotherapy lies in the application of scientific knowledge such that conducting psychotherapy entails *complementary* modes of thinking: *empathizing* and *systemizing.* The activity of mentalizing is an art that cannot be reduced to rules or procedures; hence there is a limit to which psychotherapy can be manualized beyond the statement of general principles.

- *Moments of meeting:* The art of mentalizing in psychotherapy—on the part of the patient as well as the therapist—is best exemplified by Stern and colleagues' description of *moments of meeting;* these spontaneous interactions cannot be planned, and they make a significant contribution to therapeutic movement.

- *Foundation for mentalizing:* Therapists' humanity as exemplified in mentalizing is the fundamental basis of their effectiveness in psychotherapy; yet the *formal structure* of therapy—especially the maintenance of professional boundaries and the psychological space that provides time to reflect—provides an essential foundation for therapists to sustain mentalizing in the process.

Chapter 6

Mentalizing Interventions

As we proposed in elaborating the art of mentalizing, it is one thing to have a good theory about mental functioning and yet another to apply it in a fruitful way to help people with psychological problems. This chapter continues the project of the second part of this book: translating theory into practice. We describe how you can enhance your skill in your everyday clinical practice by learning about interventions that are likely to increase mentalizing—in your patients and yourself.

Albeit an overview, this chapter is intended to be useful in your clinical practice at least insofar as it might help you begin paying attention to the process of mentalizing in your daily work. You will know that you are beginning to make use of the guidance we provide here under the following circumstances: when you feel yourself struggling to assist your patient in mentalizing; when you become aware that you are having difficulty mentalizing with respect to your patient or yourself; when you realize belatedly that you have just derailed your patient's mentalizing with a non-mentalizing intervention; or when you catch yourself operating on the basis of grossly distorted perceptions, interpretations, and assumptions. Ironically, when you become aware of your non-mentalizing interventions, you are mentalizing. A further irony: when you start obsessing about mentalizing in the middle of a session, you have lost mentalizing, because you are no longer paying attention to your patient. With respect to all forms of impaired mentalizing—in clinical practice and in daily life—we speak from extensive personal experience; conducting workshops and writing books provides no immunity from non-mentalizing interactions.

When aspiring to adhere to it, you will find the mentalizing approach to be a mixed blessing: on the one hand, you will be freed from the pressure to provide answers or insights; on the other hand, you will be challenged to develop and maintain a consistently reflective therapeutic process, that is, keeping yourself and your patient in the mentalizing mode. In the sections that follow, we point out that much of what you have been doing naturally is promoting mentalizing, even though you may not have thought about it as such; we encourage you to refocus the aims of treatment; we illustrate a mentalizing case formulation; we offer advice on refining your technique; we advocate maintaining a mentalizing stance; we encourage you to adapt your interventions according to a moment-to-moment assessment of your patient's mentalizing capacities; we describe how we think about mentalizing in the transference; we enumerate some tips on practice; and we offer some questions for self-assessment with respect to treatment adherence. We are especially fortunate to be able to conclude this chapter with a patient's first-hand account of what it is like to experience mentalizing-focused therapy.

To reiterate the theme of the last chapter: although we provide some concrete examples of the kinds of clinical interventions that can promote mentalizing, you will find in reading this chapter that we are mainly articulating a *way of thinking* about conducting psychotherapy; we are more concerned with attitude than technique. Hence learning this approach is unlike mastering a laboratory technique; ironically, teaching and learning it requires mentalizing. Wittgenstein (1953) beautifully captured this spirit in his comments about learning to interpret emotional expressions accurately:

> Is there such a thing as "expert judgment" about the genuineness of expressions of feeling? —Even here, there are those whose judgment is "better" and those whose judgment is "worse."
>
> Correcter prognoses will generally issue from the judgments of those with better knowledge of mankind.
>
> Can one learn this knowledge? Yes; some can. Not, however, by taking a course in it, but through *"experience."*—Can someone else be a man's teacher in this? Certainly. From time to time he gives him the

right *tip.* —This is what "learning" and "teaching" are like here. What one acquires here is not a technique; one learns correct judgments. There are also rules, but they do not form a system, and only experienced people can apply them right. Unlike calculating-rules. (p. 193, emphasis in original)

In the spirit of Wittgenstein, we offer general guidelines and some tips. To provide readers with a quick overview of the spirit of the approach we detail in this chapter, Table 6–1 lists interventions that are likely to promote mentalizing and those that are liable to undermine it. Taking basic mentalizing capacity for granted, we aspire primarily to draw your attention to mentalizing in the treatment process with the conviction that if you pay attention to it, you will find a way to do it.

As readers should well appreciate by this point, we are construing mentalizing as a generic approach to psychotherapy. Consistent with our presentation of mentalizing-focused therapy as the least novel approach to treatment, we assume that interventions of the style highlighted in Table 6–1 simply represent what most clinicians would consider to be good technique (as always, easier said than done). Accordingly, within this mentalizing framework, we are not concerned about your underlying model of therapy, and we are disinclined to move you away from your professional base in psychiatry, psychology, social work, or any other domain of counseling. Rather, we encourage you to reframe your interventions, whether interpretive or cognitive, in relation to mentalizing. That is, we advocate *superimposing* a mentalizing stance on your particular therapeutic approach while reducing any non-mentalizing interventions inherent in your work. As we already have stated, we are convinced that skillfully conducted treatments ranging from psychoanalysis to cognitive-behavioral therapy can promote the psychological process of mentalizing, as long as they are tailored to the patient's mentalizing capacities. Yet generic as our approach may be, we introduce a caveat: although we are advocating the extension of a mentalizing focus to a range of treatment modalities and patient populations, we must acknowledge that the general style of interventions we are espousing has been influenced by our experience of treating patients with borderline personality disorder—the wellspring of mentalization-based therapy (Bateman and Fonagy 2004, 2006).

Thus, insofar as we are particularly attentive to precarious mentalizing, we are advocating a relatively structured and supportive approach to treatment that focuses primarily on the present. In taking this tack, we do not deny that insight-oriented interpretive techniques—as emphasized, for example, in psychoanalysis—can promote mentalizing in patients with more robust mentalizing capacities. Indeed, we believe that

TABLE 6–1. CHARACTERISTICS OF INTERVENTIONS THAT INFLUENCE
MENTALIZING

Promoting mentalizing

- Maintaining an inquisitive, curious, "not-knowing" stance
- Providing a secure-base experience that facilitates patients' exploration of mental states—their own and yours
- Promoting a level of emotional engagement that is neither too hot nor too cold
- Engaging in a mirroring process in which your contingently responsive, "marked" emotions represent the patient's mental state back to the patient
- Offering interventions that are simple and to the point
- Maintaining a balance between engaging patients in exploring mental states of self and others
- Engaging patients in viewing interactions and self-experience from multiple perspectives
- Acknowledging when you do not know what to say or do and enlisting the patient's help in moving the process forward
- Working with transference so as to help patients understand how their mind is working in the room
- Validating the patient's experience before offering alternative perspectives
- Challenging patients' unsubstantiated assumptions about your attitudes, feelings, or beliefs
- Engaging in judicious self-disclosure regarding your interactions with the patient
- Letting patients know what you are thinking so as to permit them to correct your distorted mentalizing
- Acknowledging your own mentalizing failures and endeavoring to understand misunderstandings
- Acknowledging mistakes and actively exploring your contribution to the patient's adverse reactions

Undermining mentalizing

- Striving to be clever, brilliant, and insightful
- Offering complicated, lengthy interventions
- Engaging in protracted discourse in the pretend mode ("psychobabble" or "bullshitting")
- Attributing mental states to the patient based on your theoretical preconceptions

TABLE 6–1. CHARACTERISTICS OF INTERVENTIONS THAT INFLUENCE MENTALIZING *(continued)*

- Presenting your ideas about the patient to the patient with a sense of certainty
- Focusing excessively on relationship structure and content instead of relationship processes
- Attributing the patient's experience of a relationship to a general pattern rather than exploring the experience and its basis in more detail
- Using the transference to explore unconscious repetitions of past behavior
- Allowing prolonged silences
- Encouraging free association and elaboration of fantasies about the therapist
- Responding to the patient with intense, "unmarked" emotion

insight-oriented psychotherapy may be the treatment of choice for patients with psychiatric disorders in the neurotic spectrum. For such patients, we construe distorted mental *representations* rather than distorted mental *processes* as being the core problem (Fonagy et al. 1993). From our vantage point, a wide range of therapeutic approaches, including cognitive and psychodynamic therapy, have the potential to address distorted mental representations insofar as they provide the patient with alternative perspectives that the patient is able to hold in mind. Finally, we add that improvements in mentalizing capacities, regardless of the therapeutic means by which they are brought about, will enable the patient to derive benefit from more insight-oriented treatment.

You Are Doing It Already

We have predicated this book on our premise that—unrecognized as it may be—mentalizing as a process is a key aspect of all effective psychotherapeutic work. Accordingly, in adopting this approach, you need not learn yet another long and complicated method of psychotherapy; rather, we invite you to reexamine your current practice from the perspective of a different conceptual framework, namely, the attachment framework for mentalizing that we described in Chapter 3 ("Development").

Implicit mentalizing is perforce the foundation of any therapeutic work. In conducting psychotherapy, you construct and reconstruct in your own mind an image of your patient's mind. You label feelings, explain cognitions, and spell out implicit beliefs. Importantly, you engage in a mirroring process, highlighting the "marked" character of your verbal or nonverbal mirroring display in which you reflect back your patient's mental state in a modified form. Your training and experience has further honed your natural capacity to show that your reaction is related to the patient's state of mind rather than exclusively to your own.

To reiterate the developmental perspective, since Bowlby's (1988) work, it has generally been agreed that psychotherapy invariably activates the attachment system and thus generates secure-base experience. Accordingly, self-consciously or not, you are necessarily working within an attachment framework. In our view, the attachment context of psychotherapy is essential in creating the synergy between the recovery of mentalizing capacity and secure-base experience. That is, you provide the experience of being understood, which generates an experience of security, which in turn facilitates mental exploration. That mental exploration includes your patient's exploration of *your* mind—and finding of himself or herself in the process. This typically rapid, non-conscious implicit process enables the patient to apprehend what he or she thinks and feels.

In conducting psychotherapy, you are mentalizing in the sense of engaging your patients in a process of joint attention wherein their mental states typically are the focus of your shared attention. In our view, the shared attentional processes entailed by all psychological therapies strengthen the interpersonal interpretive function of mentalizing (Fonagy 2003a). Although your mind is likely to be focused on the content—your patient's apprehension about a job interview—the ultimate therapeutic value of the interchange stems from the joint focus on the patient's subjective experience in the context of one mental content after another. As it does in childhood, this joint attentional process enhances mentalizing capacity and, concomitantly, strengthens the patient's sense of self.

The explicit content of your intervention will be mentalistic, regardless of your theoretical orientation—whether you are principally concerned with transference reactions, automatic negative thoughts, or reciprocal roles. All these approaches entail explicit mentalizing insofar as they succeed in enhancing coherent mental representations of desires, feelings, and beliefs. As we described in Chapter 2 ("Mentalizing") in the context of mentalizing the self, such efforts at mentalizing explicitly will not succeed unless you draw your patient into being an active collaborator in any explication; your job is to help your patient make up his or her mind.

Finally, driving home our point that you are already doing it, owing to the dyadic nature of therapy, you are naturally fostering your patients' capacity to generate multiple perspectives. For example, when you interpret transference, you are presenting an alternative perspective on the patient's subjective experience. In so doing, you are freeing the patient from being locked into the reality of one view and, accordingly, you are enabling your patient to move from the psychic equivalence mode (world=mind) to the mentalizing mode (mind represents world in many different ways).

> Operating in the psychic-equivalence mode, a patient was utterly convinced that his therapist was so frustrated with his slow progress that the therapist was merely biding her time until she could figure out how to terminate the therapy without hurting his feelings too badly. In bringing his convictions to light, the therapist was able to acknowledge her frustration while explaining that she considers frustration to be a natural part of trying to help people with difficult problems, that she generally has fairly good tolerance for feelings of frustration, and that—as a matter of fact—it never occurred to her to consider terminating the therapy.
> In the course of this exploration, the patient came to see that his mind worked differently from his therapist's mind. Being depressed, he quickly gives up whenever he feels frustrated. By contrast, his therapist was accustomed to persisting in the face of frustration.

Thus whatever you construe the mechanisms of therapeutic change to be—creating a coherent narrative, modifying distorted cognitions, providing the emotional experience of a secure base, giving insight, or simply rekindling hope—the effectiveness of your interventions will depend on your patients' capacity to consider their experience of their own mental states alongside your therapeutic re-presentations of them (Fonagy and Bateman 2006a). Your patients' appreciation of the difference between their own experience of their mind and that presented by another person is a key element of mentalizing interventions. Integrating their current experience of mind with the alternative view that you present is the foundation of the change process; mentalizing is essential for the achievement of this integration.

Refocusing the Aims of Treatment

Table 6–2 lists three basic aims of the approach we are advocating (in which the discerning reader will identify a common theme) and the general means by which these aims are achieved. In the service of promoting mentalizing, your therapeutic tasks include stabilizing mentalizing in the context of an attachment relationship; reinstating mentalizing at any point at which it is lost; minimizing the likelihood of adverse effects associated with non-mentalizing interventions; and allowing your patients to discover themselves by means of your consistently having their mind in mind. Careful focus on your patient's current state of mind will achieve these aims. As one patient said, "Before I did all this, it never even occurred to me that what I did or thought had any effect on anyone else. Sometimes I still think that life was better, because sometimes I don't like what other people think. But it does make life more interesting!"

Successfully refocusing the aims of treatment around mentalizing requires that the therapy be organized around providing structure; developing a therapeutic alliance and adequately repairing ruptures; focusing on the interpersonal and social domain; and exploring the patient-therapist relationship. In conducting this treatment, you will need to 1) identify and work with the patient's limited mentalizing capacities; 2) focus on internal states in yourself and your patient and represent these internal states to your patient; and 3) sustain this focus in the face of continual challenges by your patient over a significant period of time. In order to achieve this level of focus, mentalizing interventions need to be consistently applied over time in the context of an attachment relationship; and they need to be employed to reinforce your capacity to develop and sustain mental and emotional closeness with your patient.

To conduct effective psychotherapy that offers the patient a prospect of moving forward, all of us therapists need a conceptual framework to make sense of what is often confusing and seemingly random dialogue or behavior within the interaction; this is the systemizing facet of our work. In this respect, however, mentalizing-focused approaches face a paradox: imposing a theoretical structure on the patient's experience is

---

TABLE 6–2.   AIMS OF TREATMENT

- To promote mentalizing about oneself
- To promote mentalizing about others
- To promote mentalizing of relationships

by means of

- Identifying and working within your patient's mentalizing capacities
- Focusing on internal states in yourself and your patient
- Representing these internal states to your patient
- Sustaining this focus in the face of continual emotional challenges by your patient

---

antithetical to our model to the extent that it entails imposing the therapist's mind on the patient's mind; this imposition would diminish exploration and discovery. Yet we cannot avoid doing it: we all try to make sense of what our patients tell us, and to do so, we use our own constructs and ideas. In itself, this inferential process is not a problem; yet, at the risk of over-egging the cake, we need to remind you that the danger lies at the moment that you start to give back your understanding to your patients in your own, fully digested form. When you do so, you must remain aware that *your* digestive processes and juices have done the work—not the patient's. Hence, unless you help your patients use their own digestion, you risk forcing your ideas onto them, which can shut down their mentalizing.

Yet in our systemizing mode, we must have a framework within which we work, and the trajectory of mentalizing treatment must be structured so as to move forward with respect to the agreed-upon goals. Nevertheless, in the trenches of the process at any given moment, we are not advocating application of a theory but rather hewing to the singular goal of maintaining mentalizing—even amidst emotional states. Thus, conducting mentalizing-focused treatment entails walking a tightrope. Inside or outside therapy, we all lose mentalizing when we become highly emotional in some way, for example, upset, excited, or embroiled in an argument. As stated at the beginning of this chapter, this mentalizing treatment approach was developed in the context of working with patients with borderline personality disorder, who are particularly prone to losing mentalizing capacity at times of stress in attachment relationships. Yet all of us therapists and patients are liable to struggle to some degree with mentalizing accurately and flexibly when we are in the throes of strong emotions in close relationships. Nonetheless, if therapy is to help strengthen mentalizing capacity, therapy itself must stimulate an emotionally meaningful process that potentially *induces* struggles with mentalizing ability. Accordingly, the treatment must stimulate the very problem that it is trying to treat—but under controlled and deftly managed conditions.

Thus, in promoting mentalizing, you will be focusing to some degree on your relationship with your patient, but in so doing, you will need to ensure that your patient's emotional state is neither so "hot" that mental collapse occurs nor so "cold" that mental rigidity and intellectualization preclude the significant development of mentalizing. Inevitably, by stimulating an attachment relationship that is meaningful to you and your patient, you risk creating adverse side effects. Careful attention to the patient's mentalizing capacities mitigates these risks.

A Mentalizing Case Formulation

Inasmuch as the nature of your interventions must be tailored continually to your patient's mentalizing capacity, it will be worth your while to assess your patients' mentalizing capacities and vulnerabilities at the outset of treatment. We recommend conducting a detailed evaluation of mentalizing vulnerabilities within the first few sessions. We explicitly identify patterns of mentalizing failure and success with the patient and incorporate these into a written formulation; this formulation represents the therapist's understanding of the patient's problems in developmental and mentalizing terms. Yet the term "formulation" might be misleading inasmuch as the written material often merely summarizes the initial interviews with an emphasis on mentalizing. The following is an example of the kind of formulation we find helpful; in addition to summarizing the presenting problems, it includes commentary on both weaknesses and strengths in mentalizing in a way that we hope is meaningful to a patient. The first part of the summary is commonly written in a factual way for referrers, and the second part is aimed more specifically to the patient and treatment team.

> **Reason for referral.** Anthony, now 23, was referred with complaints of recurrent depression, impulsivity, self-harm, and difficulty managing and negotiating life's everyday interactions. Notably, he felt he'd had a bad start in life, which he believed had left him with his current problems.
>
> Anthony dates his difficulties date back to an early age; he remembers beginning to harm himself when he was 10, and he continued to show distress throughout his childhood, getting into trouble with his parents and with the police for reacting aggressively at school and in public. His first contact with psychiatric services occurred five years ago. He had sought help for panic attacks on a number of occasions over several months, but he was repeatedly sent away without further help. On one occasion the police were called because he refused to leave after the clinic staff had tried to reassure him that there was nothing wrong. He took an overdose and cut his wrists a few hours later, which precipitated an admission to a psychiatric hospital. In the hospital, Anthony received a diagnosis of borderline personality disorder and recurrent depressive disorder. He describes being relieved that people seemed to know what was wrong with him. He was prescribed antidepressants and antipsychotic medication, but he reports that they did not help and he stopped all medication after a few months. He is now reluctant to take medication again.
>
> **Family and personal history.** Anthony's parents both have had longstanding, major drug and alcohol problems. As a consequence of his parents' drug habits and the associated unstable home environment, Anthony had a very unsettled and disrupted childhood, characterized by several moves of home and school along with severe emotional and

physical neglect. He feels his parents were only interested in their drugs and spent most of their time seeking supplies. His parents separated when Anthony was 12, due to his father's ongoing violence toward his mother. Anthony remained with his mother, but it seems that it was at this time that he became more aggressive and began taking drugs himself. He did not fit in with his peer group at school and was subjected to bullying. He has some fond memories of playing soccer as a child, which served as an escape from his disturbed home life. He played as goal keeper for a local boys' team, but this activity eventually was curtailed by repeated moves. He recalls feeling close to one of his cousins who also suffered some mental health problems, but this was the only positive memory of friendship. Anthony left school at 16 with minimal qualifications.

At 16, Anthony was physically attacked by one of his mother's boyfriends, which led to a hospital admission for a broken wrist. He left home at this point and lived on the streets for a time before moving in with an acquaintance. Shortly thereafter, he met a girl and they spent a period of time living together. After the relationship with the girl broke down, he was eventually given emergency housing through social services, where he continues to reside now while awaiting re-housing.

Anthony has been in a relationship with a new girlfriend whom he describes as being on the whole supportive; yet at times he feels misunderstood by her, and the relationship can be stormy to the point of occasional violence.

Summary. Anthony, as I understand it, you feel profoundly that, as a consequence of your parents' inability to take you seriously during your childhood, you feel "defective" in that you feel you do not have the basic tools for managing your interactions with others and for managing life in general. I realize that you are unclear what it is that you lack, but you describe a feeling that other people know how to interact with and relate to others, but you feel that you do not. In particular, you feel that you lack the ability to negotiate conflicts with others. When you feel this in group therapy, we ask you to mention it so that you can contrast your understanding of yourself in the group with how other members of the group see you.

You complain that you do not understand others' motives and that you find it hard to trust others. More specifically, you have become preoccupied with situations where you either feel disrespected and provoked by others, or where you are faced with asserting what you want. You recognize that you have reacted aggressively and violently in such situations in the past, and that your behavior has gotten you into trouble with the authorities. More recently, you have started backing down from potential conflict, which leaves you with the experience that you are being exploited. This backing down evokes powerful feelings which you identified as being humiliation. This feeling of humiliation compounds your sense of being defective, leaving you feeling hopeless and depressed. At these times, you have a tendency to isolate yourself and ruminate over things in the past. Your state of mind can rapidly spiral to a point where you feel suicidal. You describe in these moments being plagued by images of your parents looking at you with faces full of disgust and hatred. You will need to let your individual therapist know if you are plagued by threatening images in the session (or in group therapy) so that you can immediately consider what is happening in your mind at that time. You might also find that you feel your therapist is disrespectful or that you feel provoked by him. These are times when we encourage you to mention this to the therapist so it can be explored further.

Engagement in therapy. We have talked about the problems that you might have discussing what is on your mind in therapy. This is probably because you will feel the uncertainty that you have about others' motives when you talk to us. The other concern when you start therapy will be "backing down" and agreeing with your therapist when you are uncertain or even disagree. You have said that you avoid conflict, but we do not see exploring disagreement as conflict, so please let us know if you do not agree with something we say or suggest.

Initial focus. The initial focus for therapy seems to be around your own sense of being "defective," as you have called it, and also about understanding other people's motives. From our discussion it seems that you cannot understand how your parents could have behaved as they did. In this respect, it might be helpful to consider this difficulty in your individual therapy sessions—at least about how it is affecting you now. We have an idea that sometimes people stop thinking about things when they find them incomprehensible, and if this happened to you, it might have been a problem for you to make sense of your own emotional states. This problem of self-awareness could leave you feeling defective; that is, it is difficult to identify what you feel and why you feel it. You might be able to try to make sense of this in your group and in your individual therapy.

Mentalizing. In our interview we noted when your mind went blank and when you found that you did not want to talk any more about a topic. We discussed this as a problem in mentalizing.

Non-mentalizing. You frequently and rapidly lost the capacity to reflect when you were emotional and when talking about your relationship with your girlfriend. For example, you quickly stopped and said, "Oh, it doesn't matter," at one point when you felt upset. This is something that we all do, but we can do it too much. We consider this to be a non-mentalizing aspect of your way of managing your emotional states which we discussed in the meeting. This problem seems especially to be evident when you are upset. In your therapy we will try to capture those moments to see if we can work with you to find out what has happened.

We aim to help you manage the feelings without too quickly switching your mind away from what might be important. You mentioned that you often walk out on your girlfriend when she gets difficult. Again, this is an aspect of not being able to do anything else with what you feel at that moment.

At other times, you have cut yourself badly—and on a number of occasions you have cut your neck. Again, these actions occur at times when you feel that your mind has become, in your words, "like vomit." In exploring this experience we discovered that you meant there were no coherent thoughts at all but only a buzz and a mass of feeling. We need to work to anticipate these times so that you have a chance to manage what is happening without resorting to destructive actions.

Rigid mentalizing. You described a profound sense of grievance about what has happened to you, which is understandable. This seems to inform a lot of your current experience and it might interfere with your ability to see things from a fresh perspective. When this happens we explore the rigidity, as it can prevent us developing alternative ways of interacting with the world.

Sensitive mentalizing. Your relationship with your girlfriend is an area in which you find you can understand her to some extent and feel that she understands you. You gave a number of examples in which you felt that talking to each other about what was happening in your minds was helpful. This sensitive capacity to consider yourself and others is a focus for our therapy with you. You have tried living with your girlfriend, but your mind "turned to vomit" too often, so you find it better to live apart but see each other regularly. This is important because you feel that when you are with her too much you can't think. You might feel the same way when you start therapy, so we want you to talk to us if you feel that your mind is "turning to vomit." We can then try to help you to keep your thinking going for a bit longer before we decide together that you should have a bit of time on your own.

Positive indicators. You have engaged well with the program, attending both the group and individual sessions regularly. After initially presenting in a rather emotionally flattened and impassive way, you seem to be able to discuss traumatic and disturbing experiences without rapidly moving to an "It doesn't matter" attitude.

The depth of your belief that you are defective, and the pervasiveness with which you continue to interpret events from this perspective, remain something that needs to be worked out. The perseverance, resilience, and motivation that you continue to show in treatment and in your relationship with your girlfriend—despite the problems you encounter—are continuing positive indicators.

Even in this apparently simple process of providing a seemingly straightforward written summary of the central problems and some statements about the patient's mentalizing capacities, a lot can go wrong. With limited mentalizing capacities, patients who lose the sense of separateness between their mind and your mind can be easily thrown into the pretend mode; then they take on your perspective without fully understanding it or integrating it into their sense of self. Not uncommonly, for example, patients latch onto the diagnosis of borderline personality disorder and start accounting for their actions accordingly; after an impulsive breakup, the patient declares, "There goes my borderline stuff again!"—as if this were an explanation. When the patient is operating in the pretend mode, the therapist's formulation is internalized as an alien influence. Alternatively, your formulation can throw the patient into confusion if his or her mentalizing capacities collapse in the face of your well-crafted narrative.

Thus, in devising a developmentally based mentalizing formulation to provide a focus and a sense of direction for the treatment, the greatest danger is that you may become too clever—cleverness is a cardinal sin in mentalizing therapy. Accordingly, we do not employ written formulations to demonstrate our singular abilities as therapists—for example, to show our patients how extensively we understand them. Rather, as we reiterate continually, we are more concerned with establishing an interactive mentalizing process than with getting the content just right at any given moment. Hence the patient's active mentalizing collaboration in developing a formulation is critical.

Providing a formulation in writing is helpful for patients who have difficulty holding your mind in mind; they benefit from having something tangible and physical—something real. The written formulation can be a basis for mentalizing inasmuch as it can be reworked conjointly; the patient can question or challenge your view, or simply correct factual inaccuracies. This is an example of explicit mentalizing work: you present to your patients the representation that you have of them in your mind; your patients in turn represent their view of themselves back to you; and then you can demonstrate your own ability to reappraise your understanding of them.

Identifying the Pretend Mode

We recognize that despite our recurrent references to the pretend mode, readers might yet be struggling to apply the concept to psychotherapy. Here is a tip: your patients are likely to be operating in the pretend mode when you have the feeling that they are merely *bullshitting*. Thanks to Princeton philosopher Harry Frankfurt's (2005) incisive thinking, "bullshit" now has been transformed into a term of art.

As Frankfurt understands it, the essence of bullshitting is being "unconstrained by a concern with truth" (p. 38). As such, bullshitting is best understood as distinguished from lying. Unlike bullshitting, lying requires a keen concern for the truth; moreover, lying requires mentalizing, that is, being aware of the other person's factual knowledge so as to adapt one's lies accordingly. The bullshitter does not deceive about facts but rather misrepresents his intentions:

> This is the crux of the distinction between him and the liar. Both he and the liar represent themselves falsely as endeavouring to communicate the truth. The success of each depends upon deceiving us about that.

But the fact about himself that the liar hides is that he is attempting to lead us away from a correct apprehension of reality; we are not to know that he wants us to believe something he supposes to be false. The fact about himself that the bullshitter hides, on the other hand, is that the truth-values of his statements are of no central interest to him; what we are not to understand is that his intention is neither to report the truth nor to conceal it. This does not mean that his speech is anarchically impulsive, but that the motive guiding and controlling it is unconcerned with how the things about which he speaks truly are. (pp. 54–55).

Thus there is a pretend or "as-if" quality to bullshitting; intellectualizing, rationalizing, and using psychological jargon all might qualify. In our field, "psychobabble" is a good synonym for bullshitting, and it is indicative of the pretend mode.

We have a serious point to make here: identifying bullshit as such requires mentalizing, and doing so is crucial. If we fail to recognize when our patients are operating in the pretend mode, we and they may have an *illusion* of work being done; then we and they will be blindsided and disillusioned when our ostensible work has no impact on their functioning. Moreover, we run the danger that our patients will employ our own formulations and interpretations in their bullshitting, in which case our interventions remain disconnected from their reality or sense of self—thought but not felt.

To complicate matters further, we therapists also are in danger of bullshitting (operating in the pretend mode). As Frankfurt recognized, "Bullshit is unavoidable whenever circumstances require someone to talk without knowing what he is talking about" (p. 63). Accordingly, he made the point that politicians are at high risk for bullshitting because they are "frequently impelled—whether by their own propensities or by the demands of others—to speak extensively about matters of which they are to some degree ignorant" (p. 63). As mental health professionals, we run the same risk when our patients ask such questions as, "How long will it take me to pull out of this depression?" "Should I go through with the divorce?" "Should I give up on reconciling with my mother?" "Do these images that keep coming to mind mean that I was really sexually abused, even though I can't remember it?" In the face of patients' desperate sense that they must have answers, refraining from bullshitting and maintaining a mentalizing stance can be challenging indeed.

Frankfurt ends his essay with an ironic twist that reveals his deep appreciation for the mentalizing stance:

there is nothing in theory, and certainly nothing in experience, to support the extraordinary judgment that it is the truth about himself that is easiest for a person to know. Facts about ourselves are not peculiarly solid and resistant to skeptical dissolution. Our natures are, indeed, elusively insubstantial—notoriously less stable and less inherent than the natures of other things. And insofar as this is the case, sincerity itself is bullshit. (pp. 66–67)

Tweaking Your Technique

We know of no other way to stimulate mentalizing—inside or outside of therapy—than to be doing it yourself. Your ability to stimulate a mentalizing process is a core aspect of interacting with others, and thinking out loud about yourself in the therapy gradually will influence your patient through a process of identification: over time, the patient will internalize your ability to use your mind, along with your demonstrating delight in changing your mind when you are presented with alternative views and better understanding.

> A patient in a psychotherapy group commented that the therapist always appeared relaxed and calm and very even-tempered. The therapist looked slightly puzzled and said that he thought that others might have a different view, so he would think about it. After a few moments reflection, the therapist mentioned that he thought that the patient's description of him was correct in the current circumstances of the group; yet, at the same time, he suggested that it might be worth thinking about what it was about the group that allowed him to be like that—because he knew full well that he was not always in this calm state of mind. This reflection allowed the patient, the therapist, and the other group members to try to clarify their own experience of the group.

Following such leads, your patients will be more inclined to reappraise their thinking about themselves and their understanding of others. Yet greatest change will occur when the continual reworking of perspectives and understanding of oneself and others takes place in the context of attachment—that is, where attachment needs are stimulated. Accordingly, it is necessary to work more with current than past experience insofar as treatment aims to foster mentalizing in the midst of active problems in attachment relationships.

To repeat, your task is to maintain mentalizing while simultaneously ensuring that emotional states are active and meaningful. This process can go awry in two ways. On the one hand, excess emotional arousal will reduce mentalizing and potentially lead to disruptive action; on the other hand, inadequate emphasis on current attachment relationships—including your relationship with your patient—will allow avoidance of emotional states and thereby narrow the range of interpersonal and social contexts in which the patient can mentalize effectively.

We find that adding group therapy to individual sessions increases dramatically the contexts in which mentalizing emotion can take place; ideally, therefore, mentalizing-focused treatment combines individual and group modalities.

We recommend avoiding some therapy techniques with patients whose mentalizing capacity is precarious. First, we suggest that therapists avoid allowing excessive free association, a technique that can promote imagination without adequate anchoring in reality and thus can lead to distorted mentalizing or disorganization—often in the therapist as well as the patient. Free association relies on therapists continually trying to make sense of the patient's associations in their own mind (i.e., employing free-floating attention), which they are unlikely to be able to continue doing after a short time. This effort may reinforce therapists' inclination to remain silent in the hope that they will understand things if only they keep listening longer. In sitting silently while trying to make sense of another mind so as ultimately to be able to make an insightful pronouncement, the therapist has lost the key to mentalizing: stimulating inquiry in a continually *interactive* process between minds.

> A patient with long experience in psychotherapy was accustomed to therapists' silence. Accordingly, in the first session, he launched into a long monologue, oblivious to the therapist's nonverbal moves to try to get a word in edgewise. After mounting frustration, the therapist barged into the monologue: "I need to interrupt you. I've discovered that in order to be of help to my patients, I need to talk to them." The patient was a bit taken aback, and the therapist explained, "I think I'll get to understand you best if I let you know what I'm thinking about what you're saying, and then you can let me know if I'm on the right track."

Second, and for the same reason, we do not encourage active fantasy about the therapist. Another reason for downplaying free association and fantasy relates to the fact that developing insight is not our primary aim. Working with fantasy is a technique used in insight-oriented therapy as a way of understanding unconscious mental activity. In promoting mentalizing in attachment relationships, we are most concerned with preconscious and conscious aspects of mental function within the interpersonal domain.

> When talking about her own father, a patient told her therapist that obviously, he was a good father to his children. Rather than immediately exploring this comment further, the therapist asked the patient, "Where on earth did that idea come from?" The patient had no idea of the therapist's qualities with his children, fatherly or otherwise—or even if he had children for that matter. The patient responded that it was obvious,

a response suggesting that she was operating in the psychic-equivalence mode, since there seemed to be nothing particularly obvious about it. So the therapist focused on what it was in the current session that had led the patient to make such a remark, rather than encouraging further development of the idea itself.

Fantasy easily becomes too detached from reality, and spinning out fantasies about the therapist is liable to evoke the pretend mode rather than elaborating mental representations linked to reality—that is, mentalizing. Alternatively, in fantasizing, the patient is liable to regress into the psychic-equivalence mode, wherein the fantasy is experienced as being real, losing its as-if quality. In this context, it is helpful to identify when your patient is operating in the psychic-equivalence mode, in which case his or her understanding will be characterized by a conviction of being right; when the patient is in this state, you will find that entering into debates will be unhelpful. Rather than converting the patient to a different way of thinking, you should aspire to help the patient to appreciate that there *are* different ways of thinking about the same outer reality.

Patients commonly assume that they know what you are thinking. Assuming that they are off the mark, and responding from a mentalizing stance, you might make a clear statement about not being aware of such thoughts, and then you might explore how your patient has come to that belief. You might also engage in some authentic self-exploration about whether such thoughts had been present in your mind at a different time or in a different form. Or you might recognize only belatedly that there was some truth in the patient's assumption and, at some point, validate the patient's belief. For example, "Could we go back a bit? I wasn't aware of feeling angry when you brought it up but, now that you've mentioned it, I recall that I *was* feeling frustrated about your not remembering what we had talked about in our last session. Maybe you were picking that up...." Such an intervention models mentalizing, including the fact that we therapists do not always know our own mind. Problems for you and your patient will arise if either one of you claims primacy for introspection; that is, if either one of you declares knowing your own or the other's mind better. This conviction will lead to fruitless debates. Finally, as the example just given implies, in contrast to many therapies which counsel against self-disclosure, we believe that judicious and tactful disclosure about what you are thinking and feeling is essential to promote mentalizing.

In addition, we believe that putting too much effort into identifying relationship patterns—for example, on the model of schema-focused therapy (Young et al. 2003)—might reduce the development of patients' curiosity and ability to seek their own understanding. In our experience, relationship patterns tend to multiply, and in psychometric terms, they are liable to have sensitivity without specificity: the patterns fit the patient, but they are not distinctive—indeed, many are downright universal. We are more concerned about the patient's developing the mental resources to identify and deal with problematic, recurrent patterns of behavior and relationships than with delineating the array of patterns. This emphasis is non-trivial clinically. Mentalizing therapists do not get involved in discussing the structure or nature of the relationship that the patient brings but rather focus more on the patient's capacity to think about the relationship. For example, you might address the rigidity of schematic representations or roles rather than the roles or schemas themselves; the goal is to enhance and facilitate flexibility by means of generating alternative perspectives.

> A patient was aware that she saw herself as a victim in many different contexts, and she also recognized that she commonly saw herself as a victim in relation to the therapist, whom she felt was in a powerful position in relation to her. Specifically, she felt powerless owing to her persistent conviction that the therapist might decide to end the therapy at any time and that she would have no influence over his decision. She felt that he played with her feelings by holding the possibility of ending the treatment as a weapon to use against her if she were to become difficult. It was unclear what "difficult" meant.
>
> The therapist was concerned more with the unquestioning rigidity with which the patient maintained her conviction than he was with its accuracy. The patient was unable to question her viewpoint until the therapist tackled the way in which her insistence on a powerful-powerless relationship distorted much of their therapeutic work. He explored the rigidity of the conviction in an affectively charged moment of the session; he emphasized how difficult it was for her to talk openly if she believed that she had to be a good patient all the time in order to remain in therapy. At the same time, he highlighted his own difficulty in saying things when she seemed only to be listening for hints that he was going to stop seeing her. Their conjoint lack of flexibility contributed to distortions about the relationship, and it was this sense of both of them being in straitjackets that needed exploring, more than the power dynamic itself.

Although every process needs a content, the specific role relationship was not foremost in the therapist's mind: while ostensibly endeavoring to tease out the actual roles (content), the therapist understood that the *mental act* of teasing out (process) is more crucial than understanding any particular role.

Maintaining a Mentalizing Stance

We advocate maintaining a mentalizing *stance* as providing the best chance of achieving mentalizing goals. That is, in conducting psychotherapy, we strive to maintain an inquisitively curious, *not-knowing* attitude—which requires tolerance for ambiguity and uncertainty in the therapist, just as the mentalizing stance requires of patients. Table 6–3 lists the essential elements of the mentalizing stance.

Initially, we had failed to mentalize in setting out to train therapists to mentalize; we believed that learning this therapeutic stance would be easy and that we would need to devote only a small part of the training to teaching it. On the contrary: this has become the most important and most difficult skill to get right. And without a mentalizing stance, all other interventions are unlikely to be helpful. A mentalizing climate is essential for patients to do anything useful with therapists' interventions. We can best convey the difficulty in maintaining the mentalizing stance by describing our experience in conducting training.

We have found that all therapists—whatever their primary therapeutic orientation—say that they already take an inquisitive, not-knowing stance. Unsurprisingly, as the training makes plain, there appears to be a difference between what we say we do and what we actually do. At the very least, we have difficulty translating declarative knowledge into procedural knowledge. At the beginning of the basic training module, therapists are confident about their abilities to not-know. Contrary to all good training manuals, which suggest that trainees should finish training feeling well prepared and more confident, by the end of our training, their confidence has been undermined; indeed, they feel de-skilled!

In training, we move from knowledge-based discussion to viewing videotaped sessions to engaging in role-playing. We have a five-minute test: in role-playing, if you can maintain an authentic mentalizing stance for a full five minutes in the face of a patient presenting extreme challenges, then you are trained! Under these conditions, few therapists maintain mentalizing for more than a few minutes. Yet all is not lost: after training, therapists feel adequately equipped to go away and practice, and they are more confident about trying something even if they feel stupid doing so. Taking counsel from a Roman Stoic philosopher, Epictetus, we are not averse to bumbling:

> To do anything well you must have the humility to *bumble around* a bit, to follow your nose, to get lost, to goof. Have the courage to try an undertaking and possibly do it poorly. Unremarkable lives are marked by the fear of not looking capable when trying something new. (Lebell 1995, p. 87, emphasis added)

TABLE 6–3.   KEY ELEMENTS OF THE MENTALIZING STANCE

- Inquisitiveness, curiosity, and open-mindedness
- Uncertainty, not-knowing, and interest in understanding better
- Consistent focus on the mind of the patient
- Adaptation of interventions to the patient's mentalizing capacity
- Orientation toward generating alternative perspectives
- Authenticity

Use of videotapes of actual sessions and role-playing is in keeping with guidelines for training in complex tasks, and conducting psychotherapy is a complex task indeed (Binder 1999). Initially, participants are anxious and reluctant to expose themselves in front of others; hence we employ an exposure-based approach: flooding. The training leaders enact some of the first role-plays, portraying such difficult personality-disordered patients that the therapist is quickly silenced or thwarted. This ritual humiliation in front of colleagues demonstrates that it is not so bad, really, to be temporarily reduced to helpless incompetence. We all know the feeling: all of us experience the collapse of mentalizing in intense relationships—inside and outside of psychotherapy. Gradually, participants become more secure, and we divide them into small groups. We ask a pair to role-play patient and therapist while the other group members assess their adherence to the task of mentalizing. Not only is this a useful way to get clinicians to practice skills but also, as long as participants who role-play the patient are attentive to their *responses* to the interventions, they quickly realize which interventions open up mentalizing and which ones close their mind down. Derailed from process to content, some groups begin to discuss the history and difficult clinical presentation of the patient being enacted rather than focusing on the task of maintaining a mentalizing stance; the leaders routinely caution against this.

The mentalizing or not-knowing stance is not synonymous with having no knowledge. Not-knowing captures a sense that mental states are opaque and that you can have no *more* idea of what is in the patient's mind than the patient has and, in fact, you will probably have a lot less of an idea. Mentalizing, you demonstrate a willingness to find out about patients, what makes them tick, how they feel, and the reasons for their underlying problems. The mentalizing stance is respectful and devoid of assumptions. Maintaining this mentalizing stance is more difficult than it sounds. Yet the authors' extensive personal experience suggests that it does not take long to become uncertain of what a patient is talking about or trying to convey. This is excellent news for the not-knowing therapist, who can then encourage the patient to explain more and to expand on the details of his experience—not as a factual reporting but as a creative experiential elaboration.

Again, this stance is harder to maintain than you might believe. To do this, you must become an active, questioning therapist, not in a debating style but rather in an inquisitive and interested manner—especially when inquiring about feeling states. You will be discouraging patients from excessive free association in favor of detailed monitoring and understanding of interpersonal processes and how interpersonal interactions relate to their mental states. This does not mean that you simply explore or that you must agree with exactly what the patient experiences. Rather, when taking a different perspective from the patient, you should verbalize it and explore it in relation to the patient's perspective—making no assumption about whose viewpoint has greater validity.

> A patient said that he thought he had overreacted when he had spoken sharply to one of the department receptionists when he arrived late for a session. The therapist expressed some surprise inasmuch as he had understood the patient to be reacting to what the patient considered a surly attitude on the part of the receptionist; thus the therapist wasn't so sure if the patient had overreacted. Accordingly, the therapist said, "Tell me more about how you have come to the sense that you overreacted rather than responding reasonably to what you described as an unwelcoming reception?"

This example is one-sided to the extent that the therapist does not have his own experience of the actual event and must rely solely on the patient's processing of what happened. Mentalizing is stimulated more potently when the patient and therapist experience something jointly and then have an opportunity to explore it together—a principal reason for the value of transference work, which we will discuss shortly.

To summarize, your conjoint task is to determine the mental processes which have led you and your patient to alternative viewpoints and to consider each perspective in relation to the other, accepting that diverse outlooks may be acceptable. When genuinely incompatible perspectives are clear and cannot readily be resolved, they should be identified, stated, and accepted until resolution seems possible. To this end we ask therapists to share their own mind with their patients to the extent that they demonstrate how they have come to a particular understanding—or that they are muddled and unable to understand something. On one occasion a patient suggested that the therapist seemed "a bit slow in the head"—which suggested that the therapist was keeping to the mentalizing model!

Adapting Your Interventions to the Patient's Mentalizing Capacity

Patients' mentalizing capacities vary considerably within and across sessions; hence, as a mentalizing therapist, you will be monitoring the patient's state of mind continually and intervening accordingly. A basic principle: the more fragile the patient's ability to mentalize, the simpler your interventions must be. This simple principle can be difficult for therapists to follow, because most of us tend to become more complicated in our interventions as we understand less. We forget to monitor our own mentalizing capacity, and we need to do this while interacting with the patient—and not while we are sitting back listening quietly, but rather when we are actively engaging in the relationship.

Because mentalizing capacity is affected primarily by the level of emotional intensity and extent of attachment security, we recommend paying particular attention to the level of emotional arousal and being especially mindful of the patient's feeling threatened in the therapy relationship—for example, perceiving you as being hostile or obtuse. With regard to attachment, the detached-avoidant pattern requires more therapeutic work to be done within the patient-therapist relationship using mentalizing transference interactions, whereas the enmeshed-preoccupied pattern calls for careful titration of the emotional state and the intensity of the relationship.

We aspire to adapt our interventions to the patient's mentalizing capacity by organizing the interventions along a spectrum, with more supportive interventions being required at times when the patient's mentalizing capacities are impaired and more interpretive interventions (aimed at enabling the patient to shift perspectives) being appropriate when the patient's mentalizing capacity is stabilized. Transference-related interventions, in particular, require skilful mentalizing on the part of both patient and therapist.

Two additional basic principles: first, go slowly; second, when in doubt, be more supportive and less challenging of the patient's perspective. We have found in training that therapists try to do too much too quickly and easily get out of step with the patient. Your primary focus always must be on the current state of mind of your patient, and we therefore place considerable emphasis on understanding the patient's perspective within a validating context. Listening attentively as well as making observations and reflections on the patient's state of mind are validating interventions common to every therapeutic approach. Before introducing alternative perspectives, you must first demonstrate your understanding of the patient's experience as being justified, at least in the context of how the patient's mind is working at the time. The patient must feel understood—that you have his or her mind in mind. Yet we are not suggesting that you settle for a simple confirmation of the patient's experience as being understandable in a specific context, although this must be your starting point. The whole point of psychotherapy is opening up alternative perspectives.

An important part of keeping your patient's mind in mind is recognizing when he or she is operating in the psychic-equivalence mode, wherein alternative perspectives are not possible. At such times, presenting an immediate challenge or defending yourself is likely to be futile.

> A patient told his therapist that the crisis plan that had been arranged for him was "a sham." He reported that he had called the telephone number he had been given and that no one had answered. The therapist expressed some puzzlement about this and asked when the patient had made the call, because no message had been received. The patient replied that he had not left a message because if no one answered the telephone, the "so-called help" was useless as far as he was concerned.
>
> The therapist responded by pointing out immediately that the crisis plan explicitly stated that messages should be left if no one answered the telephone. He reminded the patient of the policy that all calls would be returned within two hours during the work day or within one hour of the start of the next working day if the call was received during nonworking hours. The therapist's intervention only inflamed the patient's anger: "What does that have to do with anything? No answer equals no help! Don't you even understand that?"
>
> At that point, the therapist recognized his error and regrouped by accurately identifying the patient's affective state: the therapist expressed his understanding that not only had the patient felt alone and in considerable danger of self-harm or violence at the time he telephoned but also he had just experienced something similar in the session when he felt that the therapist did not understand him and thus was not available to help. Once they had achieved this mutual understanding, the patient and therapist were able to collaborate on refining the crisis plan.

As this example illustrates, without a mentalizing stance, the process will go nowhere. The aim is to move gradually toward exploring and elaborating multifaceted representations of the self, others, and relationships—including the therapy relationship. Yet in moving toward alternative perspectives, tentativeness is appropriate; for example, "I'm getting the impression that…" "I'm wondering if…" "It occurs to me that…" To underscore that you as the therapist are operating with mental representations rather than objective reality, you can frame your interventions with "I" statements: "Here is what I'm thinking…" "When you said that, I began to think this:…" "When you brought that up, I started feeling…" Hence you are offering your mental states for your patient's *consideration*, so as to expand your patient's perspective as well as to better ascertain the validity of your own perspective. And you are implying that your contribution to the dialogue has neither more nor less intrinsic validity than that of your patient—and that together you might arrive at an understanding in a process of negotiated meaning. Yet it is likely to be you who takes the lead in teasing out alternative perspectives (e.g., "Have you considered the possibility that…" or "I'm also wondering if…"). When your patient begins bringing up alternative perspectives spontaneously, you'll know that you have succeeded in getting a mentalizing therapy off the ground.

Mentalizing the Transference

As we noted earlier, we therapists like to move quickly; pacing and staging interventions is difficult to do effortlessly and smoothly, and we generally need to move slowly. Yet, ultimately, it is important to move toward work in the transference. In some respects, our approach to transference work is traditional: we employ interpretive interventions only in the context of support and, as all therapists do, we aspire to tailor the interventions to the patient (Horwitz et al. 1996). Yet we are quite specific about this tailoring process: we concentrate on the patient's mentalizing capacities. Moreover, we construe transference work as active mentalizing in the patient-therapist relationship. Our experience in conducting training indicates that helping therapists to use transference as a mentalizing intervention has proven challenging. Table 6–4 lists central components of mentalizing the transference.

We use the phrase "mentalizing the transference" to differentiate our approach from other ways of using transference, such as interpretive work that places a premium on genetic reconstructions. nonetheless, we recognize that careful interpretive work can be effective in the treatment of patients with borderline personality disorder; such work is exemplified by Transference-Focused Psychotherapy (Clarkin et al. 1999). From our point of view, transference interventions in Transference-Focused Psychotherapy are effective by virtue of being conducted in a way that helps patients remain in the mentalizing mode. Specifically, these interventions place a premium on clarity, recurrently bring

---

TABLE 6–4.   COMPONENTS OF MENTALIZING THE TRANSFERENCE

- Exploring the current patient-therapist relationship
- Validating the patient's experience of the patient-therapist interaction
- Accepting and exploring enactments, including the therapist's own contribution and the therapist's distortions
- Presenting an alternative perspective
- Collaborating in arriving at an understanding
- Monitoring and exploring the patient's reaction

---

patients' attention back to central themes, carefully link behavior to a hypothetical model of the patient's mind, maintain an interpersonal focus, and move systematically from clarifications to interpretations. Hence, albeit focused more on mental contents than mental processes, such interventions have the potential not only to maintain mentalizing but also to improve mentalizing capacity.

To reiterate, interpretive interventions have the potential to promote mentalizing in patients who are able to remain in the mentalizing mode and to hold multiple perspectives in mind in the face of strong affects. Focusing on mental representations, such interpretive work usually bolsters mentalizing—in the sense of drawing patients' attention to distorted perceptions and interpretations of present interactions in the context of understanding the basis of these distortions in past relationships. Indeed, one of the hallmarks of mentalizing is separating the present from the past—as is critical in patients who are prone to reexperiencing trauma. Such traumatized patients, however, are liable to be operating in the psychic-equivalence mode, in which case bringing them back to the mentalizing mode is the first priority. Thus, returning to our main agenda, with an eye toward working with patients whose mentalizing capacity is limited, we emphasize more here-and-now-oriented transference work as contrasted with genetic reconstructions.

The major difficulty in conveying the distinctiveness of our approach boils down to our understanding of the term *transference*. We are often asked if we use transference, and mentalization-based therapy has been characterized as "A dynamic psychotherapy that specifically eschews transference interpretation" (Gabbard 2006, p. 1668). Here we need a clarification: asked if we use transference, our standard reply is, it all depends on what you mean by "transference." Do we focus on the therapist-patient relationship in the hope that discussion concerning this relationship will contribute to the patient's well-being? The answer is a most emphatic "Yes." Do we use the transference to provide an explanation of present behavior as based on unconscious repetition of past behavior? The answer is an almost equally emphatic "No." While we might well point to similarities among the therapy relationship, current attachment relationships, and childhood attachment relationships, we do not aim to provide patients with an explanation (insight) that they might be able to use to control their behavior pattern. Rather, transference provides an opportunity to address how the patient's mind is working with us in the room. Fundamentally, we hope to evoke the patient's curiosity in considering relationship patterns as just one of many other puzzling phenomena that require thought and contemplation as part of our general inquisitive, not-knowing stance aimed to facilitate the recovery of mentalizing.

Thus, *mentalizing the transference* is a shorthand phrase for encouraging patients to think about the relationship they are in at the current moment. We aim to focus the patient's attention on another mind, the mind of a therapist, and to assist the patient in the task of contrasting his own perception of himself with how he is perceived by others—by the therapist or by other members of a psychotherapy group. We emphasize using the transference to show patients how the same behavior may be experienced differently and thought about differently by different minds. For example, the patient's experience of the therapist as persecutory and demanding, destructive and cruelly critical, is one perception among many others. It may be a valid perception, given the therapist's behavior; but there may be alternative ways of construing the therapist's behavior. Once again, the aim is not to give insight to patients as to why they are distorting their perception of the therapist in a specific way but rather to engender curiosity as to why, given the ambiguity of interpersonal situations, they choose and stick to a specific version. In wondering why they might be doing this, we help them give up the rigid, schematic, psychic-equivalence mode of interpreting their subjectivity and others' behavior.

Nowhere is the injunction to move slowly more applicable than in the domain of working with transference. We employ the concept of *transference tracers* to refer to hints of transference responses—that is, subtle indications that what the patient is saying might be pertinent to the patient-therapist relationship. In keeping with our axiom that more complex interventions require careful groundwork, we suggest that transference tracers be used prior to exploring the potentially more conflict-laden arenas entailed in mentalizing the transference. We use transference tracers to point a way, to suggest that the therapist's mind might be different from the patient's and that the therapist might like to consider an alternative perspective. For example: "It seems that we don't quite see that in the same way. Maybe that's something we can come back to at some point. I'm not sure exactly why we see it so differently." Another example: when a patient declares that her relationships never last longer than three months, the therapist might mention, conversationally, "We'd better watch out for this relationship around that time, hadn't we?" Such transference tracers can be employed judiciously to nudge the patient gently in the direction of work in the transference. Accordingly, we use transference tracers early in the process of therapy to highlight potentially problematic areas, especially different perspectives between patient and therapist, without overheating the emotional relationship.

> The patient was talking about her feeling that while most of her boy-friends seemed to like her, at the same time she worried that all they really wanted was to use her to look after them. She always felt that she must do what they asked; hence she ended up doing their washing, cleaning, and cooking—and yet she was unable to tell them that she resented doing so. After some discussion of this problem, the therapist commented that it occurred to him that she might also feel that he was using her for his own purposes by asking her to fill in research forms all the time. The patient said that she didn't mind doing that, because it was for a greater good: to improve treatments for other people. Nonetheless, he suggested that perhaps if she found herself beginning to resent the research, she should let him know.

At this moment, the therapist could have continued to press the link between the patient's sense of doing things for others and her silent resentment about—and compliance with—research in order to help others. But he left the intervention as a hint at something by suggesting, "At any time you feel like that about the research forms or something else that I am doing, let me know if you can." The patient agreed, and then they moved on in the session. As the therapy progresses, you can focus increasingly on the patient-therapist relationship, increasing use of mentalizing the transference and challenging the patient's assumptions as you try to highlight how the patient perceives you. In this example, the therapist might return to the topic later as further examples of the patient's acquiescence to others' demands accumulate.

As our use of transference tracers illustrates, we routinely focus on here-and-now aspects of the patient-therapist interaction. We should note, however, that we would not regard all instances of focusing on the here-and-now aspects as exemplifying ideal mentalizing. For example, Strenger (1991) maintains that "most actual interpretations given in psychoanalytic practice refer to the patient's present mental states without reference to the patient's past" and that such interpretations are "easy and straightforward in their structure" (p. 63). Yet consider the clinical vignette he gives in this context:

> After a vacation a patient comes back to therapy and greets his therapist happily. After he sits down his mind goes blank, he cannot think of anything to say, and he feels distinctly uncomfortable looking at his therapist. A possible interpretation would be, "You know, I felt before that you were quite happy to see me again, and your way of expression was quite affectionate. Now it looks to me that you are terribly embarrassed by your feelings—maybe because you think I feel that your feelings are ridiculous." (pp. 63–64)

Out of context, it is risky to characterize an intervention as "non-mentalizing," but from the information provided, the interpretation seems a bit too definite given the data—the "maybe" notwithstanding. A more exploratory approach might go as follows: "At first you seemed happy to see me again, and now you look uncomfortable—have I got that right? If so, what changed?"

Specifics aside, Strenger's emphasis on "present mental states without reference to the patient's past" is entirely consistent with our approach to mentalizing the transference.

> A severely depressed patient in her mid-thirties who was very sensitive to her physical appearance complained to the therapist about how terrible she looked. She commented that her hair looked "awful," but it looked perfectly fine to the therapist, who naively said as much. The patient pointed out that if the therapist were to see pictures of her when her hair was done properly, he would appreciate the difference. The therapist replied that fortunately, the appearance of her hair was a "solvable problem," as she had managed some weeks previously—despite her anxiety about doing so—to go to the hairdresser. This rather desperate attempt at reassurance was not entirely ineffective; the patient perked up somewhat.
>
> Yet the patient persisted in the rather daunting challenge of getting the therapist to appreciate how miserable she felt by coming up with a less obviously solvable problem: she complained that her eyes made her look like a robot. She stated that her pupils were way too dilated such that her ordinarily attractive blue eyes were hardly noticeable and that, moreover, her eyes looked "glazed over" in a way that gave her a "dead-looking" appearance.
>
> The therapist responded by leaning forward and looking closely at her eyes for quite a long time, striving especially to discern the glazed-over, dead-looking appearance. He commented that while her pupils were large, the light in the room was dim and the blueness of her eyes was clearly visible. In addition, he was unable to detect any glazed look despite making a concerted effort to do so; he let her know this and added that he was very familiar with glazed-looking eyes.

Mentalizing, the patient exclaimed, "There's something wrong with my mind!" The therapist simply stated that if his experience was any guide, it was likely that others did not see her the way she saw herself.

To consider this interaction as mentalizing the transference is using the term *transference* only in the loosest sense; the patient was generalizing from others to the therapist in assuming that he, like all other persons in her life, perceived her in the same way she perceived herself. Terminology aside, the patient-therapist relationship provides an opportunity to examine interpersonal assumptions through straightforward discussions of what is on each individual's mind. This comparative examination of assumptions is what we consider *basic mentalizing* in the patient-therapist relationship.

Once basic mentalizing has been well established within the therapeutic process, we recommend further work on emotion-laden attachment concerns within our frame of mentalizing the transference.

In the middle of a session, a patient told the therapist directly that she felt he didn't care about her. The therapist quickly asked if there was anything he had just done in the session that had brought this into her mind. The therapist was keeping to our model by trying to understand the current state of mind of the patient within the affective context of the patient-therapist relationship; his intervention focused the issue. The patient initially said that there was nothing in particular; rather, it had "just occurred" to her. Her breezing over the instigator for this serious concern alerted the therapist to a possible break in mentalizing, so he engaged in a "stop-and-stand" maneuver, asking the patient to consider it a bit more.

The patient reconsidered and suggested that she had thought for a moment that the therapist was stifling a yawn and that this behavior indicated that he was bored with her. This observation allowed the therapist to validate her understanding, as it was easy to see how she might have come to that conclusion in those circumstances. He pointed out that, if he were her, he also would have been upset in the same circumstances. Yet, at the same time, he had neither been aware of being bored nor of having stifled a yawn. He stated openly that although he wasn't aware of stifling a yawn, he had been aware of having looked at his watch; he wondered if looking at his watch might have contributed to her sense that he was bored. To some extent, this interaction began to move away from mentalizing the transference, as it offered an alternative explanation, which was not the focus of the work at that point. Nonetheless, the therapist continued to suggest that the patient seemed quickly to have reached her conclusion of what was behind his action. Accordingly, the therapist was holding to the mentalizing model inasmuch as he focused on the process within the session: the rapidity with which the patient came to a conclusion was the issue for mentalizing, not the content of the interaction.

At this point, the therapist hoped that the patient would engage in further exploration but, as is commonly the case, the patient merely repeated what they had already asserted. Then her settling for a simple explanation became the subject of inquiry: the therapist emphasized his puzzlement that the patient was so certain; in so doing, he identified his own attempt to consider alternative explanations. He suggested that if someone else looked at their watch when he was talking, he also would think they might want to be elsewhere rather than with him. He added, however, that perhaps he would need to reflect on that inference and even try to validate it by staying engaged in the interaction while continuing to reflect on it rather than simply reacting on the basis of his initial assumption. The patient agreed with this reasoning and said that she often felt as if the therapist would prefer to be elsewhere; moreover, she acknowledged that this assumption made her feel unwanted. Empathizing with her experience, the therapist tried to identify the patient's current state of mind, given this understanding, and he said that he could now see how difficult it was for her to remain in the session with someone whom she felt didn't really want to be there.

The session moved on from this point to link to the patient's more general feeling of difficulty in being with people inasmuch as she was so keenly alert to any possible rejection. Thus the session moved from mentalizing the transference, to identifying an interpersonal process, to an exploration of its importance within other relationship contexts. It became increasingly apparent that this patient's rapid conclusions about other people's motives led her to become very angry suddenly or to leave interpersonal situations very quickly; these were self-defeating responses that only added fuel to her sense of isolation and her feeling of being unwanted.

In sum, while we explore the patient's motivation for manifesting a particular type of transference, the reason for the exploration is always to encourage thinking and feeling; we direct patients' attention to the working of their mind in all its vicissitudes and complexity. To beat an increasingly moribund horse, we do not attend primarily to the *content* of insights or cognitive distortions; rather we aspire to increase patients' *ability to generate* insights and to identify and ameliorate their distorting mental processes.

Top Tips

We have acknowledged the limit to which a mentalizing approach can be prescriptive. In a sense, the best we can do is offer general guidance and, in the spirit of Wittgenstein, some *tips*. An overview of these is provided in Table 6–5.

TABLE 6–5.   TOP TIPS FOR THERAPISTS

- Beware of certain words (e.g., "just," "clearly," "obviously," "only")

- Be active rather than passive

- Make contrary moves:

    —When the patient is excessively introspective, invite the patient to consider another mind

    —When the patient is excessively focused on others, invite the patient to focus on his or her own mind

- Be ordinary and non-expert; remember that you are not an expert about the patient's mind, even if you are an expert in psychotherapy

- Use the "mentalizing hand" along with verbal interventions to de-escalate affect storms

---

Be Mindful of Certain Words and Phrases

Certain words and phrases, however well intentioned, can alert you that you are moving away from mentalizing (Munich 2006). You may have stopped mentalizing if you hear yourself using such words as "clearly," "obviously," or "'only," or if you use such phrases as "What you mean is…" or "It seems to me that what you are *really* saying is…." Few things in mental life are obvious, and almost no mental state is "clearly" or "only" anything. Once you recognize that you are telling your patient about what your patient's underlying experience *really* is, then it is highly likely that your interaction is losing an exploratory focus. In such cases, you should move away from the interaction and reappraise what is happening in your relationship. Are you trying too hard? Does the patient need you to tell him things about himself, thereby structuring his self-experience, rather than trying to work them out for himself? These are some of the questions that, as a mentalizing therapist, you need to ask yourself.

We have come to pay special attention to what we call the "j-word"—*just* (Allen and Munich 2006). Alert to this word, the therapist in the last vignette we presented was mobilized by his patient's remark that the idea that he didn't care about her had "just occurred" to her. But "just" is ubiquitous in our speech. To the depressed person: "Just stop thinking so negatively," or "Just get out and exercise." To the traumatized person: "Just put the past behind you," or "Just move on." Notoriously, to the addict, "Just say no to drugs!" In such contexts, the j-word always calls for a question: "How?" Your depressed patient will say, "I just need to stop being so hard on myself." Your anxious patient will say

"I just need to relax." How? "Just" is often a non-mentalizing word in the sense of being *minimizing*. Typically, patients with psychiatric disorders will have enormous difficulty doing whatever follows the j-word. Exemplifying denial, the j-word closes off mentalizing.

We commend attention to language in the service of advocating a not-knowing stance. Again, we acknowledge that this stance is counterintuitive: understandably, as a therapist you may be inclined to move quickly into wanting to advise or do things to help your patient. But telling patients what their mind is like or what to do is, in a sense, taking their mind over; if they accede, they are allowing you to do their reflection for them or to live their life for them—including their mental life. Taking over does not stimulate the patient's own mentalizing capacity but rather reduces it. Patients have only two choices when told what is "really" in their mind or, for example, that they are "just" catastrophizing: they can accept the therapist's view uncritically, or they can reject it outright. Both responses are anti-mentalizing.

Be More Active and Less Passive

In the role of therapist, you are naturally pulled into excess passivity or activity. You might tend either to sit back and listen or to become controlling—in the latter case, for example, in trying to follow a particular model of treatment. Mentalizing entails striking a balance in which you are actively testing assumptions by questioning, probing, exploring, and reacting. Mentalizing also entails active challenging of non-mentalizing dialogue, therapy fillers seemingly used in the service of avoidance, and patients' unquestioned assumptions. It is especially productive to challenge patients' unreasonable assumptions about you, because you are present to represent your own mind to them from an alternative perspective.

Moreover, to promote mentalizing, sometimes you might need to be downright forceful:

> The third author, responding to a patient who was on the brink of storming out of his office, exhorted: "Sit down and shut up for a moment!" Startled, she did so, and some mentalizing was reinstated.

We would hardly call "Sit down and shut up!" a "mentalizing intervention." Yet had the patient stormed out of the office, no further mentalizing could have taken place. The patient was "held" by the intervention, such that conditions for mentalizing could be reinstated. Hence it was a mentalizing-promoting intervention. Plainly, to be effective, any such dramatic intervention requires a suitable relationship context.

And, more than any other example we could give, the effectiveness of this intervention demonstrates that mentalizing—in this case intuitively—is an art.

Consistent with our emphasis on therapist activity, we do not encourage long silences, which are liable not only to escalate anxiety but also to evoke excessive fantasizing. Grunts and nods might imply that you are lost and probably indicate that you have become muddled. At these moments you must retrieve your mentalizing capacity; to do so, you will need to identify your current state of mind and suggest a solution: "I am muddled and not quite sure what to say. Can we go back and explore a bit further what we have been talking about?" In this way, you model your own mentalizing while stimulating further elaboration of the patient's current problems. As we already have stated, we are not averse to bumbling; as long as it remains authentic—which it generally will be—we encourage a Columbo-like approach: the mentalizing therapist is a bumbling detective.

Make Contrary Moves

We do not recommend that you become contrary in your relationships with your patients but rather that you consider moving patients outwards when they are self-focused and inwards when they are other-focused. We envision a balancing act as you and your patient see-saw up and down, moving forward the areas of reflection and dialogue. At some points your patient will become self-focused, and this is often to be commended; yet this self-reflection may begin to take on a ruminative quality or become rigidified in a negative, shameful, self-condemning mode. At such times, you should try to move your patient out of his or her mind and into another person's mind: "How do you think that affects her?" "What was going on for her that led him to do that?" You should not be deflected from this task once you have decided that it is an appropriate move in treatment. Many patients respond by saying they don't know, and then they quickly return to their ruminative concern about their own state of mind. Then you may need to be more insistent: "Bear with me a bit—I was wondering what you made of what was happening for him that made him respond like that."

You also will need to make the converse move at times. Patients who are preoccupied with understanding others and what they are like may need pushing to reflect on their own state of mind: "What did *you* feel about that?" "How do you understand *your* reaction?"

Such moves reflect the balance between self and others inherent in the concept of mentalizing. This balance also must be mirrored in the movement between the patient and therapist within a session; a reciprocal flow of attention moves back and forth from your patient to you and vice versa. You must demonstrate your own capacity to reflect on the process at any given moment, once again exemplifying the active stance. As we discuss next, your reflectiveness in the process captures our view of the use of countertransference, which we place in the framework of "being ordinary."

Be Ordinary and Use Common Sense

We think of "using countertransference" broadly as mentalizing in the role of the therapist: knowing and speaking your mind. We think of "being ordinary" in the sense of considering what you would say or do if your friend told you this or behaved in this way toward you. We do not license you to behave in any way you please or to say whatever you like—any more than you would do in a respectful relationship with a friend. Rather, we advocate openly working on your state of mind in therapy in a way that moves the joint purpose of the relationship forward, keeping mentalizing online. To do this you often will have to speak from your own perspective rather than from your understanding of your patient's experience.

As we noted earlier in this chapter, therapists practicing mentalizing use "I" statements more often than is apparent in other therapeutic approaches. Initially, you own the experience rather than using it immediately to highlight further understanding of your patient's experience. At the simplest level, you might express your emotional reaction to something so as to normalize the patient's reaction and help the patient recognize that feelings are to be explored: "If that happened to me, I would have felt upset too." "I would be pleased about that." At the more complex level, you use your emotional responsiveness to the patient to further your joint work. To promote mentalizing, it is sensible not to push things back to the patient immediately.

Therapists are often pleasantly surprised to realize that if they talk about their own experience of the current problem without attributing it to the patient, the patient will often take on the therapist's understanding and develop it further.

> *Therapist:* I was thinking that the sessions seem a bit repetitive, and I am not sure quite why. It occurs to me that my mind just seems to go over the same old stuff and I can't think outside what we have already said.
> *Patient:* You do seem to repeat things, and I don't think I have got any further at all with the problem. Mind you, I'm not much good at

talking about what's going on a lot of the time. Sometimes I think
I don't want to get much further.
Therapist: That's interesting…so maybe both of us are keeping things
the same—anything for a quiet life!

Potentially in the throes of theory-based prescriptions and supervi-
sor-related superegos, therapists all too easily lose track of common
sense. In the course of training, recognizing that it can be an *advantage*
not to know what to do or say is a particularly freeing moment for therapists. Many therapists freeze when they don't know what to say to a
patient's question, particularly when the question is a challenging one
and especially when it is a personal one. Common sense suggests that
if you do not know how to respond in an interpersonal interaction, it is
probably best to acknowledge it openly so that it is understood. Many
clinicians in training ask us, "What do I do when this happens?" Or
they tell us, "I couldn't think of what to say!" These moments in therapy
should not be a problem if you adopt the not-knowing stance. If you
don't know what to do, you should ask yourself what you would do if
this happened and you were not a therapist; this reflection is likely to
yield an answer. For example, you might respond empathically or question further. Or you might openly state your current understanding of
your own internal state in relation to the question. If a patient challenges you to *do something* and you don't know what to do, you might
say, for example, "I'm not sure what to say or do about that. Perhaps I
don't understand it enough. Can you help me a bit more?"

If the patient demands to know what you are feeling, you should
find a tactful way of expressing it so that it is meaningful to the moment:

Patient: You're fed up with me, aren't you?
Therapist: I would say I'm more frustrated than fed up, and part of it is
that we don't seem to be able to get anywhere with this discussion, and I'm concerned that we might not be able to sort it out in
the short time we have left in this session.

The therapist's task can become more difficult when the patient
makes a practical request:

A patient asked if she could borrow a book that was on the therapist's
bookshelf. She pointed out that she could not find the book anywhere
and that it would help her in her current education project. The therapist
was taken aback by this sudden request, but he had the mentalizing
model in mind: when in a corner, point out that you are in a corner
rather than coming out fighting with your cherished techniques. Accordingly, the interaction unfolded as follows:

Patient: That's OK then, just say "Yes." I'll give it back to you next week.

Therapist: But I don't lend books, and yet of course I would like to be of help with your project.

Patient: That's a bit mean that you don't lend books. Don't you trust anyone?

Therapist: As I said, I'm in a difficult position, because I can see that it looks mean, and yet I rarely lend books because so often I don't get them back.

Patient: I'm not just anyone though, am I?

Therapist: I suppose that is part of my discomfort about it. Is this about more than borrowing the book or, in this case, is a book just a book?

Patient: Let's just treat it as a book.

Therapist: OK.

In this situation, the therapist decided not to go further in exploring the actual process of borrowing and lending the book but rather acquiesced to the request with the intention of promoting the therapeutic alliance. Nevertheless, when the patient returned the book as promised, the therapist could not refrain from asking the patient what she had found helpful in it!

Commonsense responses when emotions are high are generally safer than technique-driven interventions or interpretations. Psychotherapy research reveals a low correlation between sheer concentration of interventions and treatment outcomes; this might be explained as a result of therapists increasing their use of cherished interventions when they are floundering, in the desperate hope that more of the same will bring about change (Ogrodniczuk et al. 2000; Piper et al. 1993). In practice, this overkill strategy probably makes things worse.

De-escalate Affect With the "Mentalizing Hand"

When your patient is in the midst of an affect storm or you encounter some other uncontrolled situation in therapy, you should assume that you are the unwitting cause of the problem until proven otherwise. You should become self-referent as soon as you notice a developing problem within your interaction with the patient—one that looks likely to lead to overwhelming emotion, a paranoid state, or more simply a behavioral response such as walking out. Being self-referent in such circumstances is another counterintuitive maneuver for therapists. You might say, for example, "What have I just said or perhaps implied that might have offended you?" "What have I done that has agitated you in this way? Tell me about it so that I can understand what I have done."

You can combine such verbal interventions with a slight raising of your hand, palm out—a gentle maneuver often used by the police suggesting that it is sensible to stop whatever the person is doing. We have dubbed this gesture the "mentalizing hand." It is extraordinarily effective, and when it is coupled with a remark about your own role in provoking the problem, most escalating crises can be de-escalated. Then you can allow exploration of your contribution to the problem in order to understand your patient's perspective, which brings your patient back to our model of mentalizing the mind. You are then on track to validate your patient's experience, to work in the current relationship, to understand your contribution, to work on your patient's understanding and, only later, to consider whether your patient was perceiving you or interpreting you in distorted ways that contributed to the emotional crisis. Once these steps have been negotiated, you and your patient can develop an alternative perspective within the transference.

Self-Assessment

In this chapter, we have provided an overview of the style of interventions developed initially for mentalization-based treatment (MBT) for patients with borderline personality disorder (see Chapter 9, "Borderline Personality Disorder"); further details regarding these interventions are available elsewhere (Bateman and Fonagy 2004, 2006). As an aid to assessing your adoption of the principles we have outlined in this chapter, Table 6–6 presents an MBT-adherence checklist (Bateman and Fonagy 2006), which clinicians can adapt to the particular treatments they are conducting. The extent of adherence is scored by adding up the number of "yes" answers multiplied by the item weights and dividing by 64; we consider 80% adherence to be the standard. You may find it most helpful to use this checklist with a colleague to evaluate audiotapes or videotapes of your sessions.

A Patient's Perspective

We are grateful to a patient whose anonymity we have elected to maintain for articulating her experience of mentalization-based therapy for borderline personality disorder. The patient's short guide to this form of treatment follows (see pp. 203–207). While this piece is addressed to prospective patients, in the spirit of mentalizing, we clinicians also can benefit from this patient's perspicacious take on the treatment process.

TABLE 6–6. SELF-RATING OF MBT ADHERENCE

Framework of treatment

Yes	No	DK	My treatment is offered in a clearly structured context that is transparent to patients and treaters. (2)
Yes	No	DK	I have a clear hierarchy of therapeutic goals agreed with patient. (2)
Yes	No	DK	I have a crisis plan identified. (2)
Yes	No	DK	A case discussion has been organized where roles of other staff have been identified and the limits of confidentiality agreed. (1)
Yes	No	DK	My patient appears to understand the rationale of treatment and the purpose of group and individual therapy. (1)
Yes	No		I have explained the boundaries of therapy. (2)
Yes	No		I have arranged supervision in either peer group or with a senior practitioner. (1)
Yes	No		I have reviewed the patient's current relationships and social support network. (2)
Yes	No		I have reviewed medication or arranged for review with a colleague. The limits of medication prescribing have been defined. (1)
Yes	No		Assessment of mentalization has been completed. (1)
Yes	No		Diagnosis has been discussed with the patient. (1)
Yes	No		My formulation has been completed and has been discussed with the patient and modified accordingly. (2)

Max=18

Mentalization

Yes	No	I am taking a genuine stance of "not knowing" and attempting to "find out." (2)
Yes	No	I ask questions to promote exploration. (1)
Yes	No	In the session I ask about patients' understanding of motives of others. (1)
Yes	No	I use transference tracers in this session. (1)
Yes	No	I use transference interpretation to highlight alternative perspectives and not to give insight. (1)
Yes	No	I challenge unwarranted beliefs about me and patients' experiences of self and other. (1)
Yes	No	I do not present the patient with complex mental states. (2)

TABLE 6–6.   SELF-RATING OF MBT ADHERENCE *(continued)*

Yes	No	I avoid simplified historical accounts of current problems. (2)
Yes	No	I avoid confrontation with patient when he is in psychic equivalence mode. (2)
Yes	No	I consider if the pretend mode of mentalization is present in the patient. (2)
Yes	No	I address reversibility of mental states. (1)

Max=16

Working with current mental states

Yes	No	I attend to current emotions. (2)
Yes	No	I focus on appropriate expression of emotions. (1)
Yes	No	I link affect with immediate or recent interpersonal contexts. (1)
Yes	No	I relate understanding of current interpersonal context to appropriate recent past experiences. (1)

Max=5

Bridging the gaps

Yes	No	My reflections aim to present the patient's internal state in a modified form. (2)
Yes	No	I give examples to the patient of his experience of psychic equivalence. (1)
Yes	No	I focus attention of patient on therapist experience without being persistently self-referent. (1)
Yes	No	I negotiate ruptures in alliance by clarifying patient and therapist roles in the rupture. (1)
Yes	No	I am trying to develop a transitional "as if" playful way of linking internal and external reality in sessions. (1)
Yes	No	I judiciously use humour. (1)

Max=7

Affect storms

Yes	No	I maintain a dialogue throughout the emotional outburst. (2)
Yes	No	When emotions are aroused I attempt to clarify the feeling and any underlying emotion without interpretation. (1)
Yes	No	I only begin to address possible underlying causes of the affect storm within patient's current life as the emotional state subsides. (2)

TABLE 6–6. SELF-RATING OF MBT ADHERENCE *(continued)*

Yes	No	I identify triggers for the storm in patient's construal of their interpersonal experience immediately prior to it. (1)
Yes	No	I link affect storm to therapy process only after storm has receded. (2)

Max = 8

Use of transference

Yes	No	I build up over time to transference interpretation. (2)
Yes	No	I only use transference interpretation when therapeutic alliance is established. (1)
Yes	No	I do not use transference as simple repetition of the past. (1)
Yes	No	I use transference to demonstrate alternative perspectives between self and other. (1)
Yes	No	I avoid interpreting the therapeutic relationship as part of another relationship that the patient currently has or has had in the past. (1)
Yes	No	My transference interpretations are brief and to the point. (1)
Yes	No	I refrain from use of metaphor when the patient's mentalizing capacity is reduced. (2)
Yes	No	I do not focus on apparent conflict. (1)

Max = 10

Source. From Bateman A, Fonagy P: *Mentalization-Based Treatment of Borderline Personality Disorder: A Practical Guide.* Oxford, UK, Oxford University Press, 2006, pp. 174–176. Reprinted by permission of Oxford University Press.

❖ What is Mentalization-Based Therapy?

Mentalization-based therapy is a type of talking therapy created to treat people with borderline personality disorder. It's also been found to be useful for people with other types of mental illness. As the name suggests, it centers on the concept of mentalization. I struggled to understand what exactly this is, which could be further evidence of my need for this therapy or just that I'm a bit dim. But I finally grasped that it's unscarily straightforward. Mentalization is simply about recognizing what's going on in our own heads and what might be going on in other people's heads.

So what's the big deal? Surely we're all pretty in touch with what we're thinking, and have got as good a chance as anyone else of guessing what others are thinking? Er, no. Unfortunately those of us with borderline personality disorder are unlikely to be top scorers in the Thoughts Awareness League. Not great at accurately identifying what's happening in our own minds and even less likely to correctly work out what's in other people's minds. Especially if we're feeling stressed out.

And there's an even more fundamental problem here. When we're feeling like crap, we're likely to shut down (or at best tone down) our ability to mentalize. Thinking becomes a real effort, and reasoned thinking about thinking nearly impossible. Certainly for me, when things are tough I often self-harm specifically to avoid thinking, as that's too painful. Self-harming gives us something very concrete to focus on, which links with another aspect of borderline personality disorder. Apparently, if we've got this disorder, we tend to find it easier to believe things that we can see rather than imagining what might have led to a particular situation. (No money under the pillow, definitely no tooth fairy.)

Mentalization-based treatment is intended both to help us sharpen up our ability to mentalize and to be willing to use it, especially when we're feeling intense emotions. For example, in a session the therapist might ask us to consider what the other person in a difficult situation might have been thinking, and help us move past our initial assumption, especially if it's a really negative one.

❖ What's the Difference Between Mentalizing and Thinking?

Thinking is thinking. Mentalizing is thinking about thinking, our own thinking and other people's. Obviously it's often best just to get on and have thoughts. About whether *Borat* is the funniest film ever made or a shocking and trashy piece of sexist and racist rubbish. About whether there's something we can do as a non-punitive alternative to self-harming.

I've found it helpful looking at mentalizing from the perspective of people with autism. Perhaps it's because I've struggled to understand what mentalization is about that it's been useful to me to consider a group of people with a totally different disability to mine. People with autism live very much in the here and now. They have been described as having no "theory of mind," as most are unaware of their own thinking processes and have even less recognition that other people think or have feelings. Clearly people with autism think. (An inordinate amount of the time, it seems, about Thomas the Tank Engine, at least when they're kids.) But it's a very automatic experience, and reflecting on their own thoughts just doesn't arise. And the way they see the world is such that, although they may notice the manifestation of others' thoughts and feelings—for example, they can see that someone is smiling or hear them shouting—they don't connect that with the emotions that produce those observable responses. People with autism find it almost impossible to imagine themselves "in someone else's shoes."

For those of us with borderline personality disorder rather than autism, mentalizing is an acquirable skill, and one that can give us valuable extra perspective on a situation. Sometimes it helps to take one step further back. For example, if I'm planning to take an overdose, just thinking about it tends to take me along a route that lets me confirm this is the "right" thing to do. But if I have to mentalize, I have to look at my thinking. It's hard for me to do this without concluding that I'm not thinking straight. That my thoughts and feelings about the overdose are caused by feeling seriously like crap and that I should at least try to hold off any decision until I'm feeling more settled.

And if I then move on to thinking about others' thoughts, it takes me to the painful place of knowing how traumatized my friends are going to be if they find out that I've taken an overdose. None of this mentalizing necessarily stops me from taking self-damaging action, but it at least gives my self-protective side a decent shot at introducing some logic to the situation.

❖ What's It Like Having Mentalization-Based Therapy?

You might expect that a therapy with mentalization at its heart would involve the therapist endlessly asking "And what was in your mind? And what was in their mind?" But, luckily, this hasn't happened. It's all much more nuanced than that. Similarly, although the approach is very non-directive, when I ask for advice or need help in practical problem-solving with something I'm wrestling with, my psychiatrist often will respond in a normal way and help me out.

I had cognitive-behavioral therapy with a psychologist before I ended up being sectioned [i.e., hospitalized involuntarily]. At that stage, I was taken on by a personality disorder unit as an outpatient and have had mentalization-based therapy weekly with a psychiatrist for about 18 months. Both types of therapy feel very similar, despite the psychologist and psychiatrist being very different types of people. Both approaches have felt supportive, non-judgmental and focused on what I'm thinking. I've been able to see issues, especially painful ones, from a different perspective and to understand what might be fuelling the tough stuff. Both have made me feel like I'm setting the agenda about what we talk about and that I can say anything, however embarrassing or ridiculous I feel it is. And I know that the self-protective part of me, which tries to resist my self-destructive tendencies, gets crucial reinforcement.

The most noticeable difference in style is that my psychiatrist has very firm boundaries, so I know almost nothing about him and his life, other than what I can pick up from clues around his office. (He either rides a motorbike or is excessively worried about getting a head injury when driving his car.)

Perhaps the most tangible difference I experience is that I've only once self-harmed after a session with the psychiatrist, whereas I used to do so regularly after my previous sessions. This really puzzled me until I read a couple of books about mentalization-based treatment. These books made me realize that while the sessions feel quite normal and spontaneous, they're carefully designed to be at a level of intensity, or intrusiveness, that I can comfortably cope with. (This relates back to the business about us closing off if things become too painful.) This doesn't mean that I'm never moved outside my comfort zone—most sessions we cover things which make me cry. But somehow, overall I don't end up feeling completely jangled or bursting with feelings I don't know how to or don't want to deal with.

❖ Does It Work?

Well, I've been able to survive 18 months of pretty consistent suicidal feelings and still be around to write this. And studies have shown that it certainly works for a lot of, but not all, patients. One very reassuring thing is that it's been designed as a result of careful research into both the causes of borderline personality disorder and the impact of mental-ization-based treatment.

I don't really understand all the stuff about how borderline disorder develops, but it goes something like this. If mothers have problems connecting well with their babies, they respond differently from other mothers. One thing that the research shows is that when the babies are really upset, these mothers don't calm the babies in a way that helps the babies to understand or learn what's their own distress and what's the mother's. It's a bit like the baby's distress is magnified and bounced back at the little thing rather than being soothed and dissolved by the mother. As well as emotional mishaps like this, it's been found that many people who develop borderline personality disorder often have early experiences of abuse or neglect by parents. These things lead to many of us being unable to soothe ourselves in ways that are conventional, or not self-destructive, again reinforcing our tendencies to self-harm.

Another central proposition of mentalization-based treatment is that when we're babies and our mothers aren't able to comfort us in an effective way, we sort of bung onto our mother the parts of ourselves we can't cope with. This results later on in life with us coping particularly badly with the loss of someone close to us, partly because we might have assigned over to them the painful parts of ourselves. This contributes in a rather complicated way to our tendencies to self-harm and be suicidal, apparently to feel reconnected to the outsourced part of ourselves.

The quality of attachment in our earliest years continues to affect how we feel and think right through our lives, and if they've got off to a bad start we'll have difficulties with other close relationships. Including potentially the one with our therapist. The mentalizing-focused therapist, then, will be very aware of this and will be careful that we don't just slot back into a pattern of feeling overwhelmed by intensely painful feelings which make us close off thinking, especially about our own and the therapist's thoughts. Feeling understood by someone we trust (the therapist) is a sound place to be able to move into a calmer, safer way of coping with difficult stuff.

Recapitulation

In this chapter and the last, we have emphasized that focusing on mentalizing in the psychotherapy process builds on a natural human capacity—indeed, the capacity that *makes* us human. We therefore consider mentalizing-focused treatment to be a relatively commonsensical approach. When we are adhering to the model, we are behaving naturally; we do not transform ourselves into being "a therapist." Yet, interacting naturally in the role of a therapist, we have work to do, and it is hard work—just as mentalizing in other fraught relationships can be. Thus, as the patient's short guide to mentalizing therapy attests, although the treatment is "unscarily straightforward" as well as being "normal and spontaneous," it is also "nuanced" and—most importantly—mindfully modulated in emotional intensity.

The sheer straightforwardness of mentalizing-focused treatment ensures that the principles are relatively easy to learn. This chapter has provided a general orientation; for elaboration and further detail, we refer you to our practical guide to treating borderline personality disorder (Bateman and Fonagy 2006), the context in which the approach has been most refined and systematically researched (see Chapter 9, "Borderline Personality Disorder"). Yet we recognize that technical skill is not acquired from reading books; thus we recommend that if you wish to become proficient in the mentalizing approach, you undertake systematic training.

Fortunately, being good-enough mentalizers to begin with, therapists can become reasonably adept at delivering the treatment without extensive training. Our treatment trials all have been undertaken using mental health professionals who are trained in three-day workshops and then provided with follow-up supervision. Adherence measures using audiotapes suggest that these clinicians adhere to the model, or at least re-find it relatively quickly when they lose it. We are encouraged that adherence and effective implementation also can be maintained outside our own treatment center. For example, several members of a group of clinicians in the Netherlands undertook three-day training with follow-up supervision for a short time while the team leader received some additional problem-focused supervision. Initial independent scrutiny of treatment implementation and patient outcomes has indicated successful results. Thus we are becoming hopeful that the model of treatment can be generalized easily and remain effective in various mental health services.

While undertaking formal training is the ideal way to learn the mentalizing approach, we are keenly aware that routine consultation and supervision promotes mentalizing, simply by virtue of bringing in multiple perspectives. In this regard, we have been especially impressed by the impact of a weekly peer supervision group at The Menninger Clinic. The group is unstructured and members are encouraged to talk about their particularly difficult cases. Rarely does anyone have any useful practical suggestions; often the group is quite stymied about how the clinician might proceed; not uncommonly, the discussion, albeit lively, ends in a muddle. By the next week, the clinicians typically report that things are going much better, such that the group seems to have had a magical effect. But there is nothing magical about it: typically, the clinician has become stuck in one perspective and the group discussion opens up multiple perspectives, promoting greater flexibility and creativity in the process. Consistent with the attachment perspective we have maintained throughout this book, however, the value of this group depends entirely on a safe climate in which members are comfortable speaking freely. Thus the group is merely another instance of the principle that mentalizing (in the group) promotes mentalizing (in the treatment).

Yet we do not want to oversell the ease of conducting a mentalizing-focused treatment. Being keen on multiple perspectives, we have acknowledged the other side of the coin: it has become apparent that the mentalizing stance that we believe is central to effective treatment is harder to maintain than we first thought. Following training, for example, many therapists move from "We already do this," which is such a common theme in the first morning, to "This is hard—Help! How can we make sure we keep doing this? It's so easy to go off model!" So: join the training and feel de-skilled, read Iris Murdoch and feel humbled, and become a mentalizing therapist! Above all, it is challenging, sometimes downright fun and, to the extent we have researched it, apparently effective.

Key Clinical Points

- *You are already mentalizing.* Regardless of their theoretical orientation or professional discipline, therapists promote mentalizing in psychotherapy to varying degrees; specifically, mentalizing interventions are intended to focus therapists' attention on this process such that they can maintain a mentalizing stance more consistently and avoid unwittingly undermining mentalizing.

- *The therapist sets the tone.* Inasmuch as mentalizing begets mentalizing, it is both the therapist's and the patient's job to mentalize; yet the onus is on the therapist to take the lead and to foster a level of emotional engagement—neither too hot nor too cold—that optimizes mentalizing for both parties.

- *Mentalizing is highly interactive.* Particularly for patients whose mentalizing capacities are precarious, prolonged silences as well as encouragement of fantasy and free association are to be avoided; mentalizing treatment is a highly interactive process aimed at clarifying mental states in self and others, largely in the here and now.

- *Mentalizing compares the patient's and therapist's perspectives.* Mentalizing the transference entails examining and comparing the patient's and therapist's differing perspectives on their relationship and specific interactions; for this purpose, mentalizing therapists are relatively transparent in articulating their thoughts, feelings, and intentions in the process. They routinely acknowledge their own role in disagreements. To underscore the differences in perspectives, therapists frequently use "I" statements. The aim of discussing the patient-therapist relationship is not to offer the patient insight into habitual patterns of representing relationships but rather to use the therapeutic setting as a forum for improving the patient's mentalizing capacity.

Chapter 7

Treating Attachment Trauma

We already have laid the groundwork for treating trauma in highlighting the importance of mentalizing in the context of secure attachment relationships. In this fundamental sense, we consider trauma-related interventions to be ancient: trauma treatment came into existence when, with the advent of language, someone who was terrified after going through some horrific experience managed to talk it through with a trusted companion who provided comforting through understanding. As we also have implied, mind-minded mothers are good trauma therapists: when their child has been through a frightening experience, they help the child convey it and make sense of it in a reassuring way, restoring a sense of safety. Thus, ordinarily, the best resource for coping with potentially traumatizing experiences is the natural community (Ursano et al. 1996), as we presume has been the case since antiquity.

Unfortunately, as we also have conveyed, this natural healing process in which mentalizing is fundamental not only may fail to occur but, even worse, may be actively undermined in attachment trauma. To reiterate, trauma in attachment relationships, particularly in childhood, not only evokes extreme distress but also impedes the development of emotion-regulation capacities that would ameliorate the distress (Fonagy and Target 1997a). The greatest problem from a clinical perspective is that patients with a history of attachment trauma are liable to have profound difficulty developing and making use of what they most need to heal: secure attachments. Then they need professional help. Yet professional help is challenging to provide in light of their fear of attachment relationships coupled with impaired mentalizing capacity (Allen 2001).

Fortunately, despite the obstacles, most patients who have been traumatized in attachment relationships have not entirely given up hope in relationships (Allen et al. 2001). As the French existentialist Simone Weil (1943) stated eloquently,

> At the bottom of the heart of every human being, from earliest infancy until the tomb, there is something that goes on indomitably expecting, in the teeth of all experience of crimes committed, suffered, and witnessed, that good and not evil will be done to him. It is this above all that is sacred in every human being. (p. 51)

But Weil also appreciated the obstacles to what we are construing as mentalizing in attachment relationships; putting traumatic experience into words for others is not easy, and the others—including us clinicians—are all too likely to fail to comprehend:

> Affliction is by nature inarticulate. The afflicted silently beseech to be given the words to express themselves. There are times when they are given none; but there are also times when they are given words, but ill-chosen ones, because those who choose them know nothing of the affliction they would interpret. (p. 65)

Moreover, for friends, parents, romantic partners, and us clinicians, mentalizing trauma goes straight against the grain. Weil put it starkly:

> Thought revolts from contemplating affliction, to the same degree that living flesh recoils from death. A stag advancing voluntarily step by step to offer itself to the teeth of a pack of hounds is about as probable as an act of attention directed towards a real affliction, which is close at hand, on the part of a mind which is free to avoid it. (p. 65)

In sum, our ability to promote healing from trauma—whether it be for loved ones or for patients—stems from our humanity and our ability to provide a secure attachment, which rests on our mentalizing capacity. Yet, as Weil fully appreciated, offering this opportunity for healing is by no means easy, and those who have been traumatized in close relationships have an extraordinarily hard time making use of it. They are likely to need professional help, and we professionals who aspire to provide it are likely to need professional guidance and support.

This chapter distinguishes among various forms of traumatic experiences, emphasizing attachment trauma; elucidates two core trauma-related problems, namely, intrusive memories and reenactments; and describes the central role of mentalizing in treating these core problems. Consistent with the previous chapters on the art of mentalizing and mentalizing interventions, this chapter is not concerned with technique; rather, we focus on mentalizing as a way of thinking about treating trauma that is superordinate to technique. To reiterate, we do not aspire to convert other clinicians to yet another brand of trauma treatment. To drive home this point, we conclude the chapter with a discussion of the ways in which we view established evidence-based trauma treatments as promoting mentalizing of traumatic experience. We will continue expanding upon these trauma-related themes in the next two chapters as well, when we discuss child-parent therapy (Chapter 8) and treating borderline personality disorder (Chapter 9). We touch on mentalizing failures conducive to *inflicting* trauma in this chapter and elaborate this theme in conjunction with our consideration of violence prevention in social systems (Chapter 11).

Attachment Trauma Revisited

We find it helpful to distinguish potentially traumatic stressors along a spectrum of interpersonal involvement (Allen 2001). At the low end of the spectrum are *impersonal* stressors, most prominently natural disasters and accidents. In the middle *interpersonal* realm are traumatic stressors associated with deliberate or reckless behavior that is injurious to other persons. Interpersonal trauma stems from such diverse events as criminal assault, rape, sexual harassment, combat, and terrorism. At the other end of the spectrum, *attachment trauma* (Adam et al. 1995; Allen 2001) encompasses a subset of interpersonal trauma wherein the trauma is inflicted in an attachment relationship, whether it be in childhood (e.g., maltreatment) or adulthood (e.g., battering). Whereas interpersonal trauma instills fear of persons, attachment trauma instills fear of emotional closeness and dependency. As this whole book attests, we believe that attachment relationships are critical for healing from potentially traumatic stressors; thus, by virtue of undermining the capacity for attachment, attachment trauma most profoundly blocks the major vehicle of healing. Attachment trauma in childhood is especially pernicious in hampering development, including the development of resilience that would promote the capacity to cope with later impersonal and interpersonal traumas.

Abuse

Attachment trauma takes many forms, broadly subsumed under abuse and neglect, the various forms of which have been conceptualized well by Bifulco and colleagues (1994a, 1994b), as outlined in Table 7–1. In addition to considering physical and sexual abuse, Bifulco sharpened the relatively vague concept of emotional abuse by distinguishing between antipathy and psychological abuse. *Antipathy* entails parental rejection and hostility, which may take the form of criticism, disapproval, verbal abuse, coldness, ignoring the child, or favoritism. *Psychological abuse*, by contrast, entails cruel and sadistic treatment of the child, often with malevolent intent (Bifulco et al. 2002; Moran et al. 2002). As Bifulco and colleagues demonstrated, psychological abuse potentially takes many forms, including deprivation of basic needs or valued objects; callous

TABLE 7–1.   CORE FORMS OF ATTACHMENT TRAUMA

Cause of trauma	Severity of trauma
Abuse	
Physical abuse	Depends on age, frequency, degree of force, implements employed, part of the body involved, extent of injury, and mental state of the perpetrator (e.g., enraged, out of control)
Sexual abuse	Depends on age, frequency, extent of an attachment relationship with the perpetrator, degree of contact (e.g., penetration), and such contextual factors as secrecy enforced with threats to others
Antipathy	Depends on the pervasiveness and harshness of criticism, rejection, scapegoating, and favoritism
Psychological abuse	Depends on age, frequency, pervasiveness, and extent of sadism, terrorizing, and humiliating
Neglect	
Physical neglect	Depends on the extent of failure to provide for basic needs (e.g., food, shelter, healthcare) as well as the extent to which lack of supervision places the child in physical danger
Psychosocial neglect	Depends on the pervasiveness of lack of concern with, lack of interest in, and lack of attentiveness to the child's emotional states, cognitive and academic interests and development, and friendships and other relationships

inflicting of marked distress or discomfort; cognitive disorientation; humiliation; extreme rejection; cruel threats of abandonment; terrorizing; emotional blackmail; and corruption. Of all the possible forms of maltreatment, psychological abuse perhaps impinges most directly on mentalizing, inasmuch as it is a direct assault on the mind.

Often intertwined with being abused is witnessing the physical, sexual, and psychological abuse of other family members; moreover, children who witness violence between parents also are likely to be physically abused as well (Ross 1996). But the relation between witnessing domestic violence and being physically abused is only one facet of a broader pattern: maltreated children typically are exposed to multiple forms of abuse. Zanarini and colleagues (1997), for example, concluded that sexual abuse is not only traumatic in its own right but also is a *marker* for severe dysfunction in the family system within which the sexual abuse occurs. Similarly, psychological abuse rarely occurs in isolation from other forms of maltreatment (Bifulco et al. 2002). Consistent with the pervasively observed dose-response effect, the greater the compounding of different types of abuse in childhood, the higher the likelihood of adulthood psychopathology (Bifulco and Moran 1998; Bifulco et al. 2002). Perhaps most pernicious—and not uncommon—is *complex abuse*, construed as the co-occurrence of multiple forms of abuse in the same incident (Bifulco et al. 1994b; Stein et al. 2000); for example, when a child is deliberately terrorized in the course of sexual violence.

Neglect

A common and critical instance of the compounding of adversity is the combination of abuse (acts of commission) and neglect (acts of omission). Ironically, in comparison with abuse, neglect has been relatively neglected, not only in the research literature (Bifulco and Moran 1998; Wolock and Horowitz 1984) but also in referrals for child protective services (Ards and Harrell 1993) and mental health services (Garland et al. 1996). Such neglect of neglect is especially disturbing in light of the evidence that its traumatic impact may equal or exceed that of abuse (Egeland 1997), and its effects extend into adulthood—for example, doubling the rates of depression in one sample (Bifulco and Moran 1998). Of particular significance for clinicians, van der Kolk and colleagues (1991) found that while sexual abuse was the strongest predictor of self-destructive behavior, neglect was a potent predictor of the failure to give up self-destructive behavior despite ongoing intensive treatment.

Like abuse, neglect takes many forms that are usefully distinguished. Barnett and colleagues (1993) distinguished two forms of physical neglect: failure to provide for physical needs (e.g., food, clothing, shelter, health care, and hygiene) and lack of supervision that places the child in danger. Compared to physical neglect, emotional or psychological neglect are more challenging to define and assess (O'Hagan 1995). As contrasted with physical neglect, we have conceptualized psychosocial neglect as a superordinate term that encompasses three broad forms: *emotional* neglect, a lack of attunement and responsiveness to the child's emotional states; *cognitive* neglect, a failure to support and nurture cognitive and educational development; and *social* neglect, a failure to support interpersonal and social development (Stein et al. 2000).

Egeland and Erickson (Egeland 1997; Erickson and Egeland 1996) pinpointed *psychological unavailability* as a cornerstone of emotional neglect; the term characterizes the behavior of parents who are unresponsive to their child's pleas for warmth and comfort. Psychologically unavailable mothers, for example, are relatively detached and unresponsive, interacting mechanically. These authors' longitudinal research revealed that psychological unavailability had a greater adverse developmental impact than physical neglect and other forms of maltreatment; ironically, this form of maltreatment was the most subtle yet the most pernicious.

Mentalizing Failures

The term "psychological unavailability" captures well the converse of optimal parental mentalizing that we delineated in Chapter 3 ("Development"). The essence of optimal mentalizing is emotional engagement coupled with contingent responsiveness as evident, for example, in "marked" emotional responses: the parent is attuned to the child's emotional state and expresses the emotion along with cues that convey that the emotional expression is a reflection of the child's state, not the parent's unalloyed emotional state. As we described, such marked emotional responses have a pedagogical function in promoting the development of a sense of self and self-awareness of emotions in particular; concomitantly, marked emotional responses provide the psychosocial foundation for emotion regulation. Hence psychological unavailability is a bedrock mentalizing failure.

Yet not only neglect but also abuse and traumatizing actions more generally also entail mentalizing failure, a failure that Baron-Cohen's (1995) term, mindblindness, captures well (Allen 2007). Abusive behavior represents egocentrism at the extreme; in the face of passionate rage or lust, the abusive parent is oblivious to the child's mental states or emotional needs. Like psychopathy, however, many forms of psychological abuse entail a partial failure of mentalizing, inasmuch as the abusive parent must be somewhat attentive to the child's mental state for the purpose of effectively inflicting psychological pain. Here too, Baron-Cohen's (2003) concept of mindreading without empathy is helpful: the appropriate emotional response to the child's pain is chillingly lacking in psychological or sadistic abuse. Plainly, egocentrism also is involved in distorted mentalizing associated with abuse; for example, the physically abusive parent misperceives the child as being malevolent or the sexually abusive parent misreads the relationship as being gratifying to the child while remaining mindblind to the child's aversion.

The all-too-common conjunction of abuse and neglect (psychological unavailability) is traumatizing by virtue of leaving the child emotionally alone with unbearable emotional states that the child is unable to regulate (Allen 2001, 2005). Ironically, the most traumatizing impact of the mentalizing failures evident in attachment trauma might be their undermining of the development of mentalizing capacities in the child, one outcome of which is the intergenerational perpetuation of trauma.

Trauma-Related Psychopathology

Just as various forms of abuse and neglect are often intertwined over the course of development, the ensuing psychopathology is equally multifaceted. The psychiatric disorder uniquely associated with a traumatic etiology is posttraumatic stress disorder (PTSD), but, crippling as it may be, PTSD is merely the tip of the iceberg of trauma (Allen 2001; Herman 1992a). Traumatic stress also contributes to a host of clinical syndromes and symptoms, including dissociative disorders, depression, substance abuse, deliberate self-harm, suicidal states, eating disorders, and psychotic disorders. Moreover, attachment trauma contributes significantly to personality disorders—most conspicuously, to the disturbances of affect regulation, identity, and relationships evident in borderline personality disorder. In this chapter, we focus on two facets of complex posttraumatic psychopathology for which mentalizing interventions are especially pertinent: intrusive memories associated with PTSD and reenactments of traumatic relationship patterns associated with the wider impact of trauma on personality functioning.

Intrusive Memories

PTSD is a cruel form of trauma: having undergone horrifically painful events, its victims develop an illness that repeatedly puts them through the events in imagination, inasmuch as the core symptom of PTSD is reexperiencing the trauma (e.g., in flashbacks and nightmares). Concomitantly, persons with PTSD experience chronic anxiety and hyperarousal, which lowers the threshold for intrusive memories. Understandably, in an effort to block intrusive memories, persons with PTSD engage in strategic avoidance strategies, not only by trying to avoid people and situations that might remind them of the trauma but also by trying to avoid thinking, feeling, and talking about the trauma—that is, mentalizing. Yet as research on ironic mental processes attests (Harvey and Bryant 1998; Wegner 1994), thought suppression paradoxically *increases* the likelihood that the warded-off thoughts will come to mind. Moreover, posttraumatic avoidance is especially problematic insofar as it is associated with a wide range of destructive and maladaptive nonmentalizing behaviors, such as suicide attempts, deliberate self-harm, substance abuse, bingeing and purging, dissociation, and somatization (Brewin et al. 1996).

At the extreme, intrusive memories of trauma entail reliving the traumatic events in the form of flashbacks. Flashbacks also have a dissociative quality in that the individual is profoundly detached from current reality in the midst of reliving the trauma (Chu 1998). A patient in the midst of a flashback of physical abuse, for example, might pull himself up into a ball with his arms covering his face and head, whimpering and pleading, "Stop! Stop!" Such episodes are paradigmatic of the prementalizing *psychic-equivalence* mode (see Chapter 3, "Development") in which the sense of representingness of mental states is lost and external reality is equated with the mental state. Hence the goal of treatment is to move from excruciatingly painful *reliving* (psychic equivalence) to bearably painful *remembering* (mentalizing).

In psychoeducational groups on trauma (Allen 2005), we provide patients with a cognitive cue to help them identify when they are conflating past and present, namely, what we have dubbed the "90–10" reaction: because they have been sensitized, 10% of their emotional reaction is based on the current stressor and 90% is based on past traumatic stressors (Lewis et al. 2004). When patients can bring this cue to mind in the midst of an intense emotional reaction to a current provocation, they can mentalize the emotion, endeavoring to discriminate the past from the present. Here we are addressing the core of PTSD, namely, context-inappropriate responding (Davidson et al. 2003). As we explain it to patients, there is nothing wrong with their fear response, which is all too obviously intact; rather, the response is occurring in a nontraumatic context that is comparatively safe. Awareness of this context inappropriateness, which we aspire to promote with the "90–10" cue, requires mentalizing emotion.

Distorted mentalizing in the sense of inaccurate mental elaboration also comes into play in the context of the notoriously controversial and complex problem of *false memories* of childhood maltreatment, particularly in the context of sexual abuse (Allen 1995; Brown et al. 1998). Especially alarming is the prospect of therapists' non-mentalizing interventions contributing to such distorted mentalizing in their patients:

> Consider a worst-case scenario. A suggestible and fantasy-prone patient with a penchant for highly vivid visual imagery presents with psychiatric symptoms (e.g., depression, nightmares, panic attacks, low self-esteem, and social isolation). The therapist—without any evidence other than such ubiquitous symptoms with a host of possible etiologies—infers childhood sexual abuse to be the cause. Over the patient's protest, the therapist insists that memories of such childhood sexual abuse must be recovered though aggressive exploration. Gradually, images consistent with this putative trauma history begin coming to the patient's mind (e.g., a shadowy figure entering the bedroom), and eventually, personal event memories are constructed—essentially out of whole cloth. Unfortunately, this process is not a fictional scenario; clinical horror stories akin to it have been documented in the literature. (Allen 2001, p. 133)

Avoiding such scenarios requires that clinicians be knowledgeable about memory and its vulnerability to distortion (Schacter 1999) as well as the wide range of factors that can impair autobiographical memory for trauma (Allen 1995, 2001; van der Kolk 1994). As Fonagy and Target (1997b) describe, not only do cognitive-developmental limitations in early childhood potentially blur the fantasy-reality distinction, but also the family context specific to maltreatment is liable to undermine the child's sense of reality (e.g., through minimization and denial or through forcing the child to accept responsibility for the abuse). Yet clinicians, while remaining aware of the potential for distortion and confabulation, should be aware that systematic research documents the global accuracy of memory for childhood trauma (Brewin and Andrews 1998; Widom and Morris 1997; Widom and Shepard 1996; Williams 1995). Given the evidence for robustness of memory, coupled with myriad factors that can impair memory, clinicians are advised to keep in mind the potentially wide spectrum of accuracy in memories of extensive and multifaceted childhood maltreatment, both between and within traumatized individuals (Allen 1995). This complexity calls for the mentalizing stance: an open-minded attitude toward the accuracy of memories for the patient as well as the clinician. This stance is undermined by stereotypical assumptions about symptoms associated with abuse and by regarding natural doubts about the accuracy of memories as an indication of defenses or resistance. Yet maintaining a mentalizing stance is not necessarily easy for trauma therapists:

> While the interpersonal situation created by those patients who desperately need external validation is certainly difficult, even for experienced therapists, it must be wrong to collude with the patient's attempt to use the therapist to reduce the unknowable to a fact. The task of the therapist is to contain the patient and to show both genuine understanding of the patient's state of uncertainty and the resulting hopes and conflicts. It is far more difficult to empathize with the patient's not knowing than to reduce uncertainty by pretending to know. (Fonagy and Target 1997b, p. 205)

Reenactments

Freud's (1914) dictum that reenacting can substitute for remembering is nowhere more glaringly evident than in the reenactment of childhood attachment trauma in subsequent attachment relationships (van der Kolk 1989). Reenacting instead of remembering is a failure of mentalizing *par excellence*.

In addition to the intergenerational transmission of trauma, which we will continue to discuss, reenactment is evident in well-documented patterns of *revictimization* (van der Kolk 1989). Cloitre and colleagues, for example, documented how a history of childhood sexual abuse increases the risk of sexual assault in adulthood (Cloitre et al. 1996). Yet the repetition need not be so direct; Widom's (1999) prospective study showed that *all* forms of court-documented maltreatment (sexual and physical abuse as well as neglect) were associated with a heightened risk of rape in adulthood. Beyond the repetition of the familiar, the vulnerability to such assaults also might reflect a defensive compromise of alertness to danger associated with childhood trauma (Cloitre 1998); such a failure to identify interpersonal cues also can be understood as a trauma-related mentalizing failure (Fonagy and Target 1997a).

The sheer perniciousness of attachment trauma is evident in traumatic bonding, wherein abusive behavior cements the attachment. Traumatic bonding is evident in animals (Scott 1987), and it is evident in human relationships ranging from childhood maltreatment (Bowlby 1982) to hostage-taking situations (Strentz 1982). Yet traumatic bonding is perhaps most bewildering in battering relationships in adulthood (Walker 1979): how can the battered woman be unwilling to leave the relationship? Plainly, there is a wide range of reasons for women to remain in such relationships, not least the credible threat of being killed or having their children killed. Economic dependence also plays a prominent role. Yet relationship dynamics also are conspicuous (Dutton

and Painter 1981; Herman 1992b); these dynamics include a gross im-
balance of power, isolation from other sources of support, and low self-
esteem (including a feeling of deserving no better).

The seeming paradox of traumatic bonding is explained quite simply: the threatening behavior heightens fear, and fear heightens attachment needs (Allen 1996). Isolation from other sources of support
cements the tie to the abuser—in Walker's (1979) words, as if by miracle
glue. The bond is solidified further by the periods of loving respite that
typically follow the battering episode. Commonly, women not only remain in battering relationships but also return to them after leaving. Not
surprisingly, such behavior is associated with a pattern of ambivalent-
preoccupied attachment, itself commonly associated with childhood
maltreatment. Henderson and colleagues (1997) found that, after separating, women with ambivalent attachment continued to feel love for
the abusive partner, remained sexually involved with him, and felt a desire to get back together with him. Of course, there are two sides to these
relationships, and battering men also are liable to be insecurely attached,
using their overt power to hide their covert dependency; their jealousy
and possessiveness, abetted by coercive intimidation and violence, stave
off their own fears of abandonment (Dutton and Painter 1981).

Reenactment and intrusive posttraumatic symptoms are thoroughly
intertwined: reexperiencing is commonly evoked by reminders of
trauma, and the most potent reminders of past trauma are present interactions that resemble it (Allen 2005). Many patients with a history of
childhood trauma function at a high level for many years in adulthood
and then develop delayed PTSD (Brown et al. 1998). Naturally, they
wonder, "Why now?" For patients who present with such eruptions of
PTSD, it is always clinically useful to consider the possibility of current
reenactments; in the face of ongoing reenactments, striving to desensi-
tize patients to intrusive symptoms is liable to be futile. Moreover,
given the impairment of mentalizing associated with attachment
trauma, these patterns are liable to be opaque to the patient, who, unaware of the reenactment, is bewildered by delayed memories that
seem to come out of the blue. At worst, as depicted in Figure 7–1, vicious circles evolve when efforts to cope with posttraumatic symptoms
through destructive behavior (e.g., substance abuse or self-cutting) escalate conflicts in relationships that replicate the earlier attachment
trauma, which constitute reminders that evoke the symptoms of PTSD.

Trauma therapists also should be alert to mentalizing failures associated with more subtle forms of reenactment. Trauma notoriously
leads to sensitization to stress—that is, to heightened reactivity (Post et
al. 1997). Thus ostensibly minor reenactments can trigger major emo-

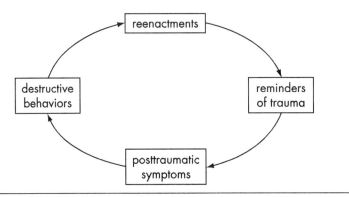

FIGURE 7–1.   REENACTMENT AND POSTTRAUMATIC SYMPTOMS.

tional reactions (i.e., what we have dubbed the "90–10" reaction). If *the core of trauma revolves around being sensitized to the experience of feeling emotionally alone in a state of high emotional distress,* the possibilities for re-experiencing childhood trauma in ordinary adult interactions abound (Allen 2001): a man who has become anxious and depressed after losing a job becomes panicky and enraged as his wife responds to his increased neediness with frustration and impatience; a woman who is frightened about her adolescent son's escalating alcohol abuse becomes infuriated by her husband's seeming retreat into working longer hours and traveling more; or a therapy patient abruptly terminates in the midst of an unfortunate coincidence between a marital crisis and the therapist's unexpected absence.

Mentalizing Trauma

Hardly an innovation, our fundamental intervention is this: "What happened? Tell me about it." By virtue of promoting the patient's mentalizing capacity, the therapist's mentalizing capacity, rather than any particular techniques, will determine the success of the treatment. For reasons we have already described, this venerable and straightforward—albeit painful—strategy of encouraging mentalizing will be challenging for persons who have experienced attachment trauma in childhood. Not only are memories liable to be confusing or clouded but, more importantly, distrust, shame, and guilt feelings will inhibit confiding. At worst, the traumatized person may lack confiding or secure attachment relationships altogether.

Moreover, for persons with PTSD, trauma treatment entails a paradox: reminders of trauma evoke symptoms of PTSD, and PTSD treatment entails talking about trauma, which perforce generates reminders. Given the combination of sensitization and impaired mentalizing, we should not be surprised that persons with a history of attachment trauma can get worse rapidly in excessively expressive treatment approaches that focus exclusively on talking emotionally about traumatic experiences. Accordingly, trauma treatment requires that therapists deftly balance *processing* trauma—mentalizing in the form of thinking, feeling, and talking about it—with *containment*. We distinguish four elements of containment (Allen 2001, 2005) as summarized in Table 7–2.

Sadly, the most critical facets of containment—supportive attachments and the concomitant competence in emotion regulation—are deficient for persons with a history of attachment trauma. Whereas the literature on treating PTSD might lead one to infer that the value of containment (secure attachment and emotion regulation) is to enable processing (mentalizing), we would argue the reverse: as developmental research attests, mentalizing has value largely insofar as it promotes containment in the form of secure attachment and emotion regulation. Ironically, although we say that the four elements of containment are essential to promote mentalizing, we are dealing with a synergy: mentalizing *is* the ultimate means of containment.

With a history of attachment trauma, mentalizing in the context of a secure attachment is challenging to achieve; yet Main's (1991, 1995) research with the Adult Attachment Interview demonstrates that it is possible. As she summarized, this interview presents the participant with "two central tasks: (1) producing and reflecting on memories involving early relationships as well as any potentially traumatic experiences *while simultaneously* (2) maintaining coherent, collaborative discourse" (Main 1995, p. 439, emphasis in original). Such discourse reflects metacognitive

---

TABLE 7–2. CORE COMPONENTS OF CONTAINMENT FOR PROCESSING TRAUMA

Knowledge about trauma and its treatment, as provided, for example, through psychoeducation

A therapeutic alliance and solid treatment frame with clear and agreed-upon expectations regarding the roles of patient and therapist

Supportive relationships as exemplified by secure attachment and, ideally, a network of such relationships in which conflicts and disruptions in any given relationship can be buffered by other relationships

Emotion-regulation and stress management strategies that can be employed by oneself (supplementing reliance on supportive relationships)

monitoring in the context of remembering, which includes mentalizing emotion (see Chapter 2, "Mentalizing"). As Main (1995) described it,

> Interview transcripts are classified as *secure-autonomous*...when the presentation and evaluation of attachment-related experiences is coherent and internally consistent, and responses are clear, relevant, and reasonably succinct. For secure-autonomous speakers, the focus of attention appears to shift fluidly between interviewer queries and the memories that are called on. Notably, it is not only individuals whose experiences appear to have been supportive who are classified secure-autonomous. Many individuals who describe difficult backgrounds are coherent when discussing and evaluating the effects of their histories and are also therefore placed in this category. (p. 439)

In this passage, Main articulated the goal of trauma treatment, namely, establishing narrative coherence—talking about the trauma without becoming entangled in the past and emotionally overwhelmed. Catch-22: the security of attachment that promotes such discourse is precisely what eludes many patients with a history of trauma. Little wonder that for such persons trauma treatment is slow and painstaking as well as painful. Phase-oriented treatment is the standard (van der Kolk et al. 1996): the treatment initially emphasizes safety and developing a therapeutic alliance as well as establishing boundaries in a reliable treatment frame. Yet therapists should not have the mindset that establishing a therapeutic alliance and a solid treatment frame is preliminary to the real work of processing trauma. On the contrary, the alliance and the treatment frame are subject to continual rupture and repair, owing to the dilemma entailed in providing an attachment relationship to a patient with a history of attachment trauma.

Hence, for persons with a history of attachment trauma, a solid treatment alliance—collaboration in the context of a secure attachment—could be construed as an optimal *outcome* of treatment, not a precondition for it. Accordingly, many patients also can benefit from additional support from psychotropic medication (Gabbard et al. 2006) as well as practical help in emotion-regulation strategies such as are offered in Dialectical Behavior Therapy Skills Training groups (Linehan 1993b). These skills training groups facilitate attending to emotions and labeling them, understanding their functions, accepting and tolerating distressing emotions, and promoting positive emotions. Hence these groups promote mentalizing emotion, as we construe it (Lewis 2006). Indeed, since high levels of emotional arousal undermine mentalizing (see Chapter 4, "Neurobiology"), stress-regulation methods indirectly promote mentalizing. These, too, are among our least novel interventions; as McEwen (2002) advised, the most effective steps you can take are the simplest: exercise, a healthy diet, regular sleep, moderate-to-minimal alcohol intake, and no smoking. If this sounds suspiciously like what your grandmother always told you, all I can say is that according to the most sophisticated, up-to-the-minute, cutting-edge science available, your grandmother was right. (p. 136)

From the perspective of promoting mentalizing, the core of trauma treatment is enabling the patient to have the traumatic memories and associated emotions *in mind* as meaningful and manageable experience, coupled with the capacity to put it *out of mind* voluntarily by employing emotion-regulation strategies and refocusing attention. Thus mentalizing emotion is at the center of trauma treatment, and it is the pathway out of destructive behavior.

Barbara, a highly successful advertising executive, sought inpatient treatment in her late thirties when her business partners became fed up with her erratic performance, associated with substance abuse, and insisted that she either get help or leave the firm. This ultimatum came on the heels of Barbara's being "dumped for another woman" by a man she had been seeing for three years. She had hoped to marry this man and to have a child with him—keenly aware that her "biological clock" was ticking. Although Barbara had been chronically depressed, she became utterly despondent in the midst of this crisis. She entered treatment with slim hope of being helped, but suicide seemed to her to be the only alternative.

Although she had not been hospitalized previously, Barbara had first sought psychotherapy in her early twenties while she was in college, and she had been helped considerably by it. She had been doing well academically, but she was fighting depression. She was engaging in binge drinking on weekends and embroiled in a series of passionate and tumultuous relationships that were short-lived.

With the benefit of her prior therapy, Barbara was able to articulate a history of extensive trauma in childhood and adulthood that, as she was well aware, continued to haunt her. She was the elder of two children; both parents were alcoholic and both were violent toward each other and toward her as well as toward her three-years-younger brother, whom she endeavored to protect. She recalled a vicious argument between her parents in their kitchen that occurred on her tenth birthday. In the course of the argument, her mother slapped her father and he, in turn, slammed her mother into the refrigerator, after which she fell to the floor. Her father was standing over her mother with his back to Barbara, and she retains a vivid image of picking up a butcher knife with the urge to stab her father in the back. Whether she actually picked up the knife or merely imagined doing so is unclear to her. She remembers running from the kitchen when she heard her brother screaming in the dining room, after which she ran him to his bedroom to comfort him.

Barbara recalls being more deeply wounded by verbal assaults than occasional whippings. When he was drunk, for example, her father would call her a "stupid, useless bitch." She remembered her mother screaming at her that she had been an "accident" that had ruined her mother's life, to which Barbara responded that she wished she had never been born. Inexplicably, when she started going to parties in early adolescence, Barbara's mother berated her for being a "whore." Barbara's saving grace was her aunt who lived nearby and who willingly provided refuge for Barbara and her brother; they spent as much time there as their parents would allow. Her aunt was not inclined to talk about Barbara's parents' behavior; Barbara said they had an "unspoken understanding" about their need for refuge. Her aunt not only provided comfort and affection but also appreciated and nurtured Barbara's artistic talent as well as taking a keen interest in her schoolwork and academic success. Accordingly, Barbara brought her friends to her aunt's home, not her parents' house.

In her mid-adolescence, Barbara recalled that she had a "split personality" in the sense that she was a good student and even a "teacher's pet" at school while being a "wild child" out of school, especially on weekends. She binged on alcohol, drugs, food, and sex. She also developed a knack for shoplifting, which she gave up after the first time she was caught.

Barbara was bright, talented, and ambitious, so she was able to earn a scholarship that enabled her to go to college, with supplementary help from a part-time job and from her aunt. When her "partying" in college started to interfere with her work, she sought psychotherapy at the urging of a friend who had found therapy to be helpful, and she remained in therapy for the last two years of college. For the first time in her life, she was able to talk about her traumatic experience in her family, to express her feelings about it, and to begin to put it into perspective. Better able to manage her feelings, she stopped using drugs and was able to curb her drinking. Connecting her worst alcoholic binges with her tumultuous sexual relationships, she decided on a moratorium for romantic relationships. As her aunt had done, her therapist took an interest in her schoolwork and nurtured her academic achievements.

Unsurprisingly, work was Barbara's strength while intimate relationships with men remained her Achilles heel. She gradually reverted to substance abuse as a means of managing the emotional turmoil associated with her recurrent frustration and disappointment in romantic relationships; then her work and her relationships with her business partners deteriorated as well. She became overtly antagonistic toward her senior male partner, who was relatively critical and demanding.

As she began psychotherapy again in the course of her hospitalization, Barbara expressed pessimism, stating that she had been in psychotherapy before and, obviously, "it didn't work." As evidenced by her current plight, all the work she did on her trauma had been "a waste of time," and it was therefore "pointless to dredge it all up again." Listening to her talk poignantly and coherently about her childhood experiences in the initial sessions led her therapist to a contrary view: she had worked effectively on many aspects of early trauma and had benefited from the work considerably. She had long abandoned her pattern of promiscuous relationships, but she had remained stuck; sexual intimacy was the sticking point. She "put up" with sex. She could not refrain from expressing her aversion, responding with evident tension at best and suddenly recoiling from touch at worst. She was pushing men away, not only by her physical aversion but also by bickering and fault finding. She knew she was doing so but didn't understand it and couldn't stop it.

From the trauma history sketched here, one could infer a multiplicity of reasons for Barbara's aversion to sexual intimacy. When she was discussing her desire to be pregnant and her ambivalence about it, a trauma came to mind that had been nearly impossible for her to think about and that she had never discussed before with anyone: she had an abortion in late adolescence. Although she had gone through more traumatic events than she could possibly remember or recount, she recalled the abortion as being the worst experience of her lifetime. Compounding Barbara's despondency in the aftermath of the abortion, she had become pregnant when she was intoxicated—she did not even have a clear memory of the event. Not only was she feeling ashamed, guilty, and frightened but also she felt she could not tell anyone. She believed that her parents would "kill" or disown her, and she could not bear the thought of falling out of her aunt's good graces. She had the abortion with some help from an acquaintance, but the acquaintance was helpful only with the logistics and could not provide any emotional support. She went through the abortion feeling utterly alone. She recalled desperately wanting to die, but she did not attempt suicide for a number of reasons: she feared she might not succeed; she was frightened of death; she wondered if she might go to Hell; and she knew her aunt would be devastated, whereas she believed her mother would be happy about it—the latter belief being a conscious deterrent.

Whereas with the help of previous psychotherapy she had been able to think and talk about a wide range of childhood traumas, Barbara had been unable to do so in relation to the trauma of the abortion. Although she remembered thinking about the abortion occasionally in her previous therapy, she put it out of mind and never talked about it. After the abortion, she recalled thinking of herself as a "monster," a "murderer," and "baby killer." At best, she had thought of herself as having been "selfish," putting her own needs before the life of her child.

Barbara's anguish as she talked about the impact of the abortion was excruciating for her and painful for her therapist to witness. The male therapist was keenly aware of limitations in his capacity to empathize as fully with the experience as a woman might be able to do. Yet Barbara's anguish was moving. The therapist was aware of a possible connection between Barbara's view of herself as a murderer in relation to the abortion and her image of stabbing her father in the back with a knife. He also wondered if her mother's wish that Barbara had never been born might have unconsciously motivated her to terminate her pregnancy. Instead of raising these speculations, however, he invited Barbara to reconsider her view that she had been "selfish" in having the abortion. Now able to reflect, she concluded that she had been in no position to raise a child for a host of reasons; this recognition didn't eliminate her guilt feelings, but it did ameliorate them. She no longer thought of herself as a selfish murderer, which previously had remained her only (and non-mentalizing) perspective on her action.

In retrospect, Barbara concluded that her unthinkable experiences associated with the abortion had played a significant role in her sexual aversion as well as in her relatively unconscious ambivalence about the pregnancy she had consciously desired. These concerns were a driving force in her unstable romantic relationships; and the emotional turmoil in these relationships, in turn, played a central role in her escalating drinking and deteriorating functioning.

This relatively brief psychotherapy during a several-weeks' hospitalization was, in effect, a restarting of the therapeutic process begun more than a decade earlier. Barbara had become aware of a major obstacle to intimacy, but the long work of surmounting this obstacle would await continuing therapy after discharge from the hospital, in her home community in another state. She concluded this episode of therapy with more confidence in its value as well as greater appreciation for the valuable and effective work she had done in prior therapy. Yet what impressed Barbara and her therapist more than any particular insight she derived from the therapy was this: she had learned that she could tolerate profoundly painful emotions without having to squelch them, for example with alcohol. Ironically, her avoidant pattern of destructive alcohol abuse had been obscuring a great deal of emotional strength. This was ordinary trauma therapy, but for Barbara, finding herself able to mentalize the fantasies and emotions related to the abortion and its impact on her romantic relationships was extraordinary. Learning that she could feel her most painful emotions and understand them by talking them through gave her a great deal more freedom. She had developed the capacity to mentalize the most painful emotions, and she no longer needed to flee from her own mind.

The psychotherapy process with Barbara illustrates a central theme in treatment focusing on mentalizing, namely, *the emphasis on process over content*—in this instance, the value of mentalizing emotion as contrasted with recovering explicit memories of trauma for the sake of insight. Barbara and her therapist agreed at the end of their work together that the therapy was most valuable in giving her confidence that she could tolerate, understand, and regulate extremely painful emotions— whatever their source. Hence she would be able to manage any traumatic memories that might come to mind, whatever their content; crucially, she no longer had to be so afraid of her own mind. Plainly, insight about the impact of her abortion on her conflicts about sexual intimacy and her ambivalence about pregnancy would be expected to help her understand her push-pull pattern in ongoing relationships; yet confidence in managing her anxiety as she continued to work on those conflicts would be most central to her success.

Barbara's history also exemplifies a core facet of trauma that we cannot overemphasize: reenactment of past trauma in current relationships (Allen 2001; van der Kolk 1989). The diagnostic criteria for PTSD (American Psychiatric Association 2000) include reexperiencing the trauma, but not reenacting it; again, reenacting childhood attachment trauma in current relationships should not be overlooked, inasmuch as reexperiencing symptoms are evoked by reminders of trauma and reenactments are a primary source of such reminders. The continual antagonism and associated turmoil in Barbara's romantic relationships mirrored—albeit in much toned-down form—the continual fighting she witnessed in her childhood. But the inevitable breakups were most devastating; she felt ashamed, despairing, and *alone*—an emotional state reminiscent of her experience of the abortion. Prior to her hospitalization, she had become suicidal again, in just this mental state.

The tight relationship between reenacting traumatic relationship patterns, the associated self-generated reminders of past trauma, and reexperiencing of traumatic memories and emotions has a straightforward implication for therapy: recovering memories of past trauma will be futile if the patient is embroiled in ongoing reenactments. Indeed, potentially destabilizing as it may be (e.g., when it is done without needed containment), recovering memories can add fuel to reenactments. Hence the primary focus of treating attachment trauma is *modifying current relationships* in the direction of increasing security of attachment by promoting mentalizing. Fonagy and Target (1997b) characterized this shift in focus as follows:

> If this modified psychoanalytic model is sound, then a substantial revision of the role of memory in psychotherapy is called for. Episodic or autobiographical memory can no longer be seen as directly relevant to psychic change. Change can be thought to occur as a function of a shift in emphasis between different mental models of interpersonal relationships—a change of procedures or ways of living with oneself and others, not of autobiographical memory. (p. 213)

No doubt, as Fonagy and Target (1997b) state, memories of past traumatic interactions can usefully illuminate problematic patterns in current attachment relationships. Yet the emphasis should remain on enhancing effective functioning in the present through improving not only relationships with others but also one's relationship with oneself (Allen 2005). Thus insight into the past is not the critical factor:

when more adaptive and rewarding ways of relating have been achieved in treatment (i.e., new patterns of relating created alongside the old), it is not essential for the patient to "know about" the origins of the old models. Cognitive awareness of these origins does not bring fundamental change, although the patient's knowledge of the rules on which he has relied can be useful in helping him to recognize when he is falling back on old, maladaptive patterns, and so selectively to activate more appropriate and adaptive patterns. (Hurry 1998, p. 51)

Such an emphasis comes as a relief to many patients who continue to struggle with trauma after extensive trauma therapy:

Charles had a long history of depression, substance abuse, and self-injurious behavior associated with a history of childhood sexual abuse and exploitation, coupled with extreme neglect. Owing to escalating self-cutting, he had been through months-long inpatient treatment in which intensive exploration of memories was the focus. After discharge, he continued to be depressed and suicidal in conjunction with ongoing conflict in a series of romantic relationships, and he was again hospitalized. Charles was referred to one of the authors for continuing trauma treatment. He did not bring up trauma in the first two sessions, and toward the end of the second session, the therapist asked him about its relevance to his ongoing difficulties. He said that he had "been through it all" in the last hospitalization and he saw no point in "slogging through the muck of the past." The therapist indicated that it would be helpful in understanding him to hear about his view of the impact of the traumas, and they agreed to talk about this in the next session.

Charles came to the next session mentioning that he had experienced two panic attacks during the preceding night, and he was very apprehensive about the session. Nonetheless, he was able to talk about a wide range of traumas in a way that led to his poignant and tearful expression of her conviction that "some childhood pain never goes away." The therapist expressed agreement with Charles's view that "slogging through the muck" would not be as productive as focusing on coping, that is, working with his feelings in the present and their relation to the continual problems he was having in romantic relationships. At that point, Charles breathed a visible sigh of relief.

Yet not all patients are so keen to focus on current problems, as a treatment process described previously (Allen 2006b) illustrates:

The patient had been in an emotionally intense outpatient treatment including Eye Movement Desensitization and Reprocessing (Shapiro 1995); her functioning had been deteriorating, and her marital conflict had been escalating to the point that she required hospitalization. Initially, she was relieved when the therapist indicated that her treatment would best focus on restoring her health and emotional stability rather than talking about her past traumatic experience. That is, the therapy as well as the hospital treatment would focus on containment. Yet the patient eventually felt increasingly frustrated and deprived in the therapy, perceiving the therapist as being similar to her emotionally neglectful parents; he too, in effect, wanted her to "stuff" her feelings and was indifferent to her pain. She began to repeat the angry and demanding behavior that had alienated her husband and blocked any possibility of reconciliation with her parents. Focusing on this reenactment in the psychotherapy and in the family work led to a positive shift in her current relationships that offered a pathway out of keeping her childhood trauma alive in the present.

To reiterate, we construe the archetype of the traumatizing childhood attachment relationship as being one in which the child is feeling overwhelmingly distressed and, most important, alone in the sense of having no one who has his or her mind in mind. At worst, excessively emotionally expressive treatment approaches that fail to provide needed containment replicate rather than remediate this early trauma: the patient feels overwhelmed and alone, without adequate support and without the internal capacities to regulate the distress. On the other hand, with adequate containment that supports mentalizing, psychotherapy can be reparative, providing a model for secure attachment and thereby a bridge to other supportive relationships (Allen 2001). As Emde and colleagues summarized:

> All mental health interventions involve the effects of relationships on other relationships. This is so whether we are focusing on current relationships or on future relationships, and it is so whether we are focusing on behavior or on the representational world. Traditional psychotherapy, which is not often thought about in these terms, is illustrative. It is generally referred to as a "relationship-based" form of intervention, meaning that the intervener and the client establish a working relationship with a shared goal of greater understanding so that there can be less suffering and more behavior that is adaptive and satisfying. What is less often appreciated is that traditional "individual" psychotherapy involves a goal of having the working (i.e., therapeutic) relationship influence sets of other relationships. The other relationships are both represented and actual. A goal of individual psychotherapy is to influence the client's represented relationships of self in relation to others and its internal world of problematic expectations (so as to generate more *reflective capacity with options* and less self-defeating encumbrances). Additionally, a goal is to influence the client's current world of everyday social relationships (so as to generate interactions that are more flexible and less self defeating). (Emde et al. 2004, pp. 267–268; emphasis added)

Mentalizing in Cognitive-Behavioral Trauma Treatments

We have considered the role of mentalizing in treating the complex psychopathology associated with attachment trauma, and our general approach to the problem of reenactment, including reenactment in the transference, is consistent with a range of accounts of psychodynamic and relational approaches to trauma treatment (Davies and Frawley 1994; Herman 1992b; Pearlman and Courtois 2005). Yet we also believe that more focal, evidence-based treatments for intrusive and avoidant symptoms of PTSD are usefully viewed as promoting healing through mentalizing, albeit with somewhat divergent techniques. Here we highlight the role of mentalizing in three well-researched trauma treatments: exposure therapy, cognitive restructuring, and Eye Movement Desensitization and Reprocessing.

Exposure Therapy

Exposure to the anxiety-provoking stimulus for the purpose of promoting desensitization is the most straightforward approach to treating anxiety disorders, PTSD among them. As Rachman (1980) put it decades ago, "Fear must be experienced before it can be reduced or eliminated" (p. 52). As we have noted, consistent with Rachman's assertion, mentalizing emotion entails thinking about feelings *while remaining in the emotional state*. Also consistent with this view, Foa and colleagues (1995) found that the best outcomes in PTSD treatment were associated with patients experiencing distress within sessions coupled with habituating to distress across sessions. Yet as Foa and Kozak (1986) and Rachman (1980) recognized, treating trauma by any means entails walking a tightrope: the intensity of the emotion must be kept within bounds to prevent retraumatization. From our point of view, moderating the level of emotion is essential to keep mentalizing online in the midst of experiencing the emotion.

On the basis of controlled research, Foa and Rothbaum (1998) have developed a treatment protocol for rape-related trauma that includes both *in vivo* exposure and prolonged imaginal exposure. The *in vivo* exposure entails returning to the vicinity of the rape under safe conditions and remaining there for 30–45 minutes, experiencing the anxiety until it abates. The in-session imaginal exposure entails recounting the traumatic experience as if it were happening in the present tense and doing so repeatedly over the course of the session. Sessions are tape recorded and patients are instructed to listen to the recordings as homework to supplement the in-session exposure.

Consistent with our emphasis on containment, clinicians who practice prolonged exposure emphasize the needs for safeguards to avoid retraumatizing the patient (Foa and Rothbaum 1998; Pitman et al. 1991). These safeguards include educating the patient about trauma and the treatment; teaching emotion-regulation strategies such as relaxation; ensuring that the patient is in a relatively calm state and reoriented to the present before terminating the session; and, from our point of view most crucial, conducting the treatment in the context of a strong and supportive relationship.

Although prolonged-exposure therapy is predicated on the fundamental principle of extinction (i.e., habituation to repeated anxiety-provoking stimuli), Foa's (1997) research attests to the psychological complexity of the change process. She proposed three core components of change which are applicable to any form of trauma treatment: 1) emotional engagement with the trauma memory, 2) constructing a coherent narrative, and 3) altering views of oneself and others in a more balanced and realistic direction. Each of these three components can be viewed from a mentalizing perspective. To reiterate, regarding the first component, emotional engagement is critical to mentalizing emotion; as we have described (see Chapter 2, "Mentalizing") emotion must be evoked, sustained, and modulated to be mentalized. Regarding the second component, as we also have seen in conjunction with Main's (1991) work (Chapter 3, "Development"), narrative coherence is the hallmark of resolution of trauma. Finally, regarding the third component, distorted mentalizing of oneself and others in conjunction with trauma must be rectified for the sake of secure attachments. The trauma treatment we described with Barbara in relation to her view of herself regarding the abortion illustrates Foa's (1997) point about the need to alter one's view of oneself in a more balanced and realistic direction; moreover, such changes achieved through mentalizing are pivotal to developing and maintaining intimate relationships.

Cognitive Restructuring

Extensive research documents the detrimental changes in cognitions associated with trauma. Janoff-Bulman (1992), for example, proposed that trauma shatters three fundamental assumptions needed for well-being: the world is meaningful, the world is benevolent, and the self is worthy. Correspondingly, Foa and colleagues (1999) found three domains of cognitions that perpetuate PTSD: negative cognitions about the self, the dangerousness of the world, and the blameworthiness of the self for the trauma.

All therapies will address cognitions insofar as they entail discourse about the trauma. Resick and colleagues' cognitive processing therapy developed to treat rape-related PTSD illustrates an evidence-based approach (Calhoun and Resick 1993; Resick and Schnicke 1992). Blending exposure and cognitive restructuring, the treatment begins with the patient writing a trauma narrative that encompasses the events and her reactions to them. She reads the account aloud to herself and then to the therapist. The treatment explores and challenges cognitive distortions, focusing on themes of safety, trust, power, esteem, and intimacy.

Plainly, the core therapeutic elements Foa (1997) articulated (emotional engagement, coherent narrative, altered views of the self and the world) apply to cognitive restructuring as well as to prolonged exposure, and both methods are eclectic in blending exposure and cognitive therapy techniques to varying degrees. As Foa and Kozak (1991) stated, for example, "In effect, we practice informal cognitive therapy during exposure, in that we help clients to examine ways in which they evaluate threat and to develop inferential processes that lead to more realistic conclusions" (p. 45). Unsurprisingly, controlled studies show exposure therapy and cognitive restructuring to be similar in effectiveness (Marks et al. 1998; Tarrier et al. 1999). In our view, the exposure component is critical to mentalizing in bringing the emotionally painful experience to mind, and the cognitive-restructuring component is equally critical in the process of mentalizing, that is, the development of the capacity to think flexibly about the trauma, to consider multiple perspectives, and to work actively in regulating the associated emotions.

Eye Movement Desensitization and Reprocessing

Shapiro (1989, 1995) presented Eye Movement Desensitization and Reprocessing (EMDR) as a novel treatment for trauma. Its label notwithstanding, EMDR is a multifaceted and eclectic treatment protocol that overlaps considerably with other approaches, including exposure and cognitive restructuring. The patient and therapist identify core traumatic images along with associated emotions and physiological sensations, and these traumatic images are brought to mind during the treatment. In addition, patients articulate negative views of the self in conjunction with the trauma (e.g., feelings of incompetence or self-blame), and they construct alternative positive cognitions (i.e., how they would prefer to see themselves in conjunction with the trauma). The treatment also includes containment in the form of education and emotion-regulation strategies as well as attention to the patient-therapist relationship.

The novel intervention is introduced in the context of the desensitization procedure: the patient is instructed to bring the traumatic image to mind while simultaneously moving the eyes from side to side, following the therapist's fingers moving back and forth in front of the face. Each cycle of bilateral stimulation is followed by the patient's being instructed to blank out the traumatic image and verbalize whatever comes to mind in an associative fashion. In conjunction with the sheer popularity of EMDR, the eye-movement component contributed to heated controversy about the intervention (Greenwald 1999; McNally 1999a). Outcome research supports the effectiveness of EMDR (Rothbaum 1997; Wilson et al. 1995, 1997), although controlled studies raise questions about the unique contribution of the eye movements to the outcome (Cahill et al. 1999) and do not show EMDR to be more effective than a range of cognitive-behavioral approaches (Rothbaum et al. 2005; Seidler and Wagner 2006; Taylor et al. 2003). Hence McNally (1999b) spoke for the critics in concluding that "what is effective about EMDR is not new, and what is new is not effective" (p. 619). EMDR entails brief exposure to the trauma (Rothbaum et al. 2005) as well as distancing from it (Lee et al. 2006), both of which can be therapeutic. From a mentalizing perspective, it is not the technique that is critical but rather the need to modulate the emotion sufficiently at various points in the treatment to enable the patient to mentalize while remaining in the emotionally aroused state.

Recapitulation

A focus on mentalizing proves a broad framework for understanding and treating attachment trauma. Mentalizing failures comprise the core of the trauma in two senses: first, the traumatizing attachment figure fails to mentalize the child; second, with no one holding the child's mind in mind, the child cannot mentalize the traumatic experiences in the attachment relationship. Hence the child lacks the resources to cope with the extreme distress. Accordingly, restoring mentalizing in two domains lies at the heart of treatment: first, mentalizing is the means to contend with the intrusive symptoms of PTSD; second, mentalizing is the key to interrupting reenactments of trauma.

Insofar as the natural strategy of avoidance only perpetuates the problems (Brewin et al. 1996), mentalizing is the solution: the PTSD sufferer must develop the capacity to have the traumatic memories in mind as meaningful and emotionally bearable experience. Mentalizing is the pathway out of psychic equivalence, the route to separating past from present, and thus the way to move from reliving to remembering. In addition, mentalizing is the foundation of emotion regulation. In our view, any treatment that enables the patient to think, feel, and talk about the trauma while emotionally engaged yet not emotionally overwhelmed will facilitate mentalizing. The exposure-based, cognitive-behavioral treatments for PTSD accomplish this. To the extent that they focus on trauma, psychodynamic treatments can do the same. Yet the more structured approaches have the advantage of holding the patient's and therapist's feet to the fire, in effect: the agenda explicitly entails processing the trauma. In the senior author's experience, it is easy for both parties to avoid facing the trauma in the more open-ended therapies.

As we also have described, in the absence of mentalizing, PTSD sufferers become embroiled in a Sisyphus-like cycle in which they unconsciously reenact past trauma in current relationships in a way that escalates the sense of threat, and these escalating stressors evoke memories of past trauma and symptoms of PTSD which, in conjunction with impulsive and destructive behavior, fuel the reenactments. Hence mentalizing is equally important in identifying the reenactments and associated reminders so as to separate the present from the past and to de-escalate the cycle of reenactment. Psychodynamic approaches to trauma treatment have specialized in this domain of reenactment (Davies and Frawley 1994; Pearlman and Saakvitne 1995; van der Kolk 1989). Ultimately, for patients who are embroiled in these patterns, the goal of trauma treatment is to stabilize current relationships in the direction of increasingly secure attachments. As we have been arguing throughout, mentalizing is the *basis* of secure attachments.

Not uncommonly, PTSD sufferers imprison themselves in a sheltered, isolated, and socially withdrawn lifestyle. Even worse, they live in a mental prison, terrified of their own mind, *afraid to think*. They are afraid to think because they are afraid to remember and they are *afraid to feel*. As Barbara's therapy illustrates, restoring the freedom to think and feel is the fundamental goal of a mentalizing-focused treatment. And the freedom to think and feel is inseparable from the freedom to form intimate attachment relationships. Moreover, the freedom to think and feel depends equally on one's *relationship with oneself*. Philosopher Hannah Arendt (2003) insightfully made this point: "if you want to think you must see to it that the two who carry on the thinking dialogue be in good shape, that the partners be friends" (p. 185). Accordingly, we can envision the ideal relationship with oneself on the model of secure attachment, with mentalizing as its basis (Allen 2005): you have the freedom to think and feel with the expectation that you will regard your thoughts and feelings with inquisitive interest and compassion. Ideally, founded on the mentalizing stance, the patient-therapist relationship can be a model for a more secure relationship with the self.

Key Clinical Points

- *Nature of attachment trauma:* Attachment trauma is traumatizing by virtue of mentalizing failures in the caregiver that undermine the development of mentalizing in the child.

- *Core interventions of mentalizing treatment:* The overall aim of mentalizing-focused trauma treatment is simple, and the core interventions are doubtless ancient: providing a safe relationship climate for the traumatized person to think, feel, and talk about the trauma. This task is simple but difficult: all of us are naturally averse to mentalizing profound suffering.

- *Overlap with other therapies:* Mentalizing interventions overlap exposure-based treatments (in enabling patients to have the traumatic experiences in mind) and psychodynamic approaches (in identifying patterns of reenactment in current relationships, including the patient-therapist relationship).

- *Optimal outcome:* Maintaining a mentalizing stance in trauma treatment requires that processing the trauma be supported by adequate containment, especially in the form of secure attachment and emotion-regulation skills. Through the vehicle of enhanced mentalizing, the capacity for containment is the optimal *outcome* of trauma treatment.

Chapter 8

Parenting and Family Therapy

The importance of developing increasingly effective mental health interventions for children cannot be overstated. Plainly, the most obvious reason for enhancing interventions is the sheer prevalence of psychiatric disorders among children—current estimates of which range from 12–15% to 20–30%, depending on the level of severity (Fonagy et al. 2002b). Yet early interventions also have a potentially crucial preventive role as well, inasmuch as psychopathology in childhood and adolescence is the foundation on which the bulk of adulthood psychopathology develops. In a landmark prospective longitudinal study, Kim-Cohen and colleagues (2003) found that roughly 75% of adults with psychiatric disorders had a diagnosable disorder prior to age 18, and 50% had a disorder prior to age 15; accordingly, they concluded: "Most adult disorders should be reframed as extensions of juvenile disorders" (p. 709).

To repeat Emde and colleagues' point, our mental health interventions perforce involve relationships influencing relationships (Emde et al.

2004). This principle was implicit in Anna Freud's view of treatment as developmental therapy: "as Anna Freud indicated, relationships and events in day-to-day life can provide an opportunity for change and growth at all stages. Developmental therapy provides such an opportunity for change through a relationship fine-tuned to the patient's developmental needs" (Hurry 1998, p. 34). Accordingly, Anna Freud construed child analysis as providing *developmental help.* In our terms, "fine-tuned" attention to "developmental needs" entails mentalizing, and mentalizing is the mediator of the therapeutic impact of relationships on relationships.

Just as mentalizing begets mentalizing, non-mentalizing begets non-mentalizing, as our recurrent reference to the intergenerational transmission of trauma attests. We begin this chapter by reiterating this intergenerational theme, extending our consideration of reenacting trauma in adult relationships as described in the previous chapter to reenacting trauma in parent-child relationships. We review Fraiberg and colleagues' (1975) classic work "Ghosts in the Nursery" as the clinical foundation for what has evolved more recently into mentalizing-focused interventions in parent-child relationships. In our view, the perspective of mentalizing illuminates the foresightedness of Fraiberg's earlier work, and we include clinical vignettes from other master clinicians in the same spirit. We separate this work somewhat arbitrarily into infant-parent and child-parent therapy, after which we describe a mentalizing-focused approach to family therapy.

Reenactment Revisited

Darlene was hospitalized in her mid-twenties after an overdose that was precipitated by her husband's threatening to divorce her and take custody of their 15-month-old son. Darlene began psychotherapy in despair, stating that her husband's stance showed that she was a "total failure" as a wife and mother.

Darlene's resumption of alcohol and drug abuse after a several-year period of abstinence precipitated the marital crisis. In the initial psychotherapy sessions, Darlene recounted her own history of being neglected by her mother, herself a chronic alcoholic. Darlene's father coped with his wife's alcoholism by avoidance; as Darlene put it, "he was always working or hanging out with his friends," spending time with her and her brother only on holidays and during special events. By early adolescence, Darlene did the same: she "hung out" with friends and spent as little time at home as possible. At age 16 she virtually moved in with a friend down the street. She characterized her adolescent life as being filled with "partying," by which she referred to promiscuous sexual relationships along with alcohol and drug use.

Darlene's saving grace was athletic talent. In the latter years of high school, a coach became a "father figure" and cultivated her interest in athletics. Her desire to be in good physical condition curbed her substance abuse, and participating in varsity sports gave her incentive to do reasonably well in her schoolwork. She settled down into a high school romance, and soon after graduation, she moved in with her boyfriend, whom she married after a few years spent living together. She had gone to cosmetology school after graduation and held a steady job.

Darlene resumed substance abuse about 6 weeks after giving birth to her son. She minimized the significance of this timing except to state that she had suffered from "postpartum depression" and was "bored" at having to stay at home with the baby. She resented her husband's refusal to take time off from work, and after she resumed using alcohol, he spent more and more time out of the house. As the marital conflict escalated and her depression worsened, she began using methamphetamines for the first time in her life, which led to a downhill spiral that culminated in her husband's threat to leave her and to take their then 15-month-old son with him.

As the therapist explored the stresses that led to the resumption of substance abuse and its escalation, Darlene focused exclusively on the marital tension that left her feeling abandoned, alone, and resentful. The timing notwithstanding, she denied that her difficulties were connected in any way with her relationship with her son. She stated that she loved her son with all her heart and that she missed him terribly while she was in the hospital. She was distressed that when her husband brought her son to visit, the boy shied away from her and interacted only with her husband. She feared that her hospitalization had "broken the bond." She was especially distressed that her son seemed to enjoy interacting with a young female nurse in the treatment program.

The therapist suspected that, the patient's protests notwithstanding, her difficulty relating to her son had played a role in Darlene's postpartum depression and distress; he continued to encourage her to talk more specifically about their relationship. In response to the therapist's sheer persistence, Darlene ultimately was able to acknowledge that although she took good physical care of her son and enjoyed holding and cuddling him, she did not really know what to do with him. She talked about how, when she learned she was pregnant, she feared that she would be a "terrible mother," as she considered her own mother to have been. Tearfully, she revealed that she felt extremely inadequate when it came to playing with her son or teaching him about anything. She showered him with toys but did not participate in his play. She put him in front of TV programs for children.

Reinforcing Darlene's sense of inadequacy as a mother, she was keenly aware that her husband, their babysitter, and her mother-in-law were far more comfortable interacting with her son. Moreover, whenever any one of them was in the home, her son would quickly gravitate toward interacting with them—not her. With a great deal of shame, she acknowledged that she felt rejected by her son as well as jealous and resentful of his other relationships.

Darlene had been too ashamed of her felt inadequacy as a mother to acknowledge it or to seek assistance. Her withdrawal into alcohol and drug abuse compounded all her problems and ultimately led to sufficient maternal physical neglect that her husband became alarmed. With the help of the psychotherapy process, Darlene was able to acknowledge that not only the marital stress but also her difficulties relating to her son had played a role in her psychiatric problems. She was then amenable to obtaining help and coaching from others to whom interacting with her son came more naturally.

As Bruschweiler-Stern (2004) detailed and Darlene's experience illustrates, the mother's relationship with her baby begins long before birth. Along with the physical pregnancy is a "mental pregnancy" during which the baby is actively mentalized and the mother mentalizes herself as a mother. With the birth, the imagined baby interacts with the real baby, and the mother faces an emotion-laden array of tasks: "keeping the baby alive, regulating the baby's states, answering the infant's needs, and *establishing a new relationship*. If *any* of these tasks is not fulfilled, the mother's level of anxiety rises very fast" (p. 191; emphasis added). Plainly, Darlene's difficulty began prior to the birth of her son: her anxiety about her adequacy as a mother rose during her pregnancy and failed to abate when she found herself unable to establish a comfortable relationship with him in his infancy. Darlene's relationship with her husband and son sadly reflects a direct repetition of the relationship pattern in her family of origin; as Darlene came to acknowledge, she had no "role model" for being a mother, and her fearfulness and shame about her own maternal inadequacy prevented her from facing her own developmental challenge forthrightly and coping actively with it. Hence she unwittingly and painfully reenacted a history of maternal neglect as well as reexperiencing and reenacting aspects of her parents' marriage in her relationship with her husband.

Silverman and Lieberman (1999) presented an instructive instance of a mother's unwittingly reenacting her history of abuse with her preschool-aged daughter. Laura, a 29-year-old divorced woman, and Isabelle, her four-year-old daughter, were referred to the authors' Child Trauma Research Project by the family court system owing to concerns about Isabelle's having witnessed extreme violence in Laura's relationship with her ex-husband, Jake—both before and after Laura left Jake when Isabelle was two years old. When Laura and Jake were living together, Isabelle witnessed recurrent violence, including physical battering and rape. Laura decided to leave Jake after witnessing Isabelle's fright when Jake came home drunk—handgun in hand—and boasted about intimidating a man in a bar with his gun. Some months later, during the period when the divorce decree was being finalized, Isabelle witnessed Jake beating up Laura.

As Darlene had done, Laura was unwittingly reenacting her own parents' relationship. As Silverman and Lieberman (1999) describe, Laura's alcoholic father was jealous, relentlessly interrogating Laura and her mother about their activities. In one jealous rage, he intentionally drove their car into oncoming traffic; all three were hospitalized. Laura's mother left her husband when Laura was 11 years old after Laura was forced to watch her father play Russian roulette, holding a gun to her mother's head. Laura had not appreciated her own reenactment of trauma until Jake unwittingly had terrorized Isabelle with the handgun in the course of bragging about the barroom incident. As the authors describe, "Laura suddenly felt 'horror-stricken' at the thought that she had allowed Isabelle to witness this scene" (p. 166).

Unfortunately, the reenactment of trauma did not cease for Isabelle with the end of the violence between Laura and Jake. As Silverman and Lieberman (1999) recount, Laura unconsciously continued to terrorize Isabelle despite her conscious intention to protect Isabelle from what she had gone through at the hands of violent men: "In an attempt to teach Isabelle to become self-protective, Laura exposed the child to painful and frightening situations, repeatedly traumatizing her in an effort to protect her" (p. 163). For example, Laura asked a stranger at a playground to tempt Isabelle by offering her a toy; Laura watched at a distance and then berated Isabelle after she accepted the toy, "telling her in graphic detail what 'terrible things' could happen to young children who accept gifts from strangers" (pp. 167–168). Ironically, Isabelle responded to Laura's subjecting her to such frightening situations by developing dissociative defenses ("spacing out") which not only escalated Laura's admonishments but also increased the likelihood that Isabelle would inadvertently get herself into dangerous situations.

Darlene's and Laura's relationships with their children exemplify a particularly worrisome form of reenacting trauma: children not only become traumatized as victims of reenactment but also can become embroiled in the intergenerational perpetuation of trauma. Darlene and Laura also exemplify a failure of mentalizing. While she was pregnant, Darlene fearfully anticipated that she would be an unfit mother, but after her son was born she was unable to think about her inability to relate to him, denying that their relationship had anything to do with her depression and substance abuse. Laura's failure to mentalize was even more glaring: she terrorized her daughter in the guise of protecting her—even *after* a sudden burst of insight when she linked her own childhood experience to her daughter's fright.

The reenactment of trauma illustrates Santayana's venerable insight that those who cannot remember the past are condemned to repeat it. Oliver's (1993) comprehensive review of research on intergenerational transmission of child abuse is especially telling in this regard. Reenactment of abuse from generation to generation is extensively documented, although it is not always as direct as in Darlene and Laura. Specific patterns can change from generation to generation, and abuse can alternate between generations. Although the proportions of abused parents who abuse their children vary from sample to sample, the rates are substantial:

> The crude rates of intergenerational transmission of child abuse according to the studies reviewed are as follows: one-third of child victims grow up to continue a pattern of seriously inept, neglectful, or abusive rearing as parents. One-third do not. The other one-third remain vulnerable to the effects of social stress on the likelihood of their becoming abusive parents. (Oliver 1993, p. 1315)

From the standpoint of mentalizing, Oliver's (1993) most telling conclusion is this: "The single most important modifying factor in intergenerational transmission of child abuse is the capacity of the child victim to grow up with the ability to face the reality of past and present personal relationships" (p. 1322). A characteristic failure of mentalizing is glaringly evident in one of Oliver's accounts:

> Maltreating parents frequently gave bland or idealized pictures of their own biological parents, especially their mothers, which could be so incompatible with old written records that repeated checks were necessary to make sure that we had the same family. In such cases, the records rather than current interviews gave the truth. (p. 1320)

Such "bland or idealized pictures" are typical of the dismissing-avoidant pattern of insecure attachment often evident in Adult Attachment Interviews (Main and Goldwyn 1994). Plainly in such instances a mentalizing intervention is indicated. Yet the challenges go a step beyond those in trauma therapy with individuals, described in the previous chapter: potentially reenacting parents not only must mentalize their own prior trauma but also must receive help in cultivating mentalizing relationships with their children.

Ghosts in the Nursery

Decades ago, Fraiberg and her colleagues (1975) pioneered parent-infant interventions intended to interrupt the intergenerational transmission of trauma. They characterized the typical baby who entered their Infant Mental Health Program as "a silent partner in a family tragedy…burdened by the oppressive past of his parents from the moment he enters the world" (p. 388). The ghosts reflect the absence of mentalizing: "Ghosts who have established their residence privileges for three or more generations may not, in fact, be identified as representatives of the parental past" (p. 388). Fraiberg and colleagues detail what can only be described as heroic work to bring the ghosts into the open so as to lay them to rest.

According to Fraiberg and colleagues' account, Mrs. March brought her five-and-a-half-month-old daughter, Mary, to their program after her husband refused to consent to her wish to give up Mary for adoption. Mrs. March was severely depressed, with a history of being suicidal; Mary was listless and tenuously connected with her mother:

> The mother herself seemed locked in some private terror, remote, removed, yet giving us rare glimpses of a capacity for caring. For weeks we held onto one tiny vignette captured on videotape, in which the baby made an awkward reach for her mother, and the mother's hand spontaneously reached toward the baby. The hands never met each other, but the gesture symbolized for the therapists a reaching out toward each other, and we clung to this symbolic hope. (p. 391)

Yet this hopeful sign was overshadowed by Mrs. March's typical obliviousness to Mary's distress. The authors describe a period in which Mary is "screaming hopelessly;" she is in her mother's arms but not turning to her mother for comfort: "The mother looks distant, self-absorbed. She makes an absent gesture to comfort the baby, then gives up. She looks away. The screaming continues for five dreadful minutes on tape" (p. 391). The key diagnostic question: *"Why doesn't this mother hear her baby's cries?"* (p. 392, emphasis in original).

The history revealed that Mrs. March's mother developed a postpartum psychosis shortly after Mrs. March's birth and shot herself in the face with a gun, leaving herself horribly mutilated. Mrs. March was cared for by an aunt and maternal grandmother; she was "the cast-out child of a cast-out family" in "a story of bleak rural poverty, sinister family secrets, psychosis, crime, a tradition of promiscuity in the women, of filth and disorder in the home, and of police and protective agencies in the background making futile uplifting gestures" (p. 392).

Mrs. March and Mary being their first patients, and having no models to work from, Fraiberg and colleagues improvised a treatment approach. They began with twice-weekly individual psychotherapy for Mrs. March and home visits to provide developmental guidance for the baby. Yet Mrs. March was fearful of her male psychotherapist, and the baby remained in peril. The female therapist conducting the home visits, Mrs. Adelson, began doing what they called "psychotherapy in the kitchen," which included "tactful, nondidactic education of the mother in the recognition of her baby's needs and her signals" (p. 394)—in our terms, mentalizing. Gradually and painfully, Mrs. March was able to talk about her own story of abandonment and neglect that she was re-enacting with Mary. The answer to the question as to why Mrs. March could not hear Mary's cries was all too plain: "This is a mother whose own cries have not been heard. There were, we thought, two crying children in the living room" (p. 395). The authors surmised that Mrs. March would hear Mary's cries when her own cries were heard. They illustrated what we would call a mentalizing approach:

> Mrs. Adelson's work, then, centered upon the development of a treatment relationship in which trust could be given by a young woman who had not known trust, and in which trust could lead to the revelation of the old feelings which closed her off from her child. As Mrs. March's story moved back and forth between her baby, "I can't love Mary," and her own childhood, which can be summarized, "Nobody wanted me," the therapist opened up pathways of feeling. Mrs. Adelson listened and put into words the feelings of Mrs. March as a child. "How hard this must have been…This must have hurt deeply…Of course, you needed your mother. There was no one to turn to…Yes. Sometimes grown-ups don't understand what all this means to a child. You must have needed to cry…There was no one to hear you." (p. 396, ellipses in original)

This mentalizing process led to a transformation in Mrs. March's relationship with Mary, heralded as follows: "Mrs. March, in the midst of an outpouring of grief, picked up Mary, held her very close, and crooned to her in a heart-broken voice" (p. 396). To use Meins's (1997) terminology, Mrs. Adelson was promoting Mrs. March's mind-mindedness: "When a crying Mary began to seek her mother's comfort and found relief in her mother's arms, Mrs. Adelson spoke for Mary. 'It feels so good when mother knows what you want.'" (Fraiberg et al. 1975, p. 397). Mrs. March responded to this intervention with shy pride. The treatment continued in this vein, illustrated by interventions related to Mary's problems with separation when she was a year old. When returning to work, Mrs. March had made hasty and inadequate babysitting arrangements for Mary, who became irritable and more difficult to manage. Mrs.

March viewed Mary as being spoiled and stubborn—in effect, adopting a "Get over it!" attitude. Mrs. Adelson was able to help Mrs. March talk about her own history of painful abandonment and losses. Another mind-minded intervention:

> Looking at Mary, sitting on her mother's lap, Mrs. Adelson said, "I wonder if we could understand how Mary would feel right now if she suddenly found herself in a new house, not just for an hour or two with a sitter, but permanently, never to see her mother or father again. Mary wouldn't have any way to understand this; it would leave her very worried, very upset. I wonder what it was like for you when you were a little girl." (p. 400)

After a period of reflection, Mrs. March responded, "You can't just replace one person with another...You can't stop loving them and thinking about them"; and, mindful of her own painful experiences, she concluded, "I would never want my baby to feel that" (p. 400; ellipsis in original).

Echoing Santayana and Freud (1914), and anticipating Oliver (1993), Fraiberg and colleagues commented on parents who short-circuit the process of intergenerational transmission by what we call mentalizing:

> There are many parents who have themselves lived tormented childhoods who do not inflict their pain upon their children. These are the parents who say explicitly, or in effect, "I remember what it was like...I remember how afraid I was when my father exploded...I remember how I cried when they took me and my sister away to live in that home...I would never let my child go through what I went through." For these parents, the pain and suffering have not undergone total repression. In remembering, they are saved from the blind repetition of that morbid past. (p. 420; ellipses in original)

As Fraiberg's work attests, many traumatized parents and infants need expert help to lay the ghosts to rest. Freud (1900) likened unconscious processes to "ghosts in the underworld of the Odyssey—ghosts which awoke to new life as soon as they tasted blood" (p. 592n). Using Freud's simile, Loewald (1960) commented, "Those who know ghosts tell us that they long to be released from their ghost-life and led to rest as ancestors.... as ghosts they are compelled to haunt the present generation with their shadow-life." He went on to note that in treatment, "the ghosts of the unconscious are laid and led to rest as ancestors whose power is taken over and transformed into the newer intensity of present life" (p. 29). While Freud and Loewald were working with transference onto the analyst, it was Fraiberg's genius to bring the baby into the treatment process as an object of especially intense and potentially destructive transferences. The transformation of Mrs. March's and Mary's relationship from one of mutual detachment to loving engagement well illustrates Loewald's "newer intensity of present life."

Infant-Parent Psychotherapy

Fraiberg and colleagues created the model for what is now a burgeoning field of clinical practice (Coates et al. 2003a; Maldonado-Duran 2002; Osofsky 2004; Sameroff et al. 2004). Perforce, as with all psychotherapeutic interventions, mentalizing has been implicitly central to this arena of practice (Slade, in press). A decade and a half before "mentalizing" began to appear in the English clinical literature, Fraiberg's (Fraiberg et al. 1975) work exemplified mentalizing-based interventions at their best. More recently, however, research on mentalizing has been introduced explicitly into this arena (Fonagy 2002).

Rendering explicit what has been implicit in work with parents of infants and children, Slade (2006) has developed interventions to enhance *parental reflective functioning,* defined as the caregivers' capacity to reflect on the child's current mental state as well their own mental states as they affect the child's mental states and the parent-child relationship (Slade, in press). Recognizing that skill in mentalizing varies along a continuum, and that skillful mentalizing is rare in parents seeking treatment, Slade (2006) assists parents in moving through stages of mentalizing from simple to complex. She begins by helping parents merely contemplate the child's basic mental states (e.g., a feeling); then she helps them appreciate how mental states underlie behavior (e.g., she is fussy not because she is "mean" but because she is "hungry and tired"); then she moves on to the dynamic relations between two individuals' mental states (e.g., the parent's anger frightens the child and the child's fearfulness further irritates the parent).

As Slade (in press) articulated, the mentalizing perspective clarifies the therapeutic psychological processes in Fraiberg's (Fraiberg et al. 1975) clinical approach. In Slade's view, the clinician provides a model of reflectiveness while holding the parent's mind in mind—an experience that can be relatively rare for the parent with a history of attachment trauma. Moreover, the clinician holds the child's mind in mind for the parent. Consequently, internalizing the clinician's mentalizing stance, the parent is gradually able to hold the child's mind in mind. Ultimately, the child internalizes the parent's now-realistic mental representations in a way that bolsters the development of a sense of self (Fonagy et al. 2002a). Notably, effective parental mentalizing of the child not only promotes emotion regulation in the child but also serves to regulate parental emotion by preventing mutually frustrating and aversive parent-child interactions; a calmer child makes for a calmer parent.

Employing this theoretical model in collaboration with her colleagues, Slade (Sadler et al. 2006; Slade 2002; Slade et al. 2004) has developed a mentalizing-based parenting program, "Minding the Baby," for high-risk, first-time inner city parents and their infants. This community-based program extends from the pregnancy to the child's second birthday, and it integrates the traditional nurse home-visitation model with the infant-parent psychotherapy model that Fraiberg pioneered. The interdisciplinary program is staffed by licensed clinical social workers and advanced-practice nurse practitioners. Home visitations include a multiplicity of interventions: teaching mothers about basic infant care; providing them with educational materials and toys as well as necessities like diapers and food; and offering practical help in obtaining housing and social services as well as medical care for themselves and their baby. These forms of practical help provide the foundation for the mentalizing interventions insofar as they demonstrate the clinicians' accessibility and reliability, which is essential for the establishment of a secure base in the relationships.

Minding the Baby has the explicit goal of promoting reflective parenting by enhancing the mother's mentalizing with respect to herself and her infant. Rarely have the mothers in the program had secure attachment relationships with their own mother; many have a history of maltreatment and exposure to violence, abandonment, and betrayal. Concomitantly, mothers are liable to have a range of psychiatric disorders, including anxiety, depression, posttraumatic stress, and psychosis as well as alcohol and drug abuse. Accordingly, at the time of their enrollment in the program mothers typically show significantly impaired mentalizing, especially when they have a history of substance abuse.

The mentalizing-promoting interventions begin with the clinicians helping the mothers develop greater awareness of their own mental states. Mothers typically begin the program with few words for their emotional experience. They are helped to articulate their concerns about pregnancy and delivery; this help is especially crucial, for example, for mothers whose history of physical and sexual abuse leads to fears of being restrained during childbirth. These mothers are assisted in the development of a labor plan, and this intervention illustrates a basic principle of the model that promotes agency through mentalizing: mothers are helped to identify their feelings and to develop means of regulating them.

Through mentalizing the mother, the clinician not only helps the mother mentalize with respect to herself but also provides a model for the mother's mentalizing her baby. As Sadler and colleagues (2006) observe, "Understanding that the baby *has* feelings and desires is an achievement for most of our mothers" (p. 280; emphasis in original). Clinicians foster the mother's attentiveness and responsiveness to the infant's mental states by modeling—for example, by imitating and speaking for the baby. Tactfully, they intervene correctively when the mother engages in distorted or inaccurate mentalizing:

> One mother, for instance, began to tease her child when he cried after catching his finger in the door. "You're a faker!" she exclaimed, mocking him. The home visitor gently spoke for the baby: "Ooh, that hurt. You're kinda' scared and want Mommy to make it feel better." Thus, she was first trying to help mother *accurately* perceive the child's intention. Then, once mother began to see the child's distress, the home visitor could guide her toward comforting the child. By reframing the baby's intention for the mother, home visitors can correct derailed interactions. (Sadler et al. 2006, p. 282; emphasis in original)

The program also includes routine videotaping of mother-infant interactions, which social workers review with the mother. Observing the videotapes provides an opportunity for the social worker to speak for the baby. With the support of the home visitor, the mother is able to reflect on her own feelings and intentions as well as those of her baby at some remove from their interaction. Home visitors also assist mothers in playing with their baby, an activity that many mothers initially find challenging. Play affords an opportunity for the mother to imagine her baby's desires, feelings, and fantasies in a relatively non-threatening context—to mentalize in the freest sense of playing with ideas about mental states.

Initial findings from an ongoing experimental two-group longitudinal study are encouraging (Sadler et al. 2006). Families generally develop positive relationships with the home visitors; infant health outcomes are positive; mothers improve in mentalizing capacity; and very few infants show profoundly insecure (disorganized) attachment.

Child-Parent Psychotherapy

Slade (in press) has proposed that the reflective parenting approach provides a coherent theoretical framework to enhance the process of working with parents in child therapy in a way that goes beyond the traditional child guidance model. From an attachment theory perspective, she describes how, in the course of several years of seeing a boy in twice-weekly therapy and his mother in biweekly sessions, she had endeavored to strengthen the security of their attachment and, indeed, succeeded in doing so. In hindsight she recognized that without thinking about it consciously, she had strengthened the attachment relationship by virtue of helping the mother mentalize in relation to her son. Accordingly, she views the work with the parents as central to child psychotherapy rather than adjunctive to it.

Slade gives a vivid example of helping non-mentalizing parents of a six-year-old boy to move into a reflective stance. The parents were in the midst of a brutally acrimonious divorce, and their son was disoriented, immersed in frightening fantasies. Avoiding each other, the parents alternately would take off for days on the spur of the moment. In an effort to help the parents mentalize their son's experience, Slade spontaneously used a metaphor from an interview she had seen of a firefighter who was disoriented in the immediate aftermath of the September 11, 2001, terrorist attack on the World Trade Center. The firefighter was in radio contact with his comrades who were buried under rubble; desperately trying to find them, he asked them for a landmark, which they gave (the corner of West Street and Franklin). Weeping, the firefighter described how the corner had been demolished; it was *gone*. He had no basic landmarks. Slade used this graphic metaphor to help the parents see how their son's world had exploded, leaving him disoriented and desperately in need of anchors and restored predictability (Slade, in press).

Coates and her colleagues (2003a) applied the model of enhancing reflective parenting to interventions with parents and their children traumatized by the September 11th attacks. Coates (2003) makes the point that what converts stress into trauma is its being "undergone alone," and she rightly asserts that "one can begin to think of trauma and human relatedness as inversely related terms" (p. 3). Epidemiological studies indicated that one-fourth of New York City's children showed major psychiatric disorders after the disaster (Hoven et al. 2003). Yet the children's mental health status was strongly linked to the child-parent relationship. As Coates and colleagues reported, children whose parents were depressed were far more likely to have behavior problems and, most striking:

> children whose parents did not know how their children were responding after September 11 were 11.1 times more likely to have behavior problems at ages six to 11 and 4.0 more likely at ages 12 to 17. Parents who cannot keep their children's experience in mind after a traumatic event have more behaviorally disturbed children, and this effect is nearly three times greater in younger children than adolescents. These findings provide further confirmation of the importance of reflective functioning as a protective factor for children under circumstances of adversity. (Coates et al. 2003b, p. 33)

Accordingly, Coates and colleagues (2003b) developed a community intervention, a "Kid's Corner" centrally located in the city, in which children were encouraged to express their experience in play and which also facilitated parental reflectiveness. In addition to helping the parents understand their own traumatic experiences, clinicians helped parents to understand the traumatic basis of their children's problems and symptoms. Sadly, numerous narratives in Coates and colleagues' (2003a) volume illustrate poignantly what Fraiberg (Fraiberg et al. 1975) articulated many years previously: many parents were so traumatized by the events of September 11th that they were unable to mentalize their children's experience because it evoked their own unbearable emotional pain. Yet, as the findings for behavioral disturbance attest, the failure to mentalize escalates the painful experience.

Although not using the concept of mentalizing, Lieberman has developed a form of child-parent psychotherapy that further enriches the work we have described thus far. In an effort to extend Fraiberg's (Fraiberg et al. 1975) pioneering work to the first six years of life, Lieberman's (2004) approach is intended to improve the child's mental health by fostering greater reliance on the parents as a secure base, which rests on the parents' mentalizing capacity. Addressed to treating young children rather than infants, Lieberman's approach places less emphasis on the parents' childhood experience and greater emphasis on promoting a *psychological partnership*; the parent-child relationship is the vehicle for helping the child:

> Using the format of joint child-parent sessions, the therapist relies on play, behavioral interventions, and verbal interpretation to translate the emotional experience of the child to the parent and to explain the parent's behavior to the child in order to promote empathic understanding and encourage emotional reciprocity. (p. 98)

Keenly aware of the intergenerational transmission of trauma, Lieberman addresses the pernicious impact of the child's internalizing *distorted maternal attributions* (Lieberman 1997; Silverman and Lieberman 1999):

> Maternal attributions could be described as fixed beliefs that the mother has about her child's existential core, beliefs that she perceives as objective, accurate perceptions of the child's essence but might in fact reflect the mother's fantasies, including her fears, conflicts, and wishes about the child and the child's function in her life. (Lieberman 1997, p. 282)

Illustratively, Lieberman (1997) described a mother of a three-month-old daughter who felt that she did not have as much milk as she would have expected in the morning. The mother explained this to herself by perceiving her daughter as so cunning that she jumped from her crib to breastfeed while the mother was sleeping and then jumped back to her crib. This belief fulfilled the mother's wish that her daughter could care for herself when the mother was unavailable. Lieberman gave another example of a mother's elaborate characterization of her hypersexual two-year-old daughter as a Love Goddess. Similarly, Lieberman (2004) gave an example of a mother bringing her three-year-old boy for assessment; his punk-style haircut was complemented by a black leather jacket with a skulls-and-bones insignia on the back, looking like "a diminutive gang member" (p. 108) notwithstanding his shy and withdrawn demeanor. The mother had a history of violent relationships with men and her son was conceived during a rape at gunpoint. When the child was tearful and tried to climb on her lap after she returned from the bathroom, she told the therapist, "See? What did I tell you? He just pretends to need me, but he is really mean" (p. 108).

As Lieberman (2004) articulates, the hypersexual daughter and punk-like son are recipients of negative maternal attributions in a process of projective identification. Not only are the distorted attributions projected onto the child but also the parent pressures the child to behave in a way that is consistent with the attributions; when the child invariably yields to the pressure, the distorted projections are internalized—yet they remain alien to the true self, which the non-mentalizing parent has failed to discern.

Lieberman (2004) utilizes the joint play session as an opportunity for the therapist to reflect on the child's behavior, to speak for the child, and thus to help the parent (in our terms) mentalize: "By responding flexibly to the child's and the parent's behavior and narrative, the child-parent psychotherapist conveys the message that everything has meaning and everything the parent and child say and do is deserving of careful attention" (p. 112). For example, she worked with a mother who dealt ineffectively with her three-year-old son's fear of monsters by telling him repeatedly that monsters don't exist. The therapist helped the mother to adopt his perspective, saying "You know how some things can be real for us but not for other people? That is how it is with children. They really believe in monsters and see them in their imagination" (p. 115). This intervention was the basis for creating a psychological partnership in which the mother and son collaborated to ensure his feeling protected from the monsters.

While we strive to intervene in psychopathology, we must not lose sight of factors that promote resilience (Stein 2006). Fittingly, as a counterpoint to ghosts in the nursery, Lieberman and colleagues (Lieberman et al. 2005) have drawn attention to "angels in the nursery" and the corresponding intergenerational transmission of benevolent parental influences. We must keep in mind that reenactment is not always based on distorted attributions, nor is it only associated with traumatic memories: "Akin to the unknowing replaying of ghosts...there is an *effortless recapitulation* of loving interpersonal exchanges that brings back memories long forgotten" (p. 510; emphasis in original). The angels are critical in the process of interrupting the intergenerational transmission of trauma. Parents who retain some memory of being loved by a benevolent attachment figure despite trauma have an alternative model: "Instead of having no recourse but identification with the aggressor to feel secure, these parents could model themselves after 'angels in the nursery' perceived as powerful and benign" (p. 511). Hence Lieberman and colleagues propose a health-promoting process of *identification with the protector*. Accordingly, they urge clinicians working with traumatized persons to be mindful of eliciting benevolent childhood memories in a more balanced approach that promotes mentalizing:

> A therapeutic stance that gives equal importance to supportive early memories and to memories of conflict, abuse, or neglect should be established at the outset of treatment because the initial therapeutic sessions shape the client's perception of what the therapist considers worthy of attention. Cultivating a frame of mind where experiences of joy, intimacy, pleasure, and love are considered to be as worthy of therapeutic attention as negative experiences can be of great assistance in promoting momentum toward psychological health. Constricted and rigid images of the parent may then be rounded out into more humane and flexible perceptions that incorporate an understanding of the older generations' circumstances and the conditions that shaped their behavioral intergenerational transmission may then move backward as well as forward to encompass both the older generations and the young into a process of recognition and acceptance that can result into the intergenerational transmission not only of trauma but also of forgiveness and compassion. (Lieberman et al. 2005, p. 517)

Mentalization-Based Family Therapy (MBFT)

Peter Fonagy, Mary Target, Pasco Fearon, and their colleagues developed Mentalization-Based Family Therapy (formerly called Short-Term Mentalization and Relational Therapy; SMART) as a mentalizing-focused approach to family therapy with children and adolescents (Child and Family Program 2005; Fearon et al. 2006a). As Slade (in press) articulated in relation to her reflective parenting approach in child-parent psychotherapy, the general therapeutic strategy in MBFT is not fundamentally new; yet a consistent focus on mentalizing lends coherence to the clinical process (Fearon et al. 2006a). As with family therapy approaches more generally, the therapist makes every effort to involve all relevant family members, including parents who are separated. MBFT has been conducted with children ranging from seven years old to adolescence. MBFT includes a psychoeducational component (see Chapter 10, "Psychoeducation") in articulating the treatment model to the family and educating the family about the nature of mentalizing and how mentalizing can be helpful in addressing family problems.

MBFT was designed as a 6- to 12-session intervention that is not intended to resolve all problems but rather to promote longer-term resilience by cultivating skills in mentalizing that will help family members support each other and engage in constructive and collaborative problem solving. MBFT interventions exemplify the conviction that presenting problems stem from mentalizing failures and that mentalizing failures are relationship-specific. Hence the treatment focuses on "relationship problems and mentalizing solutions" (Fearon et al. 2006a, p. 203). Broadly, as modeled by the therapist, MBFT consistently promotes a mentalizing attitude, that is, a spirit of inquisitiveness and curiosity about mental states coupled with an appreciation of the limitations of mindreading capacities. Thus the MBFT therapist focuses consistently on engaging family members' interest in understanding each others' mental states as well as correcting distortions in understanding. The seven core interventions employed in MBFT (Fearon et al. 2006a) are displayed in Table 8–1.

As in other psychoeducational approaches, MBFT incorporates tasks and games that encourage an appreciation for the playful nature of mentalizing as well as providing family members with direct experience in perspective taking. For example, in the "feeling hot-potato" game, the child picks up a card listing a basic emotion such as sad, mad, or scared. The child enacts the emotions as she or he experiences them, and then (when catching the hot-potato) each adult is placed in the position of reenacting the emotions as the child experiences and expresses them, subject to correction by the child. Another example is the "trading places" game in which parents play the role that their children play in various situations (e.g., doing chores or going to school); children coach their parents in what to think, say, and feel.

MBFT is a work in progress: it is a manualized intervention (Child and Family Program 2005) with an evolving training module (Williams et al. 2006) that is in the process of being evaluated for effectiveness.

TABLE 8–1.   CORE INTERVENTIONS IN MENTALIZATION-BASED FAMILY
THERAPY (MBFT)

- **Identifying, highlighting, and praising examples of skillful mentalizing**
  (e.g., commenting to a mother about her son's positive response to her
  demonstrated interest in his point of view)

- **Sharing and provoking curiosity**
  (e.g., showing interest in what a child feels and sharing hypotheses with an
  inquisitive attitude, reflected by phrases such as, "I'm not sure I've got this
  right, but I was wondering…")

- **Pausing and searching**
  (e.g., interrupting a non-mentalizing interaction and indicating an interest
  in exactly what each individual in the interaction was thinking and feeling
  as the interaction unfolded)

- **Identifying preferred non-mentalizing narratives**
  (e.g., highlighting repetitive conversations that characteristically lead
  nowhere, so as to move family members into a mentalizing stance)

- **Identifying and labeling hidden feeling states**
  (e.g., encouraging family members to label their feelings and inquiring as
  to what other feelings are not being recognized or expressed)

- **Using hypotheticals and counterfactuals**
  (e.g., "What if?" questions that encourage family members to play
  with ideas)

- **Therapists' making use of self**
  (i.e., communicating about their own mental states and how these are
  affected by family members' behavior and interactions)

Recapitulation

The innovative work with parents and their children that we have reviewed in this chapter exemplifies best the translation of basic developmental research into clinical practice. As we reviewed in Chapter 3
("Development"), the synergistic development of mentalizing and secure attachment begins in infancy and extends into early childhood.
What we call mentalizing has been studied meticulously in parent-child
relationships under such rubrics as mind-mindedness (Meins et al.
2002), reflective parenting (Slade 2005), and maternal insightfulness
(Oppenheim and Koren-Karie 2002). These parental mentalizing capacities are part and parcel of the evolution of attachment relationships
(Fonagy 2006) and, as such, they are natural and intuitive. As Darlene's
experience illustrates, however, early trauma in attachment relationships impairs the natural development of these capacities.

We are now well placed to implement Anna Freud's vision (Hurry 1998): we have theory-driven, research-based clinical interventions to provide needed *developmental help* for children and their parents. Central to all the interventions we have discussed in this chapter is the therapist's modeling mentalizing of the child for the traumatized parent whose capacity to do so has been compromised. The need for these interventions is all too plain. Although alleviating suffering in children and their parents will always be in the forefront of the clinician's mind, we must also keep in mind the preventive goals of interrupting patterns of intergenerational transmission of trauma (Oliver 1993) as well as heading off the highly likely development of childhood psychopathology into psychopathology in adulthood (Kim-Cohen et al. 2003).

Key Clinical Points

- *Transmission of trauma:* The intergenerational transmission of trauma is mediated by non-mentalizing reenactments in which, through externalizations, traumatized parents are liable to traumatize their children.

- *Modeling in therapy:* In mentalizing-oriented parent-infant therapy, the therapist models mentalizing for parents—for example, in the form of mind-minded commentary on the infant's behavior. In addition, the therapist helps parents mentalize their own trauma and its influence on their relationship with their infant.

- *Focus on process:* Consistent with the general tenor of mentalizing-focused treatment, the Mentalization-Based Family Therapy (MBFT) approach to family therapy focuses on process rather than content: rather than endeavoring to solve specific family problems, interventions promote family-wide mentalizing by helping all family members to recognize and articulate their varying perspectives.

Chapter 9

Borderline Personality Disorder

In this chapter we apply the concept of mentalizing to the development and treatment of borderline personality disorder (BPD). Our approach to BPD is predicated on the assumption that treatment interventions will be most effective when they address core psychopathological processes as understood from a developmental perspective. We focus on mentalizing as a core component of psychopathology and treatment. In the context of BPD, we maintain this focus not only because impaired mentalizing is central to problems with affect regulation and disturbances in attachment relationships but also because a focus on mentalizing in treatment reduces the likelihood of causing harm in a group of patients who may be particularly vulnerable to the negative effects of psychotherapeutic interventions.

We begin this chapter by placing BPD in a broader developmental framework that respects the sheer complexity of the disorder and its development. Next we articulate core developmental processes that bear on mentalizing and contribute to vulnerability to BPD, and we then review the links between disturbances in attachment relationships and impaired mentalizing. This developmental ground provides the foundation for our account of mentalizing failures in the phenomenology and symptomatology of BPD. We conclude the chapter with a description of mentalization-based treatment programs for BPD and research on their effectiveness.

Developmental Framework

In our concern with mentalizing, we should not give short shrift to the complexity of BPD symptomatology, which is characterized by numerous disturbances in cognitive, emotional, behavioral, and interpersonal functioning. Commonly, these deficits include emotional instability; feelings of emptiness; identity disturbance; impulsivity; suicidal behavior and deliberate self-harm; enmeshed, dysfunctional, and volatile relationships; inordinate anxieties about being abandoned by those one cares about; and paranoid thoughts (Lieb et al. 2004). Along with its complexity, the sheer severity of BPD bears underscoring. More than most other personality disorders, BPD has a powerful negative impact on quality of life (Cramer et al. 2006), and BPD is associated with exceptional exposure to negative life events, especially those involving interpersonal stress (Pagano et al. 2004). Compared to those with other personality disorders, persons with BPD are at higher risk for suicide attempts (Yen et al. 2003), and, not surprisingly, they use more mental health services than those with major depressive disorder (Bender et al. 2006).

Plainly, the complex symptomatology of BPD is matched by an equally complex etiology. To place our focus on mentalizing impairments in broader perspective, we view the developmental vulnerabilities to BPD as evolving in the context of *transactional dynamics in attachment relationships*. Table 9–1 enumerates the fundamental assumptions of the dynamic developmental view we embrace (Crick et al. 2005; Hughes and Ensor, in press).

Depue and Lenzenweger (2005) have proposed an influential model for the etiology of BPD that illustrates the dynamic transactional approach. They suggest that we should think of personality disorders as fluid multidimensional configurations produced by specific confluences of neurobehavioral dimensions that exist within the space of normal personality. Accordingly, BPD can be more or less stable, depending on multiple contextual factors (Gunderson et al. 2003; Morey and Zanarini 2000). As McGlashan and colleagues put it, "DSM-IV personality disorders are hybrids of more stable traits and less stable

---

TABLE 9–1.   DEVELOPMENTAL ASSUMPTIONS

• **Stage-specific manifestation of symptoms:** Symptoms of the disorder will be manifested differently at different developmental periods.

• **Stage-specific impact of deficits:** A specific influence may be critical at a certain stage of development but matter less at other stages; concomitantly, the impact of a specific deficit will relate to the child's stage of development.

• **Multiple precursors of mentalizing capacity:** A complex capacity such as mentalizing will have multiple components, and each component will have its own developmental precursors, mediating mechanisms, and related compensatory strategies.

• **Disorders in relation to developmental tasks:** Contextual determinants will moderate the relationship of risk factors and pathogenic outcomes, and thus atypical personality development can be identified only by considering the difficulties in negotiating developmentally appropriate, normative tasks that have relevance for BPD.

• **Models for disorder and recovery:** Given what we know about the natural course of BPD, and particularly its potentially reversible character, the dynamic model must explain not only the emergence of the disorder but also the process of spontaneous—and sometimes dramatic—recovery.

---

symptomatic behaviors" (McGlashan et al. 2005). Hence, while personality normally mediates complex emotional responses to interpersonal events that are likely to enhance adaptation, personality *disorder* appears when these emotional responses are *maladaptive*—either absent or inappropriately intense. Fear of abandonment, for example, can be construed as an inappropriately intense variant of a normal affiliative response.

Transactional models have the potential for change built into them: in the course of modifying their environment, individuals change their own characteristics as well as the environment in ways that potentially alter the nature of future interactions between the two (Cicchetti and Rogosch 2002). The transactional model also characterizes both the emergence of mentalizing capacity and its characteristic failure in BPD. For example, the disorganization of the attachment system might lead to a child's being increasingly manipulative and controlling, and then such controlling actions might undermine the caregiver's capacity to provide a normative playful environment for the child. Of course, transactional dynamics characterize not only the moderation of the child's interactions with the social environment but also the broader phenomenon of nature interacting with nurture. Initial studies suggest significant genetic contributions to BPD, particularly as evident in affect dysregulation (Lieb et al. 2004; Torgersen et al. 2000). Longitudinal studies indicate that children who go on to develop BPD are vulnerable not least because they are likely to bring hard-to-manage temperaments to the parent-child relationship (Depue and Lenzenweger 2001). For example, we can imagine that parents will have difficulty interacting in a manner that supports the child's autonomy when the child is high in novelty seeking, need for stimulation, reactivity, and anxiety proneness (Cloninger et al. 1993). More broadly, social experience will affect both brain structure and function—and, by the same token, brain structure and function profoundly influence subjective experience.

The dynamic developmental model we adopt implies a complex *cascade* of developmental causation. We expect early experience and early consequences of developmental processes to moderate and shape the impact of later developmental stages, be these maturational or psychosocial. For persons with BPD, we assume that the mental structures established during early phases of development are insufficiently robust to withstand the increasing challenges that later childhood, adolescent, and early adult experience inevitably bring; hence these later challenges precipitate a catastrophic collapse of functioning. The purported childhood markers of this vulnerability include a hostile-paranoid world view; intense, unstable, and inappropriate emotion; impulsivity; overly close relationships; and a lack of a sense of self (Crick et al. 2005). Baird and colleagues (2005) use a persuasive metaphor to describe the neuropathological impact of biological changes in adolescence on the brain of persons with vulnerability to BPD: these adolescent changes are "like attaching a 330 horsepower motor to a cardboard box to make a vehicle; it simply will not work" (p. 1046). The "cardboard box" we have in mind is precarious mentalizing, and we now turn to an examination of core developmental deficits that contribute to this precariousness.

Developmental Processes That Create Vulnerability to BPD

Thus far we have staked out the general territory by construing BPD as a multifaceted disorder rooted in transactional dynamics intertwined with impaired mentalizing. Next we highlight three domains of developmental research pertinent to mentalizing: affect regulation, effortful control of attention, and social cognition; as we discuss, attachment relationships play a key role in each of these three domains.

Affect Regulation

Clinicians who treat patients with BPD generally agree that excessive negative affect coupled with impaired affect regulation is central to the disorder (Conklin et al. 2006). The DSM-IV-TR diagnostic criteria include "affective instability due to a marked reactivity of mood (e.g., intense episodic dysphoria, irritability, or anxiety)" as well as "inappropriate, intense anger or difficulty controlling anger" (American Psychiatric Association 2000, p. 710). This characteristic affect dysregulation was suggested originally in the psychoanalytic literature (Schmideberg 1947) and has since been reaffirmed in writings on the subject from a variety of theoretical perspectives—biological, cognitive-behavioral, and interpersonal. In their definitive review, Siever and colleagues (2002) consider problems with affect regulation to be the hallmark of one of two endophenotypes of BPD—the other being impulsive aggression. Linehan (1993a) considers affect dysregulation to be one of three key vulnerabilities, the others being low distress-tolerance and an invalidating environment. To anticipate our argument: as depicted simply in Figure 9–1, affect dysregulation and impaired mentalizing interact in a vicious circle; furthermore, *both* of these intertwined disturbances interact in a vicious circle with a non-mentalizing attachment environment.

Several studies show persons with BPD to demonstrate high levels of affective reactivity. Individuals with BPD experience more negative affect, and negative experience tends to have higher salience for them (Brown et al. 2002; Korfine and Hooley 2000). In the 6-year McLean follow-along study, 90% of more than 300 participants endorsed affective

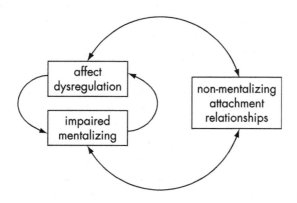

FIGURE 9–1.   IMPACT OF A NONVALIDATING ENVIRONMENT.

instability as a characteristic feature of their condition (Zanarini et al. 2003). Factor analysis of symptom presentations of 668 participants in a major longitudinal study of personality disorders (Sanislow et al. 2002) yielded three factors: disturbed relatedness, behavioral dysregulation (i.e., impulsivity), and affective dysregulation.

Going further, some specialists have construed BPD as a mood spectrum disorder or, more specifically, as a bipolar spectrum disorder with extremely rapid cycling (McKinnon and Pies 2006). Consistent with this view, there is modest co-occurrence of these disorders in terms of longitudinal course and risk for new onsets (Gunderson et al. 2006b). Yet the pattern of affect dysregulation commonly observed in BPD can be distinguished from mood variation in bipolar disorder (Goodwin and Jamison 2007); affective dysregulation in BPD is highly situational and is primarily associated with high levels of interpersonal sensitivity (Bradley and Westen 2005). Furthermore, in contrast to the relatively favorable course of BPD (Zanarini et al. 2006), the natural course of bipolar disorder is one of recurrent episodes with substantial residual symptomatology (Judd et al. 2002). Nonetheless, given the overlap between these two disorders, it is hazardous to diagnose BPD cross-sectionally during a mood episode and, conversely, it is important not to overlook the diagnosis of bipolar disorder in the context of BPD symptoms (Goodwin and Jamison 2007).

Neurobiological research buttresses clinical evidence of affective dysregulation in BPD (Gabbard et al. 2006)—and, as we discuss shortly, this dysregulation is intertwined with problems in the effortful control of attention. Patients with BPD show evidence of structural and functional impairments in brain areas normally considered to be central in affect regulation (Putnam and Silk 2005). For example, functional imaging studies show evidence of disrupted amygdala functioning in BPD, possibly associated with the salience of negative affect (Donegan et al. 2003; Herpertz et al. 2001a). In addition, imaging studies show evidence of disrupted serotonergic functioning in the orbitofrontal cortex that may link to impulsivity (New et al. 2004; Soloff et al. 2003b) and the diminished ability to modulate or control destructive urges (Skodol et al. 2002). These deficits, in turn, may be linked to increased cortisol levels associated with chronic stress and overactivity in the hypothalamic-pituitary-adrenal axis that not only blunts serotonergic activity (Minzenberg et al. 2006a) but also disrupts hippocampal functioning in a vicious circle with chronic stress (Schmahl et al. 2003). Yet we caution that the presence of neurobiological differences in either structure or function must not be equated with exclusively biological causation. Neurophysiological differences may result from social or family influences or, more likely, from complex transactional process between constitutional (e.g., temperamental) factors and psychosocial processes (Fruzzetti et al. 2005).

We have emphasized how the absence of parental mentalizing of the child's emotion contributes to impaired development of affect regulation in the child (see Chapter 3, "Development"). Evidence suggests that the absence of marked contingent mirroring at six months is associated with the development of disorganized attachment at 12–18 months (Koós and Gergely 2001). The disorganized pattern in infancy is characterized by the infants' incoherent and ineffective attempts to self-regulate upon reunion with their caregiver after a brief separation. Specifically, following separation, infants manifesting disorganized attachment exhibit such behaviors as freezing, rocking, and self-harm (e.g., head banging) as well as dissociative states (Lyons-Ruth and Jacobvitz 1999). Disorganized infants go on to develop highly controlling oppositional behavior in middle childhood (Green and Goldwyn 2002; van IJzendoorn et al. 1999) and dissociative features in adolescence and adulthood (Lyons-Ruth 2003; Sroufe et al. 2005; Weinfield et al. 2004). Disorganized attachment also has been linked to impaired self-control and affect dysregulation (Kochanska and Murray 2000; Kochanska et al. 2001). Thus we speculate that the absence of marked contingent mirroring experience in infancy creates a vulnerability to affect dysregulation by creating less robust self-representations of internal states of emotional arousal. By failing to promote the capacity to mentalize emotion, this developmental process undermines the capacity for self-regulation and contributes to the unpredictable quality and excessive intensity of emotional experience.

Although we have emphasized the caregiver's role in promoting affect regulation, the transactional model also incorporates contributions from the infant's side. One might imagine a subtype of BPD in which disturbances of affect regulation result primarily from deficits on the infant's side of the parent-infant dyad; such deficits in infant reactivity might challenge or even render impossible the establishment of parental contingent responding. For example, abnormal hippocampal or amygdala functioning could contribute to highly anxious and emotionally labile infant behavior, presenting the caregiver with an infant who is not able to benefit from the ordinary regulating qualities of the attachment relationship. This constellation might well create disorganized attachment relationships that are principally driven by the child's constitutional vulnerabilities (Lakatos et al. 2000). Yet we are cautious about overestimating the influence of constitutional factors in the infant on the parent-child relationship at this earliest developmental phase, inasmuch as security of attachment is rare among infant behaviors in showing no heritability in twin studies (Bokhorst et al. 2003; Fearon et al. 2006b). Hence we have ample reason to give thorough attention to environmental influences.

Effortful Control of Attention

Patients with BPD show evidence of general impairment of executive function (Belbo et al. 2006; Dinn et al. 2004), although the extent to which neurocognitive deficits are specific to BPD versus being associated with comorbid major depression remains somewhat controversial (Fertuck et al. 2006). We have suggested that disorganized attachment will disrupt the development of an agentive sense of self and that problems in effortful control (Posner and Rothbart 2000) may be a concomitant of lack of agency (Fonagy 2001b). Recent studies of attention processes in patients with BPD are consistent with our proposal (Hoermann et al. 2005; Lenzenweger et al. 2004; Posner et al. 2002). A comprehensive review of neurocognitive research (LeGris and van Reekum 2006) identified 36 studies of persons who were suicidal or diagnosed with BPD; regardless of the level of depression, impairment in one or more cognitive domains was typical. Most of these cognitive impairments involved some specific or generalized deficits linked to the dorsolateral prefrontal and orbitofrontal regions; these regions are closely involved with dysfunctions of self-control, particularly the effortful control of attention. Most commonly reported were problems with response inhibition and decision making along with visual memory impairment. Many studies also found impairment in attention and verbal memory along with impairment in visuospatial organization. Much of this dysfunctional cognition appears to be at the level of metacognition (see Chapter 2, "Mentalizing").

Patients with BPD show diminished ability to actively suppress irrelevant information when it is of an aversive nature; they also perform poorly in tasks that require them to inhibit or put out of their mind ideas that are peripheral to their primary focus. For example, individuals with BPD remember words that they were instructed to forget, especially when these words are of specific emotional concern to them (Domes et al. 2006; Korfine and Hooley 2000). Recent findings link these failures of selective retrieval to a constellation of brain activity that entails hyperactivation of a self-referential mode of information processing and a lack of differential amygdala, orbitofrontal, and cingulate activations in response to emotionally salient and neutral stimuli (Schnell et al. 2006). The failure to direct attention voluntarily appears to link directly to the problems of unstable affect we considered earlier, but not to self-reported impulsiveness (Domes et al. 2006); the latter may be a separate, less socially determined aspect of vulnerability in patients with BPD. In any case, combined with affect dysregulation, impaired control of attention will undermine the capacity to cope with interpersonal stress. Hence persons with BPD might appear to act rashly because they give insufficient consideration to what their social partners think or feel. More specifically, they are not able to exclude from consideration a range of hypotheses about others' thoughts and feelings for which there is little evidence and which most other persons would ignore or inhibit.

How is effortful control related to early experience? We reviewed evidence linking secure attachment to attention earlier (see Chapter 2, "Mentalizing"). Self-regulation may be modeled by the caregiver's regulation of the infant's activity. Suggestions that joint attention with a caregiver serves a self-organizing function in early development (Mundy and Neal 2001) are consistent with a well-demonstrated relation between attachment security and general intelligence (van IJzendoorn and van Vliet-Visser 1988). Research indicates that the development of self-control is rooted in mutual responsiveness, which, perforce, is predicated on mentalizing interactions. Kochanska and colleagues' longitudinal research (Kochanska et al. 1996, 1997, 2000) found that higher levels of mutual responsiveness in mother-child dyads between ages 26 and 41 months predicted greater self-control, the internalization of maternal rules, and a lessened need for maternal control and coercion. Two large longitudinal studies also showed that individual differences in effortful control were relatively stable from age 30 months onward, suggesting that effortful control may indeed be one of the capacities that can be traced back to early development. Children in Kochanska's longitudinal sample (Kochanska et al. 2001; Kochanska and Murray 2000) whose interactions with their mother were characterized by greater mutual responsiveness manifested more effortful control and were better able to follow both "Do" and "Don't" commands. A unique study by Kochanska (2001) demonstrated that infants' attachment classification at 14 months predicts their emotional developmental paths over the first 3 years, and attachment is an even better predictor than the earlier history of emotional responsiveness.

Consistent with the beneficial impact of mutual responsiveness, there is considerable evidence that the absence of controlling behavior on the part of the parent—paradigmatic of non-mentalizing interactions—predicts internalization of control in preschool children. The program of work by Ryan and colleagues has demonstrated that on the whole, parents who are controlling and less supportive of their child's autonomy have children who are less motivated to achieve, more likely to engage in risky behaviors, and less likely to experience well-being and mental health (Ryan and Deci 2003). The benign effect of parental support for autonomy persists into adolescence, evident in self-worth, identity, and self-determination (Chirkov and Ryan 2001; Ryan and Kuczkowski 1994).

In sum, we see secure attachment with the primary caregiver as predicated on mentalizing interactions; such interactions facilitate the child's capacity to coordinate and regulate internal states by effortful control of attention. By implication, such internal control relates to a sense of autonomy and agency, and it contributes to the ability to engage in adaptive and mutually reciprocal interpersonal interactions. By contrast, non-mentalizing interactions, in synergy with disturbed attachment relationships, are liable to undermine effortful control of attention as well as executive functions and self-regulation more broadly; BPD is one potential outcome of this adverse developmental process.

Social Cognition

Characteristic patterns of disturbed interpersonal relatedness distinguish BPD from other personality disorders (Livesley and Jackson 1992; Skodol et al. 2006). For example, interpersonal stressors are more likely to precipitate suicide attempts in BPD than in other disorders associated with depression (Brodsky et al. 2006). Moreover, deficits in social cognition render individuals with BPD particularly susceptible to interpersonal stressors. Observational studies consistently suggest that in interpersonal relationships, individuals with BPD exhibit not only emotional hyperresponsiveness (Herpertz 2003; Leichsenring and Sachsse 2002) but also deficits in emotion recognition and the capacity for empathy (Bland et al. 2004; Soloff et al. 2003a). Yet deficits in social cognition are context dependent; for example, impaired emotion recognition is most evident for complex emotional stimuli in the context of antagonism and threat (Minzenberg et al. 2006b). Similarly, clinical experience suggests that cognitive functioning more generally will be most perturbed in the context of emotionally self-referential information concerning abandonment, persecution, abuse, or torture (Zanarini et al. 1998). Accordingly, persons with BPD are impaired in interpersonal problem solving—for example, formulating less specific solutions on means–end problem-solving tasks and reporting higher levels of negative attitudes and a more impulsive-careless style of solving social problems (Bray et al. 2007). Work from Westen's laboratory demonstrated that compared to those with other disorders such as major depression, patients with BPD represent others' internal states with less complexity and differentiation (Baker et al. 1992; Westen et al. 1990a). Accordingly, the diagnosis of BPD is associated with impairments on mentalizing tasks (N.A. Stokes, J.D. Feigenbaum, P. Fonagy, et al.: "Theory of Mind in Borderline Personality Disorder," submitted for publication).

In sum, we interpret the clinical and research literature as showing that patients with BPD have vulnerabilities in the higher-order integration of social information; in turn, maladaptive ways of coping with these vulnerabilities generate some of the more serious symptoms of the disorder. Plainly, interpersonal problems encompass a whole constellation of difficulties, including dramatic shifts from idealization to disillusionment with others, frantic efforts to avoid perceived abandonment, and inappropriate interpersonal aggression (Raine 1993). Yet emerging literature suggests that all these interpersonal problems may share a common mechanism, namely, transient difficulties in accurately differentiating and representing the mental states of others who are significant to them as well as in maintaining a firm grasp of their own subjective experience (Fonagy et al. 2000; Gunderson 2001). Hence persons with BPD are faced with the unfortunate combination of a proclivity to experience (and actively evoke) distress in relationships *and* an impaired ability to engage in interpersonal problem solving—especially in the context of emotionally intense attachment relationships.

Attachment Disturbance and Impaired Mentalizing in BPD

Throughout this book we have emphasized the close connection between attachment and mentalizing, and central to our view of BPD is the contention that precarious mentalizing stems from disturbed attachment relationships. In the first part of this section, we review four lines of evidence for this view: 1) insecure attachment patterns in adults with BPD, 2) a history of disturbed parent-child relationships in persons with BPD, 3) intergenerational transmission of BPD in the form of parent-child concordance for the disorder, and 4) a history of downright traumatic attachment relationships in persons who develop BPD. In the second part of this section, we link BPD to impaired mentalizing in attachment relationships.

Evidence for Attachment Disturbance in BPD

Several longitudinal studies spanning 18 years or more indicate that early attachment insecurity is a relatively stable (i.e., enduring) charac-

teristic of the affected individual, particularly when the insecurity occurs in conjunction with subsequent negative life events (Hamilton
2000; Waters et al. 2000; Weinfield et al. 2000). Persons suffering from
BPD show a pattern of insecure attachment. Two longitudinal studies
that followed children from infancy to early adulthood revealed associations between insecure attachment in early childhood and BPD symptoms on follow-up (Lyons-Ruth et al. 2005; Sroufe et al. 2005). Levy
(2005) ably reviewed the relation of BPD to adult attachment patterns.
Nine of the reported studies employed the best available assessment
tool for adult attachment, the Adult Attachment Interview (Main and
Goldwyn 1994); two further studies used clinical rating scales; and over
a dozen studies used self-report measures. There is little doubt that BPD
is strongly associated with one form or another of insecure attachment;
interview studies, for example, suggest that only 6%–8% of persons
with BPD show secure attachment. More specifically, interview studies
consistently show an excess of insecure-disorganized attachment, and
questionnaire studies characteristically reveal fearful-avoidant and preoccupied attachment patterns.

Consistent with the extensive evidence of insecure patterns of adult
attachment in persons with BPD is equally consistent evidence of problematic parenting and parental bonding in their childhood history
(Johnson et al. 2001; Paris 2003; Russ et al. 2003). Yet most studies have
the limitation of retrospective designs. Hence Johnson and colleagues'
(2006) longitudinal study is especially noteworthy. These researchers
conducted a community-based investigation of 593 families whom they
interviewed during the index offspring's childhood (age 6 years), adolescence (14 and 16 years), young adulthood (22 years), and later adulthood (33 years). They employed the Structured Clinical Interview for
DSM-IV Personality Disorders (First et al. 1997) to assess personality
disorders in the offspring, and they related these diagnoses to parenting
behaviors observed during the childrearing years. They also controlled
for childhood behavioral or emotional problems as well as parental psychiatric disorders. Increased risk for personality disorders in young and
later adulthood was associated with the number of different types of
problematic parental behaviors observed in the home during the childrearing years. More specifically, low levels of parental affection or nur-
turing were associated with elevated risk for BPD as well as antisocial,
paranoid, and schizotypal personality disorder. Aversive parental behaviors such as harsh punishments also increased the risk for BPD and
paranoid personality disorder. Moreover, the findings indicated that
childhood behavior problems did not predict BPD, which argues
against a child-to-parent effect; in addition, parental psychiatric disor-

der (Axis I) did not predict BPD, which weighs against genetic media-
tion. The crucial developmental factor was problematic parental
behavior. Furthermore, the strength of the association between problematic parenting and personality does not decrease between young
and later adulthood, indicating that a long-term vulnerability has been
created by these adverse early experiences. Finally, the study suggests
that both neglect and physical abuse additively increase the likelihood
of personality disorder and, as we will continue to elaborate, are liable
to undermine the full development of mentalizing.

Several additional studies have related family disturbance to the development of BPD. In general, low family cohesion and high instability
have been shown to characterize families of patients with BPD (Feldman et al. 1995). Albeit with less methodological sophistication, some
older cross-sectional studies found that mothers of adolescents with
BPD rated themselves as being less empathic, more egocentric, and less
differentiated (Golomb et al. 1994; Guttman and Laporte 2000). Parents
of college students scoring high on measures of BPD symptoms rated
themselves retrospectively as having been overinvolved or inconsistent
(Bezirganian et al. 1993; Brennan and Shaver 1998).

Such global observations, however, do not address the interactive
processes that might dispose a child to develop BPD. A fascinating longitudinal study from Lyons-Ruth's laboratory (Lyons-Ruth et al. 2005)
examined such interactions. Albeit in a small sample, the study showed
that disrupted maternal communications in infancy correlated significantly with symptoms of borderline pathology assessed at age 18.
Disrupted communications included frightening behavior, grossly mis-
attuned emotional responding, and role reversals (e.g., seeking comfort
from the infant); these are the kinds of behaviors indicative of a significant parental failure in mentalizing the child. Moreover, the magnitude
of the effect was substantial, inasmuch as 40% of the infants of the
mothers with disrupted affective communication later displayed features of BPD, compared to only 12% of those whose mothers did not
show disrupted communication. Notably, inappropriate maternal withdrawal from the infant most strongly predicted symptoms of BPD in the
child 17 years later. Beyond disrupted communication, additional predictors of later BPD included the mother's referral to social services for
documented maltreatment of the infant as well as the total lifetime level
of abuse of the child as reported in adolescence. The specificity is considerable: half of the high-risk, clinically referred infants displayed features of BPD, compared with only 9% of matched controls.

Although longitudinal studies are few, we have a general consensus
on the transgenerational transmission of attachment behaviors, and

therefore observations of the parenting behaviors of mothers with BPD are informative with respect to the development of this disorder (Fonagy et al. 1995; van IJzendoorn 1995; van IJzendoorn and Bakermans-Kranenburg 1997). Observations of mothers with BPD reveal anomalies in their interactions with their infants. For example, mothers with BPD are unable to modulate their emotional expression in interactions with their infants in a laboratory situation that requires mothers to adopt a still-face demeanor and then to reengage with their infant; non-contingent interactions were characteristic of the reengagement phase (Danon and Graignic 2003). A carefully controlled experimental study using the still-face paradigm revealed that mothers with BPD showed more intrusiveness and insensitivity towards their two-month-olds (Crandell et al. 2003). A subsequent study also showed more intrusive mothering with 12-month-olds, who, in turn, were more likely to be disorganized in their attachment (Hobson et al. 2005).

The impact of these anomalous attachment experiences is evident in significant emotional and behavioral problems in the offspring. Children of mothers with BPD have been shown to have more psychiatric diagnoses, including symptoms characteristic of BPD (Weiss et al. 1996). When asked to make up stories with various prompts, young children of mothers with BPD provide more negatively toned narratives that include more intrusions of traumatic material (Macfie et al. 2005). We speculate that anomalies in the early experience of mirroring are pernicious in creating vulnerability for traumatic experience. Such vulnerability might amplify the impact of less intrinsically traumatic experiences or might preclude the natural capacity to heal—or both. There is one pertinent study on the transgenerational transmission of traumatic experience: the probability of combat-related PTSD was much higher in the parents of offspring with BPD than in a matched control group (Eurlings-Bontekoe et al. 2003). Yet we recognize that in the absence of later adversity (e.g., exposure to traumatic events or vicarious trauma through transgenerational transmission), anomalous early experiences might not lead to serious sequelae such as BPD (Fonagy 1999).

Traumatic experience in childhood attachment relationships represents the extreme of anomalous parent-child interactions. Extensive research has linked early attachment trauma to the development of BPD. For example, Bradley and Westen (2005) found that a childhood history of lengthy and traumatic separation or permanent loss differentiated patients with BPD from those with other personality disorders as well as from those with other Axis I disorders such as schizophrenia and depression. A meta-analytic review found that 20–40% of BPD patients experienced traumatic separations from one or both parents in childhood (Gunderson and Sabo

1993). A more recent summary of the literature (Levy 2005) estimates separation and loss at 37–64% but identifies four studies that failed to confirm these findings. Hence experience of separation and loss appears to be neither necessary nor sufficient for the development of BPD.

Numerous clinical and empirical studies have linked childhood trauma, and childhood sexual abuse in particular, to BPD (Herman et al. 1989; Zanarini 1997; Zanarini et al. 1997). Moreover, some studies have raised the possibility that particular characteristics and patterns of maltreatment may be specific to BPD; such patterns include severity of abuse, age at onset, number or types of abuse, the relational closeness to the abuser, and the number of caregivers involved (McLean and Gallop 2003; Silk et al. 1995; Yen et al. 2002). As already suggested, childhood sexual abuse is most often considered to be etiologically linked to BPD on the basis of its high prevalence in this group (Battle et al. 2004) and its association with outcome (Gunderson et al. 2006a).

Linking Attachment-Related Mentalizing Deficits to BPD

In the first part of this book (Chapter 3, "Development") we reviewed evidence linking secure attachment with robust mentalizing and attachment trauma with impaired mentalizing. Having built a case linking attachment disturbance and mentalizing impairments to possible developmental precursors of BPD, we now consider evidence linking maltreatment-related mentalizing deficits to the *diagnosis* of BPD. In two studies employing attachment narratives, we examined the relation between maltreatment, mentalizing capacity, and BPD. In a sample of 86 individuals with a diagnosis of personality disorder we found that 97% of patients who had a history of maltreatment and poor mentalizing capacity met criteria for BPD (Fonagy et al. 1996). We replicated these findings in a study of criminal violence, showing that persons with personality disorder who had a history of criminal violence were most likely to fail to mentalize in an attachment context (Levinson and Fonagy 2004). In a more recent unpublished study, we matched participants for gender, age, education, and Axis I diagnoses and found that those who met criteria for BPD performed more poorly than a group without personality disorders (or with non–cluster B personality disorders) in a nonverbal measure of mentalizing, that is, the Reading the Mind in the Eyes Test (Baron-Cohen et al. 2001). Further analyses revealed that those with a history of adversity who had low mentalizing scores also were more likely to have a BPD diagnosis.

Yet, inasmuch as many patients with BPD do *not* experience sexual or physical abuse (Paris 2004), an etiological model also must explain the development of BPD for non-abused individuals. Conversely, the majority of abuse victims will not develop a personality disorder (Binder et al. 1996; Horwitz et al. 2001). Given the high prevalence of maltreatment in the history of individuals with BPD, we easily focus on the dramatic details of the adversity and lose sight of what may be the critical causal contextual variables. We suggest that sexual and physical abuse per se may not be the most important factor in the long-term outcome; rather, contextual factors in the family environment, such as the caregivers' response to the disclosure of the abuse, may be critical (Horwitz et al. 2001). Numerous aspects of the family context of maltreatment might play an important role in undermining the robust development of the child's mentalizing capacities, including family chaos, disrupted attachments, multiple caregivers, parental neglect, alcoholism, and affective instability among family members.

To elaborate our view of the importance of family context, we have seen that the level of mental state understanding—and particularly emotion understanding—relates closely to open discussion of emotions in the parent-child dyad. We argue that maltreatment compromises unconstrained, open, and reflective communication between parent and child—or indeed between child and child (Fonagy et al. 2007). Maltreatment by a parent undermines the parent's credibility: internal states are not considered, or they are not represented accurately, and actions are not linked to accurate representations of mental states. Even in cases where the abuse takes place outside the family, its impact will depend on mentalizing within the family. For example, if the abuse is denied or minimized, or the child is blamed for it, the child will be affected by the parent's failure to have the child's subjective experience in mind. Thus ostensibly reflective discourse will not correspond to the core of the child's subjective experiences, and this discordance will impair the child's capacity to mentalize the trauma.

In sum, we believe that the central factor that predisposes the child to BPD is *a family environment that discourages coherent discourse concerning mental states.* Abusive experiences per se are not the primary cause of BPD; yet maltreatment in the family is highly likely to be associated with absent or distorted mentalizing. Indeed, consistent with our emphasis on the importance of the presence of a mirroring relationship for establishing mentalizing, some studies point to the importance of neglect, low parental involvement, and emotional abuse—rather than the presence of physical and sexual abuse—as the critical predictors of BPD (Johnson et al. 2001; Ludolph et al. 1990). Studies that have examined the family context of childhood trauma in BPD focus on the unstable, non-nurturing family environment as the key social mediator of abuse (Bradley et al. 2005). Moreover, underinvolvement is the best predictor of suicide (Johnson et al. 2002) and personality dysfunction (Zweig-Frank and Paris 1991). Accordingly, we construe *parental emotional underinvolvement with children* as most likely to impair the appropriate development of mentalizing capacity. We should also note, however, that not only lack of attunement but also consistent *mis*attunement impairs the development of mentalizing; moreover, being misunderstood in attachment relationships is highly aversive. Hence a recurrent focus of mentalizing in therapy is *striving to understand misunderstandings*.

Our formulation concerning emotional neglect converges well with theory of development that provides a base for Linehan's (1993a) Dialectical Behavior Therapy for BPD. In Linehan's view, a key factor is the *invalidating* family environment of the young person with prodromal BPD. Fruzzetti and colleagues have elaborated the nature of invalidating family interactions with deleterious effects (Fruzzetti et al. 2003, 2005). Parental invalidation not only is associated with the young person's reports of family distress, his or her own distress, and psychological problems; invalidation also relates to aspects of social cognition, namely, the capacity to identify and label emotions. This finding is not surprising inasmuch as invalidation includes undermining of self-perceptions of internal states. Examples include not accepting the accuracy or veracity of the child's self-description; treating children's reports of their reactions as invalid, inappropriate, or flawed; dismissing or trivializing children's opinions, thoughts, and desires; criticizing or punishing children's reports; and normalizing problematic or abnormal responses.

Our formulation highlights those aspects of invalidation that entail systematic undermining of the child's experience of his or her own mind; this invalidation might occur through direct disconfirmations, by minimizing difficulties, or by failing to teach the child to discriminate effectively between what he or she feels and what the caregiver feels. Our approach is consistent with Dialectical Behavior Therapy in proposing that a pervasive history of invalidating (non-mentalizing) responses from attachment figures generates skills deficits primarily in emotionally charged interpersonal situations where social-cognitive capacities are essential. The failure of interpersonal understanding further compounds the social stress, leading to major difficulties of emotion regulation and interpersonal problem solving—at worst, actively evoking chaos in relationships.

Thus, while we do not attribute an exclusive role to trauma, we nevertheless believe that maltreatment will play a key role in shaping the pathology of BPD for individuals rendered vulnerable to stressful psychosocial experiences (particularly in an attachment context) by virtue of inadequate early mirroring and disorganized attachment. Maltreatment also may play a direct role in the etiology of BPD by virtue of undermining mentalizing. We consider the impact of trauma most likely to be part and parcel of a more general failure of considering the child's perspective. This failure is manifested through neglect, rejection, excessive control, relationship incoherence, and confusion. Taken together, these adversities can devastate the experiential world of the developing child and leave deep scars evident in distortions of social-cognitive functioning.

Nonetheless, we believe that aggression and cruelty directly focused on the child, as well as the profoundly invasive boundary violations associated with sexual abuse, often will have specific effects in addition to the nonspecific influences we have just described. For example, aggression and cruelty can lead to the defensive inhibition of the capacity to think about others' malevolent thoughts and feelings about the self (Fonagy and Target 1997a). The reluctance to conceive of mental states on the part of maltreated individuals might be understandable given the frankly hostile and malevolent thoughts and feelings that the abuser must realistically hold to explain his or her actions against a vulnerable young person (Fonagy 1991). Similarly, Freyd (1996) has construed incestuous sexual abuse as *betrayal trauma,* occurring in a context in which "the person doing the betraying is someone the victim cannot afford *not* to trust" (p. 11, emphasis in original). Hence awareness (i.e., mentalizing) of the betrayal endangers the child by threatening the attachment relationship. In this context, dissociation is a common non-mentalizing defense (Allen 2001; Freyd 1996). Consistent with this line of thinking, forms of maltreatment that are most clearly malevolent and clearly target the child—such as physical, sexual, and psychological abuse—are liable to have the greatest adverse impact on mentalizing. To reiterate, such abuses also *exemplify* non-mentalizing behavior on the part of the abuser.

Unstable Mentalizing in BPD

Having made our case that impaired mentalizing plays a central role in the development of BPD, we are now in a position to describe characteristic failures of mentalizing in the phenomenology and symptomatology of BPD. We have reviewed the adverse impact of affective dysregulation on mentalizing capacity in Chapter 4 ("Neurobiology") and need not reiterate it here, except to underscore its particular relevance to BPD (Gabbard et al. 2006). In the following, we elaborate how activating attachment needs can undermine mentalizing; how prementalizing modes of experience are evident in BPD (in relation to which projective identification comes into play); and how mentalizing impairment relates to disorganization of the self in BPD.

Attachment Activation and Mentalizing Impairment

As we described in the first part of this book (Chapter 3, "Development," and Chapter 4, "Neurobiology"), attachment bears complex relations to mentalizing, and attachment and mentalizing sometimes can be activated reciprocally (Fonagy 2006). Most problematic, the hyperactivation of attachment in BPD may be a consequence of abuse and emotional neglect in attachment relationships; yet the activation of attachment needs constitutes a reminder of trauma, and trauma-related triggering of the fight-or-flight response is one potential mechanism that may inhibit mentalizing in individuals with BPD. Thus the coincidence of trauma and attachment could create a vicious circle. Trauma normally leads a child to seek proximity with the attachment figure for the sake of protection. Yet depending on a maltreating attachment figure carries the risk of an escalating sequence of further maltreatment, escalating distress, and an increasingly desperate inner need for the attachment figure. As we noted earlier in this chapter, a number of studies point to the high prevalence of enmeshed-preoccupied attachment associated with BPD, and preoccupied attachment is indicative of a hyperactivated attachment system. This vicious circle perpetuates traumatic attachments: the ready triggering of the attachment system in BPD residual to trauma is manifested in a rapidly accelerated tempo of intimacy in interpersonal relationships along with vulnerability to the transient loss of mentalizing when attachment needs are activated in these relationships—as they are often likely to be, given the hyperactivation of the attachment system.

In sum, we envision three routes by which mentalizing may be suppressed in individuals with BPD:

1. Psychological defenses against mentalizing might be mounted to protect individuals from contemplating the mental states of those who harbor malevolent thoughts and feelings toward them.
2. Trauma-related shifts in thresholds for switching from the mentalizing to fight-or-flight modes may account for precipitous losses of mentalizing in individuals with BPD, who are particularly vulnerable to high levels of emotional arousal.
3. Hyperactivation of the attachment system associated with safety seeking may drive the individual into further contact with an abusive attachment figure.

As we discuss next, the loss of mentalizing is accompanied by the emergence of prementalizing modes of experience that are also characteristic of BPD.

Prementalizing Modes of Experience and Projective Identification

We have described prementalizing modes of experience in Chapter 3 ("Development") and merely highlight their application to BPD here. Most prominent in BPD is the *psychic-equivalence mode,* wherein mental states are conflated with external reality. As psychotherapists know all too well, psychic equivalence suspends the "as-if" mode of experience: everything thought, felt, or imagined, appears—sometimes frighteningly—to be "for real." This experience can add drama as well as risk to interpersonal relationships, and patients' exaggerated emotional reactions are justified by the seriousness with which they suddenly experience their own and others' thoughts and feelings. The corresponding vividness and bizarreness of subjective experience can appear as quasi-psychotic symptoms (Zanarini et al. 1990).

Conversely, in the *pretend mode,* thoughts and feelings can come to be dissociated to the point of meaninglessness. In the pretend mode, reality places fewer limits on the creation of mental representations, and patients can discuss experiences without grounding them in reality. Several studies of persons with BPD using projective tests and other narrative methods have provided evidence of representations of others' mental states that are hypercomplex, idiosyncratically elaborated, and malevolent (Stuart et al. 1990; Westen et al. 1990a, 1990b). Hence patients with BPD are liable to oscillate between experiences that are too real (psychic equivalence) and too unreal (pretend). Attempting psychotherapy with patients who are in the pretend mode can lead the therapist to lengthy but inconsequential discussions that have no link to emotionally genuine experience (see Chapter 6, "Mentalizing Interventions").

Lastly, the developmentally early *teleological mode* entails a primacy of tangible realities over mental representations; for example, as is all too evident in BPD, actions speak louder than words. Experience is only felt to be valid when its consequences are overtly apparent. Affection, for example, is only taken seriously and felt as such when accompanied by physical expression, such as a touch or caress. Emotional pain can be expressed fully, for example, only via the sight of blood from cuts on the arms.

Mentalizing is essential for effective affect regulation; hence these prementalizing modes leave the patient with BPD either flooded with unmanageable feelings or dissociatively detached. Projective identification, the most socially disruptive feature of cognition in BPD, is a common defense in the face of unmentalized affect. Projective identification is the apparently unstoppable tendency to create unacceptable experience within the other. Externalizing the split-off parts of a disorganized self is one way of coping for the child with disorganized attachment, and externalization can feel like a matter of life and death for the traumatized individual who has internalized the abuser as part of the self. This experience is evident from the extreme levels of dysphoric affect reported by individuals with BPD—what Zanarini and colleagues characterize as the pain of being borderline (Zanarini et al. 1998). The unbearable emotional experience can include feeling abandoned, evil, betrayed, helpless, misunderstood, mistreated, victimized, inferior, permanently damaged, rotten to the core, and monstrous (Allen 2001); such feelings characterize patients' experience on a daily basis and in a relatively stable way (Bradley and Westen 2005; Zanarini et al. 2003; Zittel-Conklin and Westen 2005).

The externalization of these unbearable internal states through projective identification is widely recognized in countertransference reactions of therapists working with patients with BPD. Such reactions include anger, resentment, and hatred; helplessness and worthlessness; fear and worry; and concomitant urges to save and rescue the patient (Gabbard and Wilkinson 1994). Complications come when therapists defend themselves by emotional distancing (Aviram et al. 2006). The distancing is especially problematic inasmuch as patients with BPD are unusually sensitive to rejection and abandonment; for example, they may react by harming themselves or withdrawing from treatment when they perceive such distancing as rejection. As Aviram and colleagues (2006) point out, the stigmatizing and rejecting attitude engendered in clinicians through such externalizing of alien parts of the self can exacerbate the patient's behaviors that initially create the stigmatizing attitude. The result is a self-fulfilling prophecy and a cycle of stigmatization to which both patient and therapist contribute.

In a vicious cycle with projective identification, the patient with BPD can obtain relief from experiences of overwhelming and intolerable emotion by reverting to the teleological, action-oriented mode, for example, by substance abuse, deliberate self-harm, and suicidal behavior. Yet these self-injurious actions create a terrified alien self in the other—be it a therapist, friend, or parent—who thus becomes the vehicle for what is emotionally unbearable. The need for this other person who "uniquely understands" (and thereby suffers) the patient's dysregulated affect can become overwhelming as an adhesive and addictive pseudo-attachment develops. Not surprisingly, as we already have indicated, studies of adult attachment patterns of patients with BPD repeatedly highlight a combination of preoccupied and unresolved attachment (Fonagy et al. 1996). The therapist who is drawn into the intense attachment via projective identification then loses the capacity to mentalize—at worst, reenacting the initial trauma (i.e., mentalizing failure) and losing all therapeutic leverage in the process.

Disorganization of Self

Clinical descriptions of BPD commonly include an unstable sense of self (Janis et al. 2006; Parker et al. 2006), and the diagnostic criteria for BPD include "identity disturbance: markedly and persistently unstable self-image or sense of self" (American Psychiatric Association 2000, p. 710). In our view, mentalizing is crucial for maintaining a stable sense of self (Fonagy et al. 2002a), and in social contexts where mentalizing is impaired, a number of indications of a failure of self-organization become apparent. Mentalizing in the form of a psychological self-narrative normally maintains an agentive sense of self (Fonagy and Target 1997a). In this context, we are not construing the self as a representation but rather as a *process* with specific qualities that are closely related to autonomy and agency—that is, a consciously accessible sense of regulating one's own behavior (Ryan 2005).

Our emphasis on the self as process is consistent with changes in the phenomenology of the self associated with transient disruptions of mentalizing. To take one example, mentalizing underpins normal self-regulation via self-talk and other processes that involve thinking about internal states (Dennett 2001); given impaired mentalizing, patients with BPD resort to self-punishing negative vocalization as a strategy of self-regulation (Rosenthal et al. 2006). Moreover, in the face of negative affect, patients with BPD may feel unable to experience themselves as authors of their actions. This loss of a sense of agency leads not only to a sense of temporally diffused identity (Kernberg 1983) but also to experiences of inauthenticity or painful incoherence, feelings of emptiness and inability to make commitments, disturbance of body image, and gender dysphoria (Akhtar 1992). These alterations in self-experience in patients with BPD are confirmed by factor-analytic studies of data from clinically experienced informants (Wilkinson-Ryan and Westen 2000).

Consistent with our developmental perspective, we speculate that children who cannot develop stable and coherent representations of their own experience through the experience of being mirrored are liable to internalize the caregiver's distorted representation as part of their self-representation (Winnicott 1971). We have called this discontinuity within the self the *alien self* (Fonagy et al. 2002a), a concept compatible with Kernberg's (1975) postulation of unmetabolized introjects. Such introjects are experiences of the self in relation to the caregiver that are encoded concretely rather than as well-differentiated, abstract representations (Bradley and Westen 2005). We intend our metaphor of the alien self to capture pathological actions of the patients with BPD that are not experienced as self-endorsed—even when these actions are reasonably construed by others as intentional and conscious. Such actions are experienced as alien in the sense of being either dissociated from the self or forced upon the self as compulsions (Ryan 2005).

We understand the controlling behavior of children with a history of disorganized attachment (Kochanska et al. 2001; Solomon et al. 1995) as analogous to projective identification, wherein the experience of incoherence within the self is alleviated through externalization. This view sheds additional light on the desperate attachment-seeking behavior of the patient with BPD. Disorganized attachment has been associated with an extraordinarily intense need for the caregiver in middle childhood that is akin to separation anxiety (Moss et al. 2004). This desperate craving for closeness can be fueled by the need for the caregiver as a vehicle for externalizing the alien parts of the self.

Clinical Implications

We have been laying the groundwork for a treatment approach to BPD focusing on mentalizing by reviewing evidence that the disorder develops in the context of a wide range of adverse experiences in early attachment relationships. While outright abuse is the most dramatic form of adversity, we have proposed that the core problem is one of *omission* rather than commission, namely, the caregiver's failure to mentalize in interacting with the child. The child's failure to develop robust mentalizing capacities, in turn, is associated with developmental deficits in affect regulation, effortful control of attention, and social cognition. Unfortunately, the perpetuation of insecure attachment and correspondingly unstable mentalizing propels the individual into attachment relationships that are potentially destabilizing: heightened attachment needs evoke intense affects; mentalizing collapses; and pre-mentalizing modes of experience, coupled with projective identification, further undermine relationships and self-organization.

Hence, as we shall see next, in offering psychotherapeutic treatment, we walk a tightrope: we must provide an attachment context that will strengthen mentalizing while continually risking the possibility that stimulating attachment will undermine the very mentalizing capacity on which successful treatment must build.

Treatment

We begin this section by presenting evidence for the dilemma we just posed: persons with BPD can benefit from treatment, but treatment also has the potential to make them worse. Then we continue to press our point that clinicians treating patients with BPD must be particularly attentive to promoting mentalizing and not unwittingly undermining it. We conclude the chapter with a description of mentalization-based treatment programs for patients with BPD and research on the effectiveness of these programs.

Course of BPD and Potential for Iatrogenic Harm

Clinicians expect BPD to have an enduring quality. Early follow-up studies highlighted the seemingly inexorable nature of the disorder, not envisioning recovery but rather a disease process that ran a long-term course, albeit with a possibility of burnout (Stone 1990). At worst, therapeutic nihilism was justified by the sheer severity of symptoms—the intensity and incomprehensibility of emotional pain, the dramatic self-mutilation, and the baffling degree of ambivalence in interpersonal relationships.

Two carefully designed prospective studies have countered this pessimistic view of the course of BPD and thus highlight the inappropriateness of therapeutic pessimism which, at worst, has confined individuals with severe personality disorder to the margins of even generous healthcare systems (Shea et al. 2004; Zanarini et al. 2003). The majority of patients with BPD experience a substantial reduction in their symptoms—and far sooner than previously assumed. After 6 years, 75% of patients diagnosed with BPD sufficiently severe to require hospitalization achieve remission by standardized diagnostic criteria (Cohen et al. 2006; Skodol et al. 2006; Zanarini et al. 2006). Hence patients with BPD *can* undergo remission—a concept previously used solely in the context of Axis I disorders. A 50% remission rate is typical by 4 years, but continuing remission is steady (10–15% per year). Recurrences are rare, perhaps no more than 10% over 6 years. This trajectory contrasts with the natural course of many Axis I disorders, such as mood disorders, where improvement may be more rapid but recurrences are more common.

While improvements of BPD are substantial, symptoms such as impulsivity and associated self-mutilation and suicidality show more dramatic change than mood instability and compromised social functioning. Thus the dramatic symptoms abate, but abandonment concerns, the sense of emptiness, relationship problems, and vulnerability to depression are liable to remain present in at least half the patients. When dramatic improvements occur, they sometimes occur quickly, quite often associated with relief from severely stressful situations or abusive relationships, discontinuation of substance abuse, or effective treatment of anxiety or mood disorders (Gunderson et al. 2003). Accordingly, comorbid conditions can undermine the likelihood of improvement (Zanarini et al. 2004), and these must be treated.

Given that the vast majority of cases of BPD resolve naturally within 6 years, why have clinicians across the globe traditionally agreed about the treatment-resistant character of the disorder? Earlier surveys indicated that 97% of patients with BPD who presented for treatment in the United States received outpatient care from an average of six therapists. An analysis of outcomes measured 2–3 years later suggest treatment as usual is at best only marginally effective (Lieb et al. 2004). How can we square such findings with what we now know from new data on the natural course of the disorder?

We infer that some psychosocial treatments practiced currently— and perhaps even more commonly in the past—have impeded patients' capacity to recover in what would otherwise be the natural course of the disorder (Fonagy and Bateman 2006b). In Stone's (1990) classic follow-up study of patients treated nearly 40 years ago, a 66% recovery rate was achieved only in 20 years—four times longer than reported in more recent studies. It is unlikely that the nature of the disorder changed or that treatments have become that much more effective. The known efficacy of pharmacological agents, new and old, cannot account for this difference (Tyrer and Bateman 2004), and the evidence-based psychosocial treatments are not widely available. Sadly, it is far more likely that the apparent improvement in the course of the disorder is accounted for by harmful treatments being offered less frequently. Possibly, this change reflects diminished treatment availability owing to changing patterns of healthcare—particularly in the United States (Lambert et al. 2004)—more than clinicians' recognition of the potential for iatrogenic deterioration and, accordingly, an avoidance of damaging side effects of treatment. We must take seriously the possibility that, like medications, psychotherapeutic interventions have the potential to be harmful.

Psychotherapy requires that the patient be able to utilize alternative perspectives presented by the psychotherapist, and this is precisely the area of difficulty for patients with BPD (Fonagy and Bateman 2006b). Accordingly, we advocate that psychotherapeutic treatment of BPD be focused relatively single-mindedly on fostering mentalizing (see Chapter 6, "Mentalizing Interventions"). In this respect, our approach is broadly consistent with the aims of Dimaggio and colleagues' (2007) psychotherapeutic interventions for core metacognitive dysfunctions in BPD (inability to integrate various states of mind, inability to differentiate between fantasy and reality, and emotional dysregulation).

Mentalization-Based Therapy for BPD

In setting up the mentalization-based therapy (MBT) programs (Bateman and Fonagy 2004, 2006), we began by reviewing the literature and concluded that effective treatments share several common features summarized in Table 9–2. Helpfully, many of these attributes also characterize researchable treatment protocols.

We have developed two variants of MBT, the first being a Day Hospital Program. Initially, patients attend on a five-day-per-week basis, and the maximum length of time they spend in the program is 18–24 months. This program combines individual and group psychotherapy focused on implicit mentalizing processes with expressive therapies (e.g., involving artwork and writing) that also promote skill in explicit mentalizing. The exact structure and content of each group is less important than the interrelationships among different aspects of the program, the working relationships among the different therapists, the continuity of themes between the groups, and the consistency with which the treatment is applied over a period of time. Such nonspecific aspects probably form the key to effective treatment, and the specificity of the effects of various therapeutic activities remains to be determined.

TABLE 9–2.   COMMON FEATURES OF EFFECTIVE TREATMENTS FOR BPD

- Well structured
- Devote considerable effort to enhancing compliance
- Focus sharply on specific problem behaviors such as self-harm or problematic interpersonal relationship patterns
- Offer a coherent conceptual framework that patients and therapists can share
- Encourage a supportive attachment relationship between therapist and patient, consistent with the therapist's adopting a relatively active rather than a passive stance
- Relatively long in duration
- Well integrated with other services available to the patient

Integration within the program is achieved through our focus on mentalizing; all groups have an overall aim of increasing mentalizing within a framework that encourages exploration of minds by minds.

Entrance to the Day Hospital Program requires that the patient show at least some of the following features: high risk to self or others, inadequate social support, repeated hospital admissions interfering with adaptation to daily living, unstable housing, substance abuse, and highly unstable mentalizing. Patients who show some capacity for everyday living and who have stable social support and accommodations are more likely to be treated within the second variant of MBT, the Intensive Outpatient Program, particularly if their mentalizing processes are characterized only by vulnerability in close emotional relationships. At present we do not have a measure of the severity of personality disorder adequate to assign individuals to one program or the other on the basis of a standardized score; the primary considerations are level of risk and instability of social circumstances.

The 18-month Intensive Outpatient Program consists of once-weekly 50-minute individual psychotherapy sessions coupled with once-weekly 90-minute group therapy sessions. As in the Day Hospital Program, the group therapist is different from the individual therapist. The requirements placed on patients in the Intensive Outpatient Program are more onerous than those placed on patients in the Day Hospital Program because outpatient participants are less chaotic and have better mentalizing abilities, along with a better capacity for attentional control and affective regulation. The two components of the program, namely the group and individual sessions, cannot be separated; hence frequent absence from either one leads to discussion about continuation in treatment. We do not make a policy of discharging patients automatically because of nonattendance; yet, if patients do not attend one component of the program, then this is discussed with them in the next session they attend, whether it is the individual or group session. Patients are informed at the beginning of treatment that persistent and prolonged absence from any component of the program will lead to discharge to our low-maintenance outpatient clinic for further consideration of treatment. Return to the program remains possible after this transfer, but only following further work on the underlying anxieties.

We take this rigorous stance about attendance because many patients find the individual session more acceptable than the group session; they attend the former and not the latter. Such patients may have ostensibly accepted the requirement of group work in the assessment interviews but covertly done so only to access individual therapy. This problem must be addressed as soon as treatment starts, because we consider group treatment to be the richest forum for promoting mental-izing. Not surprisingly, patients with BPD may have an aversion to groups owing to a reduced capacity to keep themselves in mind or to recognize that others have them in mind when they are listening to the problems of others; this difficulty accounts to some degree for their anx-iety about groups and their oscillations between over- and under-involvement with others. As they become involved with others' problems, they are liable to lose themselves in the mind of the other; when they do so, they lose a sense of self, which, in turn, leads to rapid distancing from others for the sake of self-preservation.

There are three main phases to the trajectory of MBT, each of which has a distinct aim and harnesses specific processes. Overall, the initial phase aims to assess mentalizing capacities and personality functioning as well as to engage the patient in treatment. Specific processes include providing a diagnosis, offering psychoeducation, establishing a hierar-chy of therapeutic aims, stabilizing social and behavioral problems, re-viewing medication, and defining a crisis pathway. During the middle phase, all the active therapeutic work aims to stimulate ever-increasing mentalizing ability. The final phase prepares the patient to end inten-sive treatment. This termination phase requires the therapist to focus on the feelings of loss associated with ending treatment; to help the patient consider how to maintain gains that have been made; and to develop an appropriate follow-up treatment program tailored to the patient's par-ticular needs.

The initial phase of treatment includes a written formulation, which remains a work in progress (see Chapter 6, "Mentalizing Interven-tions"). All patients in the Partial Hospital Program and Intensive Out-patient Program participate in a review with the whole treatment team every three months. The group therapist, the individual therapist, the psychiatrist, and other relevant mental health professionals meet with the patient to discuss progress, problems, and other aspects of treat-ment. The practice of having practitioners meeting together jointly with the patient ensures not only that everyone's views are taken into ac-count and integrated into a coherent set of ideas but also that mentaliz-ing as manifested through the discussion of the different viewpoints is modeled as a constructive activity that furthers understanding. These regular reviews lead to a reformulation which can then form the basis of ongoing treatment.

Although the hard work for the patient of strengthening mentaliz-ing takes place in the middle phase, this phase might appear easier on the surface for the therapist: by the time the initial phase has been nego-tiated, many of the crises will have subsided, the level of engagement in treatment will be clear, patients' motivation may have increased, and the capacity to work within individual and group therapy may be greater. In addition, the therapist may have a better understanding of patients' overall difficulties and thus have a more robust image of them in mind. Concomitantly, patients also will have become aware of therapists' foibles and ways of working. Yet for other patients and therapists, the treatment in the middle phase may continue to be disrupted, so that the therapist must continue to repair ruptures in the therapeutic alliance and to sustain his own and his patients' motivation at this phase while striving to maintain a focus on mentalizing.

Although patients with BPD improve naturally over time, the improvement occurs primarily in impulsive behavior and affective instability. The problems of maintaining emotionally charged interpersonal relationships, engaging in intricate negotiations of difficult social situations, and interacting effectively with complex social systems may be less responsive to treatment. The patient with BPD who no longer engages in deliberate self-harm may nonetheless lead a life severely curtailed by an inability to form constructive and intimate relationships with others. Such patients remain incapacitated in how they live their lives unless they develop effective ways of interacting with others. Thus, along with integrating and consolidating earlier work, the final phase of treatment focuses on the interpersonal and social aspects of functioning, as long as the symptomatic and behavioral problems are well controlled.

The final phase starts at the point at which the patient has six months of treatment remaining. In keeping with the principles of psychodynamic psychotherapy, we consider the ending of treatment and the associated separation responses to be highly significant in consolidating gains made during the therapy. Inadequate negotiation by the patient of the experience of separation, potentially abetted by inadequate processing of the ending on the part of the therapist, may provoke in the patient a reemergence of earlier ways of managing feelings and a concomitant decrease in mentalizing. In such cases, social and interpersonal functioning will be compromised.

Responsibility for developing a coherent follow-up program and for negotiating further treatment is given to the patient and the individual therapist. Although most patients desire further treatment, we do not routinely offer any specific follow-up program. Some patients have had a many-year career of interacting with mental health services; to leave these services behind requires a major change in lifestyle for which the patient might not be fully prepared by the end of 18 months. The patient with a severe personality disorder who has undergone many years

of failed treatments, multiple hospital admissions, and inadequate social stability is unlikely to be able to walk away from services, never to
return, after 18 months—regardless of the success of the treatment.
Most patients require further support as they adapt to a new life.

Many patients choose intermittent follow-up appointments rather
than further formal psychotherapy. This follow-up is arranged within
the treatment team. For example, senior practitioners who have known
the patient and who are known to the patient offer 30-minute individual
appointments every four to six weeks. During follow-up appointments,
the therapist continues to use mentalizing techniques, encouraging the
patient to continue exploring their own and others' mental states in the
service of interpersonal problem solving and maintaining stable intimate relationships. The follow-up contract is flexible, and patients can
request additional appointments if they are having particular difficulty.
In general, however, the optimal trajectory over follow-up entails increasing time between appointments over a six-month period so as to
encourage greater patient autonomy and responsibility. How long a patient is seen in this manner depends on the therapist and patient, and
the duration should be mutually agreed upon. Some patients elect to be
discharged relatively early during follow-up with the proviso that they
may call and request an appointment at any time in the future. Other
patients prefer an appointment many months ahead, and this structure
provides adequate assurance within their own mind that we continue
to have them in mind, giving them greater confidence and self-reliance
to negotiate the stresses and strains of everyday life.

Research on Effectiveness of MBT

Our research on MBT is naturalistic in the sense of remaining true to ordinary clinical practice. Thus we construe our outcomes assessments as
effectiveness research rather than efficacy research, the former having
the advantage of relatively straightforward translation to other clinical
settings. The programs were developed and implemented by a team of
generically trained mental health professionals with an interest in psychoanalytically oriented psychotherapy rather than by highly trained
personnel within a university research department. Thus the research
takes place within an ordinary clinical setting and in a locality and
healthcare system in which patients are unlikely to be able to obtain
treatment elsewhere. Hence we have been able to trace patients within
the service and thus to collect accurate clinical and service-utilization
data. In addition, patients are treated at only two local hospitals for
medical emergencies, enabling us to obtain highly accurate data of epi-

sodes of self-harm and suicide attempts that require medical intervention. But this naturalistic clinical approach to research also has a downside: the partial hospital program is complex and multifaceted, leading to difficulty in pinpointing the effective ingredients. Nonetheless, we designed the program to lend itself to dismantling at a later date to determine the contribution of specific therapeutic components to the outcome.

Our own evidence base remains small as far as treatment outcome is concerned; yet replication studies are under way, and an increasing number of practitioners are using mentalizing techniques in treatment, so more information will accrue rapidly. Our original randomized controlled trial of treatment of BPD in the Partial Hospital Program (Bateman and Fonagy 1999, 2001) showed significant and enduring changes in mood states and interpersonal functioning. The benefits, relative to treatment as usual, were substantial and were observed to increase during the follow-up period of 18 months.

Forty-four patients who participated in the original study were assessed at three-month intervals after completion of the earlier trial. Outcome measures included frequency of suicide attempts and acts of self-harm; number and duration of inpatient admissions; service utilization; and self-report measures of depression, anxiety, general symptom distress, interpersonal functioning, and social adjustment. Patients who had received partial hospital treatment not only maintained their substantial gains but also showed a continuing improvement on most measures—in contrast to patients in the control group, who showed only limited change during the same period. This suggests that rehabilitative changes had taken place that enabled patients to negotiate the stresses and strains of everyday life without resorting to former ways of coping, such as self-injurious behavior.

Healthcare utilization of all patients who participated in the trial was assessed using information from case notes and service providers (Bateman and Fonagy 2003). Costs of psychiatric, pharmacological, and emergency room treatment were compared across three periods: six months prior to treatment, during 18 months of treatment, and for 18 months of follow-up observation. There were no differences between MBT and control groups in the costs of service utilization pre-treatment or during treatment. The additional cost of day-hospital treatment was offset by less psychiatric inpatient care and fewer emergency room visits. The trend for costs to decrease in the MBT group during 18 months follow-up was not apparent in the control group, suggesting that day-hospital treatment for BPD is no more expensive than general psychiatric care and shows considerable cost savings after treatment.

Unpublished findings from a recently completed 8-year follow-up of the patients in the original MBT trial compared the long-term effects of MBT with treatment as usual. In comparison with those in the control group, only a small minority of MBT patients met criteria for BPD, whereas the vast majority of the control group did so; the largest differences between groups were in the realms of impulsivity and interpersonal functioning. Patients in the MBT group also showed advantages in many other domains: significantly better global functioning, fewer suicide attempts, fewer emergency room visits and days hospitalized, less extensive utilization of medication, and substantially greater employment.

The effective components of this complex treatment program remain unclear, although the common feature of all the different treatment elements was our focus on mentalizing. Patients in the Day Hospital Program received a range of treatments in addition to individual and group therapy, including psychodrama and other expressive therapies along with some psychoeducation early in treatment. To determine whether the focus on mentalizing is a key component, and to see if a more modest program may be effective in a group of patients with less severe BPD, we conducted a randomized controlled trial of individual and group psychotherapy alone, as offered in our Intensive Outpatient Program. The unpublished results of this recently completed study showed that, compared to supportive clinical management, MBT was associated with significantly greater rates of decline in suicide attempts, deliberate self-harm, and hospitalizations, as well as numerous indices of subjective distress. Importantly, MBT also was associated with greater improvements in social functioning. Hence the effects of MBT—in relatively pure form—go well beyond reducing the more dramatic, self-destructive symptoms of BPD.

Recapitulation

To return to our starting point in this chapter, we have proposed a conceptual framework for BPD in which treatment interventions are designed to dovetail with impaired psychological processes rooted in developmental psychopathology. Our developmental model respects the intertwining of environmental adversities and neurobiological vulnerabilities. While recognizing that BPD has complex etiology and symptomatology, we have proposed precarious mentalizing as a core problem; this conceptualization provides considerable therapeutic leverage insofar as we are able to provide belated developmental help with mentalizing in individual and group psychotherapy. Accordingly, we have the potential to interrupt what often has been a long process of intergenerational transmission of psychopathology.

Our central thesis is that the phenomenology of BPD is the consequence of several factors:

1. The attachment-related inhibition of mentalizing
2. The reemergence of modes of experiencing internal reality that antedate the developmental emergence of mentalizing
3. The continual pressure for projective identification
4. The re-externalization of the self-destructive alien self— which further undermines mentalizing, affect regulation, and attachment relationships in vicious circles

As we stated in Chapter 4 ("Neurobiology"), attachment and mentalizing to some extent can be mutually inhibiting, and effective treatment must activate both simultaneously. The challenge of treatment, accordingly, is to maintain and promote mentalizing in the context of stimulating attachment needs—needs that paradoxically have the potential to undermine mentalizing and destabilize the patient's functioning. As we have described it, MBT is designed to avoid the pitfalls of an overstimulating treatment that unwittingly prolongs the course of BPD. We believe that consistent attention to mentalizing is the best safeguard against iatrogenic harm and is also an optimal focus for expediting what we now know to be the natural course of recovery from BPD.

Being research minded, we are unlikely ever to be fully satisfied with the evidence for the effectiveness of MBT, and MBT is a relative newcomer to the field. Nonetheless, we are encouraged by the evidence for the effectiveness of the multifaceted partial-hospital MBT protocol as well as the more focused intensive outpatient protocol. Meanwhile, we and our colleagues in other clinical settings are in the process of actively expanding our knowledge base.

Key Clinical Points

- *Insecure attachment and BPD:* Extensive evidence links border-line personality disorder (BPD) to insecure attachment rooted in problematic parent-child interactions that are conducive to unstable mentalizing. In turn, mentalizing failures play a prominent role in impairments in affect regulation, effortful control of attention, and social cognition—all of which are evidenced in the symptomatology of BPD.

- *Emotional unavailability and BPD:* Although abuse is common in the history of many persons with BPD, emotional unavailability and the concomitant failure to promote mentalizing is the common core; this view of BPD is consistent with the emphasis on the "invalidating environment" in Dialectical Behavior Therapy.

- *MBT, a supportive therapy:* Psychotherapy stimulates attachment needs, and heightened attachment needs are liable to destabilize the relationships of persons with BPD such that overstimulating psychotherapy relationships can be detrimental. Hence mentalization-based therapy (MBT) is a relatively supportive approach that endeavors to keep mentalizing online in the context of an attachment relationship.

- *Effectiveness of MBT:* Controlled research on day hospital and intensive outpatient treatment programs provides substantial empirical support for the effectiveness MBT for BPD. Specifically, MBT decreases self-destructive behavior and dysphoria along with lessening utilization of treatment resources; concomitantly, MBT improves social and occupational functioning, and all these improvements are maintained over a considerable period of time.

Chapter 10

Psychoeducation

Psychoeducation can be defined as "a professionally delivered treatment modality that integrates and synergizes psychotherapeutic and educational interventions" (Lukens and McFarlane 2004, p. 206). To date, psychoeducational interventions have been targeted to specific psychiatric disorders. The Menninger Clinic, with its long history in providing psychiatric training for a wide range of professional disciplines as well as public education about mental illness (Menninger 1930, 1947), has provided fertile ground for expanding and refining psychoeducational interventions (Allen 2005, 2006a; Craig 1985). Yet, most recently, we have gone beyond the traditional disorder-focused approach to psychoeducation by developing psychoeducational groups on mentalizing to enhance patients' participation in treatment as a whole; this new approach has been based on our conviction about the central role of mentalizing in treatment coupled with our belief that our patients are better able to collaborate when they understand what we clinicians are trying to do with them (Haslam-Hopwood et al. 2006).

Picking up a thread from Chapter 8 ("Parenting and Family Therapy"), we begin this chapter by describing an educational group on parenting based on mentalizing. The remainder of this chapter describes the educational groups on mentalizing that we have developed for adult patients at The Menninger Clinic. We did not design our psychoeducational groups on mentalizing to be stand-alone interventions; rather, they are integral to multimodal hospital treatment programs. Accordingly, we have not researched their effectiveness and thus we do not know the extent to which they make a unique contribution to treatment outcomes. For clinicians who wish to employ the concept of mentalizing explicitly with their patients and family members and to educate them accordingly, we include as an Appendix to this chapter our explanation of mentalizing for patients and their family members, "What is Mentalizing and Why Do It?"

Reflective Parenting Workshops

As we described in Chapter 8, Slade and colleagues' (Sadler et al. 2006; Slade et al. 2004) Minding the Baby project includes a substantial educational component—for example, educating parents about child care as well as social resources. Yet the main thrust of the intervention is fostering mentalizing interactions between parents and their infants. In contrast, we would characterize Slade and colleagues' group intervention for parents of infants, toddlers, and preschoolers as primarily psychoeducational.

Unlike Minding the Baby, which is designed for high-risk parents and infants, "Parents First" (Slade 2006) is a preventive intervention designed to be delivered in ordinary educational and childcare settings. In addition to the group intervention, the program provides mental health consultation to staff members and families, but the component pertinent to this chapter is the *reflective parenting workshops*. These workshops include a series of reflective exercises conducted across a 12-week period, and the exercises are presented in a fixed sequence according to graded levels of difficulty. Family activities intended to promote parental mentalizing also are prescribed as between-workshop exercises.

Workshop leaders are trained to model reflectiveness and to identify various levels of mentalizing as well as problems in mentalizing; they also exemplify the mentalizing stance, namely, an attitude of inquisitiveness and curiosity, with intent to hold mind in mind. Parents are helped to recognize that their children, no matter how young, behave according to their thoughts, feelings, and goals. As is true of the mentalization-based approach to family therapy described in Chapter 8,

Parents First is intended primarily to cultivate mentalizing capacity for the purpose of promoting general competence rather than to help parents solve specific parenting problems. Parents who are disinclined to reflect, however, are inclined to seek practical advice regarding specific problems with their children.

The graded series of exercises begins with having parents simply watch their children's behavior and talk about what they observe. Next they are encouraged to interpret the basis of their child's behavior in terms of desires, emotions, and thoughts. Then, moving to another level of complexity, parents are helped to appreciate the connection between their own state of mind and their child's experience—for example, considering the impact of their emotions and expectations on the child's own experience of self. In a related vein, they are made aware of differences in perspective as these are evident, for example, in disagreements between them and their children. All these steps set the stage for supporting the parents' capacity to mentalize in emotionally charged moments—what we consider to be the gold standard of mentalizing.

In the last stage of the workshop, the sheer complexities of mentalizing in parent-child relationships are addressed. Parents' attention is drawn to ambivalence, limitations in mindreading capacity, and the proclivity for parents and children to misinterpret each other's intentions. The group process helps to normalize these problems while providing support for participants' efforts, as is true in our clinic-based psychoeducational groups.

Components of a Course for Adult Psychiatric Inpatients

None of our clinical work or research has made us more keenly aware of the complexities and subtleties of this ostensibly ordinary capacity, mentalizing, than our efforts to educate patients about it. We initiated the intervention in the Professionals in Crisis program at The Menninger Clinic (Bleiberg 2006). In this program, we work with an especially inquisitive and well educated patient group composed of physicians and other health professionals, attorneys, business executives, and the like, who are in treatment for problems including mood and anxiety disorders, often coupled with addictions and frequently intertwined with a history of traumatic attachments and personality disturbance. They ask challenging questions: "How is mentalizing different from empathy?" "Can you mentalize too much? "Am I mentalizing when I'm ruminating?" "I'm learning to mentalize—now how do I get my spouse to mentalize?" Not uncommonly, after spending an hour talking about mentalizing—and aspiring to do it—an intrepid patient asks: "But *what is* mentalizing?" Oftentimes only after attending several sessions on mentalizing (and spending a few weeks in a treatment program emphasizing mentalizing) do patients exclaim, "Now I understand it!"—typically, after they have been able to use their mentalizing capacity and recognize it as such in the heat of an emotion-laden interpersonal conflict with a family member, staff member, or peer.

Helpfully, when patients new to the group are expressing their difficulty understanding the concept, patients who have been in the group for a number of sessions empathize with their perplexity and encourage them to stick with it, anticipating that they, too, will eventually understand it. The group leaders routinely acknowledge not only their continuing efforts to understand the nuances of the concept *mentalizing*, but—more importantly—their ongoing struggles to mentalize skillfully in their daily life, not only in their clinical work and relationships with colleagues but also in their primary attachment relationships.

After first establishing the psychoeducational group in the Professionals in Crisis Program, we extended it into our program for young persons who are having severe difficulty with the transition from adolescence into adulthood, many of whom present with a multitude of clinical syndromes coupled with personality disorders and addictions (Poa 2006). The groups for professionals and young adults meet weekly for 50-minute sessions, which include a combination of lectures, discussion, and group exercises. The groups vary in size but sometimes contain up to 24 patients; staff members and trainees also attend. As we will describe in more detail shortly, the group has a curriculum consisting of three sections, each consisting of 2–3 sessions. An overview is provided in Table 10–1.

The groups are open-ended, and patients attend throughout their several-week stay. By necessity, patients enter the group at various points in the curriculum; hence every session begins with a brief description of mentalizing (or not so brief, depending on the level of understanding in the group and extent of challenging questions). More experienced patients often provide the orienting descriptions for newer patients. To orient patients to the concept, and especially to help patients who enter the group in the middle or toward the end of the curriculum, we distribute at admission an article we wrote for patients, "Mentalizing as a Compass for Treatment" (Allen et al. 2003).

TABLE 10–1.   PSYCHOEDUCATIONAL GROUP CURRICULUM

Understanding mentalizing and its development:
Present the rationale for building a treatment alliance around the process of mentalizing; discuss the various facets of mentalizing and the benefits of mentalizing skillfully for self-awareness and healthy relationships; describe the optimal conditions for the development and maintenance of mentalizing in terms of secure attachment and optimal emotional arousal.

Psychiatric disorders and impaired mentalizing:
Explain how psychiatric disorders and symptoms enter into a vicious circle with mentalizing impairments, beginning with substance abuse and extending the discussion to depression, anxiety, trauma, and personality disorders.

Promoting mentalizing in treatment:
Conceptualize treatment as encompassing a range of arenas for practicing mentalizing as well as for identifying failures in mentalizing and the reasons for them; includes discussion of interactions in the inpatient milieu with peers and staff members, the assessment process, individual and group psychotherapy, and two particularly stressful treatment processes that challenge mentalizing, namely, clinical rounds with the treatment team and family work.

Understanding Mentalizing and Its Development

The first section of the course, "Understanding Mentalizing," covers the basic concept and the developmental factors that promote mentalizing. We define mentalizing as attending to mental states, and we then highlight the territory of mentalizing as covering awareness of thoughts and feelings in self and others. We contrast mentalizing with empathy, stating that mentalizing entails empathy for oneself as well as others. We also relate mentalizing to mindfulness, namely, mentalizing entails mindfulness of mind. We emphasize mentalizing emotion to dispel the misunderstanding that mentalizing is an intellectual process; on the contrary, mentalizing *is* emotional.

We explain the two fundamental types of mentalizing failures—that is, failure to engage in mentalizing and distorted mentalizing. Regarding the latter, we note the slippery slope of imagination and projection—both of which are essential to mentalizing, yet both of which can lead to distortions. We continually emphasize how mentalizing failures are rooted in egocentrism, that is, the tendency to assume without reflection that others' thoughts and feelings correspond with one's own. In contrast, mentalizing requires the effort to consider different perspectives. In psychoeducational groups, we routinely employ the concept of "excrementalizing" as a colloquialism for distorted mentalizing (see Chapter 2, "Mentalizing"); this memorable term grabs patients' attention.

We explain to patients how mentalizing develops best in the context of secure attachment relationships and, concomitantly, under conditions of optimal emotional arousal. We make the point that we endeavor to create these same conditions in the treatment milieu. That is, for mentalizing to flourish, patients must have a basic sense of safety and trust in each other as well as in us clinicians. Accordingly, we emphasize the need for fundamental benevolence and good will on everyone's part. While we inform patients that excessive emotional arousal and the fight-or-flight response impair mentalizing, we also explain that we endeavor to push the envelope in the sense of assisting them to mentalize under increasingly stressful conditions. Not infrequently, in a paranoid mode, patients believe that we deliberately provoke them for this purpose; on the contrary, we explain that inevitable mentalizing failures on the part of clinicians as well as the ordinary challenges of treatment will evoke the needed emotional challenges.

In virtually every session, we reiterate that we take some basic mentalizing capacity for granted and that we do not pretend to be teaching patients how to mentalize. Rather, we explicitly state that we are promoting a pro-mentalizing *attitude*, namely, a stance of inquisitiveness and curiosity about mental states. Hence we are aspiring to influence how patients allocate their attention as well as encouraging them to use their imagination. Indeed, in advocating this mentalizing spirit in the context of good will, we are striving to set the general tone for the treatment programs. In short, we are advocating a mentalizing stance among patients as well as clinicians.

Mentalizing and Psychopathology

The second part of the curriculum is devoted to helping patients appreciate the relations between various forms of psychopathology and impaired mentalizing. Admittedly, we are on more or less solid ground here, depending on the arena of psychopathology we are considering. As the contents of this book suggest, we have considerable knowledge about mentalizing in the context of trauma and borderline personality disorder. Under the rubric of theory of mind, some research has demonstrated mentalizing deficits in depression (Inoue et al. 2004; Lee et al. 2005) and bipolar disorder (Kerr et al. 2003). Clinical interventions addressing metacognitive deficits have been developed for anxiety disorders (Wells 2000) and a broad range of personality disorders (Dimaggio et al. 2007). Although mentalizing deficits are evident in schizophrenia

(Doody et al. 1998; Frith and Corcoran 1996), we have not yet involved patients with primary psychotic disorders in our psychoeducational groups on mentalizing.

We engage patients in a general discussion of the two-way street between mentalizing and psychopathology: most straightforwardly, psychopathology impairs mentalizing and, more subtly, impaired mentalizing contributes to psychopathology. We begin by considering substance abuse, because of the blatant relation between intoxication and impaired mentalizing. Yet this discussion underscores that addictions not only impair mentalizing in relation to the self but also tend to be associated with obliviousness to the mental states of others, attachment figures not least. Substance abuse also illustrates well the potential impact of impaired mentalizing on the development or exacerbation of psychiatric disorders: impaired capacity to mentalize emotion contributes to the rigid reflex-like pathway from intense emotional arousal to substance abuse; that phenomenon provides an occasion to explain how mentalizing provides a needed "pause button" that potentially enhances the flexibility of coping responses (Allen 2005). Lastly, we note how impaired mentalizing contributes to conflict in close relationships; these interpersonal conflicts, in turn, generate distress that can lead to episodes of alcohol and drug abuse.

The adverse impact of anxiety on mentalizing is a main theme of the psychoeducational group, inasmuch as we routinely discuss the importance of an optimal level of emotional arousal for mentalizing and the problem that excessive anxiety evokes the non-mentalizing fight-or-flight response. Conversely, we discuss how anxiety is fueled by the flawed mentalizing of rumination as well as by distorted mentalizing of others' mental states (e.g., projecting one's self-critical attitudes onto others). Attachment trauma, which is common in the patient population, plays a key role in these discussions. We explain the role of sensitization to stress as a factor that lowers the threshold for switching into the fight-or-flight mode, and we also discuss how projecting past trauma onto current relationships is a form of distorted mentalizing that exacerbates anxiety.

Patients readily identify how depression undermines mentalizing in its pervasively adverse effects on concentration and flexible thinking. We discuss how rigid patterns of negative thinking about the self and others run counter to mentalizing, and we consider the adverse impact of failure of attunement to others' mental states as part and parcel of depressive episodes. We draw patients' attention to aspects of their depressive behavior that impair their relationships (e.g., lack of emotional responsiveness and expressiveness, speaking in a monotone, lack of interest in others' experience, excessive reassurance seeking). We also discuss conflicts characteristic of depressed persons' close relationships, namely, the tendency for partners and spouses first to become frustrated, critical, and coercive and, second, when those efforts lead nowhere, to give up and withdraw; of course, both tendencies further aggravate depression. From the standpoint of mentalizing, we identify these interpersonal processes in depression to draw patients' attention to the impact of their behavior on others.

We also educate patients about recent efforts to augment cognitive therapy for depression with mindfulness practice, inasmuch as this mindfulness-based approach to cognitive therapy exemplifies the spirit of mentalizing (Segal et al. 2002). The combination of cognitive therapy and mindfulness training helps patients identify depressive states of mind as such and to regard them with some detachment, with a sense that "this too shall pass." This novel approach to cognitive therapy is effective in relapse prevention; as we understand it and explain it to patients, the intervention fosters mentalizing depressive emotion in a way that blocks rumination and distorted negative thinking. As we explain it to patients, interrupting these counterproductive thought patterns is crucial in preventing depressive *feelings* from stabilizing into depressive *illness;* mentalizing is critical in blocking this pathogenic cascade.

The mentalizing psychoeducational group provides an ideal setting to discuss personality disorders, because the setting is explicitly aimed at being conducive to open-mindedness and inquisitiveness. This spirit is crucial, because the topic of personality disorders is potentially inflammatory: rather than feeling enlightened and helped, many patients feel criticized and insulted when they are informed that they have been diagnosed with a personality disorder. We recognize these feelings and acknowledge that being told that you have a personality disorder is not a compliment. We immediately identify two common misconceptions: first, that personality disorder characterizes the whole of the patient's personality rather than a problematic facet, and, second, that personality disorders do not respond to treatment. We are emphatic on this second point, because many patients are demoralized about the diagnosis of personality disorders, believing that they are untreatable—contrary to extensive evidence (Perry et al. 1999; Target 1998). Nonetheless, we introduce a crucial caveat; effective treatment of personality disorders hinges on awareness of the problem and a willingness to change (Yudofsky 2005).

We define personality disorders generally as problematic and recurrent patterns of interpersonal behavior that primarily affect attachment relationships (Rutter 1987). We propose that, properly understood, personality disorder diagnoses potentially can be helpful in highlighting common problematic patterns for the sake of altering them. Endeavoring to promote open-mindedness, we point out that most personality disorders can be understood as exaggerations of personality traits (Parker and Barrett 2000). In moderation, these traits have a potentially adaptive function, as is evident with compulsivity, dependency, avoidance, narcissism, and even paranoia. We emphasize that rigidity is the core problem in personality disorders, and we reiterate that the central value of mentalizing is fostering flexibility. In the spirit of mentalizing, we involve patients in an open discussion of key personality disorders, focusing on how these disorders might be associated with impaired mentalizing of both self and others. In discussing narcissistic personality disorder, for example, we examine cycles of idealization and devaluation of others, both of which involve distortions in mentalizing and both of which might stem from a distorted view of the self.

Borderline personality disorder is more complex to discuss, because it cannot be construed simply as an exaggerated personality trait. We focus the discussion on insecure attachment and the associated fears of abandonment, coupled with interpersonal behavior that *evokes* rejection and abandonment. As is true of the entire psychoeducational group, these discussions are intended to circumvent defensiveness and to cultivate reflectiveness for the sake of developing a treatment alliance in relation to personality disorders.

Mentalizing in Treatment

Having construed promoting mentalizing as an overarching aspiration of treatment, we discuss how the various components of treatment provide patients with opportunities to practice mentalizing and to refine their skill. We note that the initial assessment process calls for mentalizing in the sense of challenging patients to provide a coherent narrative of their presenting problems and their historical context. Patients frequently complain that from the pre-admission contacts through the initial phase of treatment, they must keep reiterating the same story. We point out that they have an opportunity to mentalize rather than merely giving a recitation: treatment challenges them to create fresh stories with new perspectives throughout the process (Holmes 1999).

We explain to patients that we aspire to recreate in the treatment environment the same conditions that promote the development of mentalizing beginning in early childhood: secure attachments and optimal emotional arousal. Yet we recognize that insecure attachment and problems with emotion regulation strain mentalizing capacities throughout treatment. Nonetheless, most patients experience the treatment milieu—an around-the-clock opportunity to interact informally with other patients and staff members—as a *relatively* safe space for mentalizing. Yet we recognize that a continuous feeling of security—not that it is possible—would not be conducive to what patients most need: increased capacity to mentalize in the face of challenge and emotional arousal, especially when attachment needs are heightened and threatened.

Hence, as we explain it to patients, the inpatient treatment environment provides a graded series of challenges. Psychoeducational groups, the mentalizing group included, promote mentalizing; yet, owing to the high level of structure, these groups generally are not emotionally challenging. Although individual psychotherapy as Bowlby (1988) envisioned it provides a secure base for mental exploration, inevitable disruptions in the security of the relationship provide opportunities to mentalize under emotional conditions. Group psychotherapy provides a rich field for mentalizing with regard to both self and others, as there are multiple others to be mentalized and multiple others mentalizing the self. Particularly stressful are clinical rounds, 15-minute periods during which the patient meets for routine treatment review and planning with several members of the core treatment team. In clinical rounds, patients often have much at stake—for example, aspiring to influence their team members to grant them privileges and off-grounds passes, to alter aspects of their treatment program, and to support particular discharge plans. Concomitantly, team members challenge patients about treatment resistances. Particularly early in the treatment process, patients are liable to feel scrutinized, threatened, and judged harshly; accordingly, we discuss the potential for mentalizing to be distorted by paranoid processes. As we describe to patients, everyone must keep everyone else's mind in mind, notwithstanding the high levels of anxiety and frustration potentially evoked. Owing to the psychoeducational focus, patients become keenly aware of the need to mentalize in this context, even if they are not able to do it consistently, and we find that discussing these challenges in the psychoeducational context enables patients to be more reflective about their experience of clinical rounds.

Finally, we characterize family work, done routinely in telephone conference calls and occasionally in face-to-face meetings, as the most stressful aspect of treatment. As our colleague, psychologist Toby Haslam-Hopwood, tells patients, these family sessions entail "mentalizing under battlefield conditions"—remaining in the mentalizing mode in the face of threats in attachment relationships. Patients routinely observe that not only they but also their family members have great difficulty mentalizing. As we explain it, we aspire to "push the envelope," in effect, by raising the threshold of emotional arousal at which patients and their family members are able to retain mentalizing capacities.

We also take advantage of the psychoeducational group on mentalizing to address treatment resistance as a ubiquitous and understandable phenomenon. We help patients understand that resistance is a natural expression of inevitable anxiety evoked by the prospect of changing patterns of behavior that are adaptive in some sense while maladaptive in others. In this context, we encourage patients to examine their ambivalence about treatment and about change; awareness of resistance is but one instance of a hallmark of mentalizing, that is, tolerance of ambivalence and conflicting emotions, which perforce entails adopting multiple mental perspectives on the same reality.

Mentalizing Exercises

Improved mentalizing capacities depend on integrating the explicit with the implicit. Explicitly, beyond explaining the concept, we endeavor to promote positive attitudes toward mentalizing as well as paying greater attention to doing it. Yet we aspire to go beyond explicit understanding by fostering patients' capacity to mentalize implicitly in daily life. As we already have stated, treatment affords multiple arenas for practicing attentiveness to mentalizing and for cultivating greater skill, particularly under emotional conditions. Not infrequently, we use the cliché "walking the walk as well as talking the talk." Yet we do not want to minimize the value of talk—explicit mentalizing. Imagine trying to teach someone how to play the piano or to drive a car without explicit instruction: it would be possible but highly inefficient. We employ explicit instruction to draw attention to a process that also must be performed implicitly.

Following the model of psychoeducation in the Professionals in Crisis program, our colleague, psychologist April Stein, initiated the implementation of a similar group in the treatment program for young adults in transition (Poa 2006). After co-leading the group with the senior author for several weeks and identifying these young persons' need for more active involvement, she proposed that we supplement the didactic material and discussion with mentalizing exercises, tasks designed to illustrate and enhance mentalizing (Haslam-Hopwood et al. 2006). These tasks are similar in spirit to exercises incorporated in Mentalization-Based Family Therapy (Fearon et al. 2006a). The exercises help patients grasp mentalizing at an implicit level; thus we aspire to practice what we are preaching. These exercises are continually evolving; Table 10–2 highlights some of our favorites, which we discuss next.

TABLE 10–2. MENTALIZING EXERCISES

Exercise	Activity
Projective stimuli	Group members look at an ambiguous stimulus depicting an interpersonal situation, and each member constructs a story; the stories are summarized on the board and members interpret others' and their own stories.
Treatment metaphors	Group members generate a metaphor for their current experience of treatment; the metaphors are listed on the board and members interpret others' and their own metaphors.
Mentalizing situations	A group member describes an emotionally charged interpersonal situation objectively without reference to participants' mental states, and the other group members articulate inferences about the mental states likely to have been involved.
Anticipatory role-playing	A group member selects a peer to role-play an upcoming interaction (e.g., in family work) that is likely to be challenging, and the interaction is discussed in a way that promotes the group member's awareness of the other person's perspective.
Observing nonverbal interactions	Two group members volunteer to sit in front of the group and to interact without speaking for a couple of minutes; then the rest of the group members try to infer what each volunteer had been thinking and feeling.
Identify the falsehood	Each group member makes a list of five or six personality traits, one of which is not true of him or her; then other group members try to identify the false trait, giving a rationale on the basis of what they know about the person.

The richest exercise for mentalizing, we have found, employs ambiguous projective test stimuli from the Object Relations Test (Phillipson 1955; Shaw 2002). The test consists of several heavily shaded cards, most of which depict shadowy human figures in ambiguous situations. Optimally ambiguous, these stimuli elicit remarkably diverse responses from different individuals. We typically rely on two cards from the set: the first depicts a salient lone standing figure and a nearby crouching figure that may or may not be seen; the second depicts two figures facing each other, looking down in what is often interpreted as an intimate relationship. We use one card per session; we pass the card among the group members, asking each member to get a "quick take" on the card and to jot down a brief story. Then we write the gist of each patient's story on a large board.

This group-administered projective technique is extremely instructive in relation to mentalizing. We point out that, first, constructing a story is mentalizing—that is, attributing mental states to a situation. The sheer diversity of stories illustrates the multiplicity of mental perspectives on a single stimulus. We point out that mentalizing in this task is not unlike interpreting ambiguous interpersonal situations more generally inasmuch as these, too, require projection and leave much room for individual differences.

A second facet of mentalizing in this task entails inviting each patient to reflect on the basis for his or her particular story. This invitation to reflection is an especially powerful intervention in the context of the wide individual differences among stories displayed on the board; each person's uniqueness stands out starkly. Stories to the first card (with the salient individual) can range from a child being ignored by a parent to a stalker about to commit homicide. Stories to the second card (depicting a couple) can range from a loving embrace at the moment of a wedding engagement to emotional detachment in the aftermath of a breakup. Often, patients are struck by the significance of their story only after the fact; at the time of constructing the story, the meaning was opaque to them (i.e., "It just looked like that"). Thus patients become aware of the role of unconscious mental activity in their perceptions.

A third facet of mentalizing in this task, which often emerges spontaneously in the discussion, is the opportunity for patients to speculate about the meaning of other group members' stories, and this speculation is informed to varying degrees by their personal knowledge of each other from their shared experience in treatment. Alternatively, sometimes we first ask the group to infer what the story might reveal about the mind of the storyteller, and then we ask the storyteller to comment on the validity of the group members' inferences. This process is most rewarding when storytellers learn something new from the group about what is going on in their own mind.

We also devised a simple and closely related task that captures the spirit of mentalizing as "playing" with different mental perspectives: we ask group participants to generate metaphors or similes that capture something about their current mental state, illustrating with the cliché "I feel blue." Again, patients generate remarkably diverse and idiosyncratic similes (e.g., "a ship on fire in the middle of the ocean," "cleaning out the debris from the garbage disposal," "a volcano erupting in the middle of a rainstorm"). We also apply this exercise to the experience of specific treatment modalities such as clinical rounds (e.g., "I feel like a person without a law degree trying to defend my case in front of a bunch of judges"). In this task, we ask group members to speculate about the meaning of the metaphor based on their knowledge of the patient who proposed it, and then the person who generated the metaphor gives his or her own understanding of its personal significance. In the same vein, we sometimes ask group members to make a drawing, and then we ask the other group members to interpret the personal significance of the drawing. With drawings as with metaphors, the creating and the interpreting entail mentalizing.

> The psychoeducational group leaders asked the group members to come up with a metaphor for their current experience of treatment. A patient compared her treatment to a weaving, stating that the weaving was coming along well but some very complex and difficult parts were just ahead. She added that this particular weaving ultimately would be finished but that she would need to continue weaving.
>
> Group members commented on several aspects of the metaphor: that the weaver was employing skill, that weaving is part of a tradition in which skill is learned from others, that the weaver needed to keep herself in good shape to continue weaving, and that the weaver had confidence. The leaders also commented that weaving was not only a fine metaphor for treatment but also an apt metaphor for the process of mentalizing.
>
> In contrast, another group member gave a metaphor depicting a nightmare in which he was trapped at the bottom of the sea with his eyes plucked out and his soul stolen. Group members and leaders commented on the frightening quality of the metaphor as well as on the hopelessness it implied. One group leader responded that a difficult mentalizing challenge would be to find any hope in the metaphor. Brilliantly, a group member pointed out that hope lay in the fact that it was a *nightmare*—a dream, not a reality. The group leader underscored the importance of distinguishing between the mental state of hopelessness and a hopeless reality, the difference between *feeling* hopeless and *being* hopeless.

Another simple task entails asking patients to think of a recent emotionally charged interpersonal interaction and then to describe the situation entirely objectively, without including any information about the participants' mental states. For example: "My father insisted that I read a letter my mother wrote to him explaining why she left him soon after I was born." Group members are asked to share their thoughts about the mental states of all participants—not only the patient but also the mother and father in this instance. Again, after group discussion, the patient who provided the scenario comments on the accuracy of the group members' mentalizing. Not uncommonly, the patient who proposed the scenario develops a richer understanding of his or her experience in the course of the discussion.

Mentalizing is inherent in role-playing inasmuch as switching roles entails adopting different perspectives on a relationship. As a mentalizing exercise, we employ role-playing in relation to challenging interactions that patients are anticipating (e.g., a telephone call to a spouse to gauge her intentions to file for divorce). In the course of role-playing, patients are able to anticipate their own future mental states as well as to have an opportunity to consider more thoroughly their partner's point of view. Observations from other patients enrich both perspectives. Patients report subsequently that the role-playing helped them with the interaction they were anticipating.

Here is one of the most straightforward mentalizing exercises: we ask for two volunteers from the group to sit in chairs in front of the group and to interact without speaking for a couple of minutes. Then we ask the group members to state what each person was thinking and feeling during that brief time period. The volunteers then give feedback regarding the accuracy of group members' mentalizing. Even more simply, we select a single volunteer from the group to be "mentalized" and, after a minute or so of silence, patients state what they believe was on the volunteer's mind. Memorably, a young woman in one group said of her male peer who was new to the program that he was experiencing "emotional hunger" and, remarkably, of all the group members' statements, he said this observation was most on the mark.

Although we generally focus on mentalizing with respect to states of mind, we also include an exercise that involves mentalizing in relation to personality traits. Each group member writes down several adjectives characterizing his or her personality, one of which is false. Other group members are asked to identify the falsehood and to give reasons for their choice. The following is a representative list: self-conscious, kindhearted, manipulative, self-critical, and critical of others. Plainly, these characteristics might be more or less observable, and the extent to which group members can discern them will depend on the extent to which they know each other. The task is especially difficult when a member is new to the group. Generating the list also requires mentalizing in the sense of including a trait that might be relatively opaque and surprising to others. For example, the patient who included "manipulative" in his list correctly anticipated that others would not suspect this of him, and he gave convincing examples of his subtle manipulativeness.

Plainly, the number of possible mentalizing exercises is limited only by the group leaders' creativity and imagination. And group leaders need not be limited by their own imaginativeness; once patients get the general idea, they too generate instructive exercises.

Family Workshop

On the basis of our experience in patient education, our colleagues Efrain Bleiberg and Toby Haslam-Hopwood have developed a one-session, hour-long psychoeducational presentation on mentalizing for family members who attend a two-day family workshop offered routinely during each patient's inpatient stay. As is true for patients, written materials on mentalizing also are made available to family members (Allen et al. 2003).

The family workshop presentations provide a highly condensed version of the didactic material reviewed in this chapter. The presenters explain the concept of mentalizing; the developmental conditions conducive to mentalizing; the adaptive functions of mentalizing; the reasons for focusing on mentalizing in inpatient treatment; and the ways in which various treatment interventions promote mentalizing. We let family members know our view that their own mentalizing takes courage, especially when they are empathizing with the emotional pain of a loved one. As with patients, we present this material to family members with the intent of bolstering the treatment alliance: we help them understand how we clinicians are thinking about the treatment so as to engage them more effectively in collaboration. We are gratified when we hear of family members talking with patients about the importance of mentalizing. Of course, for family members as for patients, mentalizing is easier said than done, and the family work puts them all to the test.

Recapitulation

As we have discovered in other arenas of patient education (Allen 2005, 2006a), there is no better way to learn than to teach. As our colleague George Gergely (2007) has described, *pedagogy* is a uniquely human mentalizing capacity that facilitates rapid transmission of knowledge (see Chapter 3, "Development"). Like other facets of mentalizing, pedagogical interactions require that each participant has the other's mind in mind. Ironically, the psychoeducational group discussions about mentalizing demand a high level of mentalizing in appreciating patients' confusion and helping them to understand more fully.

However well intended they might be, psychoeducational groups run the risk of promoting intellectualizing. Regarding the mentalizing community we are aspiring to establish, Michels (2006) raised "the potential risks of quasi-mentalization, a collaboration between patient and therapist to pretend mentalization without the real thing," and he raised concern about how the focus on explicit mentalizing "translates into the more normal implicit capacity" (p. 331). He went on,

> We are all familiar with the humorous portrayal of the psychotherapy patient who is preoccupied with his own and others' psychodynamics, oblivious to the way in which others respond. One can envision a person, or community, in which explicit preoccupation with quasi-mentalization leads to a similar phenomenon. (p. 331)

Of course, intellectualizing—what we call operating in the pretend mode—arose long before patient education, although the kind of education we have described certainly can provide much fodder for it. This is one reason for our emphasizing that mentalizing is an emotional process and for our focus on mentalizing emotion in particular. In addition, the incorporation of mentalizing exercises into the psychoeducational groups also underscores the value of practicing, not just preaching. Yet in recognizing the need for mentalizing implicitly, we should not downplay the value of explication; to do so would be to miss the value of language and, indeed, consciousness: through the effortful regulation of attention, using the tools of language, we are able to break out of rigid patterns of ineffective behavior and respond in novel and flexible ways when nonconscious routines fail to be adaptive. Mindful of intellectualization, we should not shortchange the value of thinking.

Key Clinical Points

- *Purpose:* Psychoeducation is not intended to be a stand-alone intervention but rather is designed to enhance the therapeutic alliance in mentalizing-focused treatment, predicated on the conviction that understanding mentalizing and its value facilitates the activity of mentalizing.

- *Curriculum:* Three main components of the psychoeducational curriculum are: 1) understanding the concept of mentalizing along with the developmental conditions that promote and undermine it; 2) examining a range of psychiatric symptoms and disorders as they interact with impaired mentalizing in vicious circles; and 3) appreciating how various treatment modalities promote mentalizing.

- *Exercises:* Psychoeducation combines implicit with explicit mentalizing by incorporating group exercises that actively engage patients in contrasting different group members' perspectives on each others' mental states in the here and now. Thus many exercises are designed to highlight individual differences among group members in perceptions and interpretations of the same stimulus.

Appendix

What Is Mentalizing and Why Do It?

You are mentalizing when you're aware of what's going on in your mind or someone else's. You're mentalizing when you puzzle, "Why did I do that?" or wonder, "Did I hurt her feelings when I said that?" Your ability to mentalize enables you to make sense of behavior. You hear a car door slam shut and it draws your attention. Then you see the man who slammed the car door reaching into his pockets and coming up empty-handed. He starts to get agitated, tries unsuccessfully to open the door, looks through the car window toward the ignition, and starts cussing. All this behavior would be bewildering if you didn't automatically infer that he's frustrated because he locked his keys in the car.

Mentalizing, you automatically interpret behavior as based on mental states, such as desires, beliefs, and feelings. The man wanted to be able to drive his car, believed that he'd have a hard time getting back into it, and felt frustrated—perhaps also helpless. Sometimes you need to mentalize to interpret *your own* behavior: "How could I have been so gullible as to lend him money when I knew full well that he's totally undependable?" Often you need to mentalize to understand your emotional reactions: "Why am I *this* upset about her not calling me back right away? Why am I so sensitive right now? I've been feeling like a lot of people have been letting me down lately..."

Such questions are merely the launching point for how you might explain things to yourself. Seeing the man become frustrated about locking himself out of his car might stimulate your own memories of being locked out and a recognition that this happened to you when you were distracted. Using this further understanding from your own self-exploration will enhance the interaction if you go over to sympathize with the man and to see if you can help.

A shorthand idea for mentalizing is *keeping mind in mind*. Mentalizing requires attention and takes mental effort; it's a form of mindfulness, that is, being mindful of what others are thinking and feeling as well as being mindful of your own thoughts and feelings. Thus mentalizing is similar to empathy. But mentalizing goes beyond empathizing, because it also includes awareness of your own state of mind—empathizing with yourself. Thus, you're mentalizing when you're going in to ask your boss for some time off and you're thinking, "I'm feeling anxious. It makes sense that I'd feel anxious right now, because he might feel put out. Well, I can tolerate that." If your boss unfairly gives you grief about taking some time off, you'd be mentalizing in thinking, "I'm getting frustrated, so I need to choose my words carefully. I need to acknowledge that this makes his life more difficult and let him know how important the time off is to me." Thus you are mentalizing when you demonstrate your understanding of your boss's annoyance and try to address it while simultaneously explaining your own point of view.

The following situations call for mentalizing:

- Comforting a friend in distress
- Clearing up a misunderstanding with a friend
- Calming down a child who is having a tantrum
- Developing strategies to refrain from overeating
- Persuading an employer to give you a raise
- Proposing marriage
- Describing symptoms and problems to your psychiatrist

As all these examples attest, mentalizing is common sense; we are all natural psychologists in trying to understand behavior and figuring out why people think and feel the way they do. Mentalizing is like language in being innate: we all develop the capacity to mentalize, barring genetic conditions such as autism. Yet, like language, mentalizing develops best in an environment conducive to learning.

Like using language, mentalizing comes naturally; most of the time you don't need to think about it. You don't need to be a linguist to use language, and you don't need to become a professional psychologist to mentalize. Yet mentalizing is a *skill* that can be developed to varying degrees. Failing to mentalize can contribute to serious problems in relationships. Your friends, family members, or spouse will be unhappy if you're oblivious to their needs and feelings or if you continually misinterpret their actions. Psychiatric disorders such as depression and substance abuse notoriously interfere with mentalizing, because they compromise the capacity for flexible thinking, lead to distorted views of the self, and undermine attention to others' experience. When such disorders develop, you can benefit from learning about mentalizing, from paying greater attention to doing it, and from becoming more skillful at it.

Developmental psychologists have been researching mentalizing over the past few decades, so we now know a lot about how it develops and how we can improve it. This summary describes different aspects of mentalizing, conditions that affect mentalizing, the nature of skillful mentalizing, and the benefits of mentalizing. We conclude by revealing our main goal: to influence your attitude toward mentalizing.

Aspects of Mentalizing

Mentalizing involves awareness of yourself as well as others. Our colleague, psychiatrist Jeremy Holmes at the University of Exeter in the United Kingdom, puts it this way: mentalizing is *seeing yourself from the outside and others from the inside.* Mentalizing with regard to others takes effort: you cannot merely assume that others think and feel the way you do, although they might; you must *shift perspectives* and try to take their point of view. Thus the more you know about another person, the more accurate your mentalizing will be. For example, you are probably better at understanding a person with whom you have an intimate relationship and others who are close to you than you are at grasping the motives of more distant acquaintances. Yet, as we will discuss below, you might be aware that you also have greatest difficulty mentalizing when you come into conflict with those to whom you are closest. All of us run into circumstances that interfere with our ability to mentalize, usually when we feel threatened or find ourselves in the throes of intense emotional arousal.

You cannot take for granted your ability to mentalize with respect to yourself: even though you live in your own mind, you don't necessarily always know how your mind is working. All of us are capable of self-deception. It's common for others to see aspects of ourselves to which we are blind. Often, we know ourselves best through dialogue with others: you might start out just feeling vaguely "upset" and, over the course of the conversation with a trusted friend, come to recognize that you're feeling hurt, ashamed, and resentful. Thus others, seeing us from the outside, can help us see ourselves more clearly from the inside.

You can mentalize in different time frames. You can mentalize about specific mental states in the *present:* "I'm getting all worked up for nothing." "She's starting to get impatient with me." Also, you can reflect on *past* mental states: "Now that I've calmed down, I can see that she intended her criticism to help me, not to belittle me." In addition, you can mentalize by anticipating *future* mental states: "If I don't let her know that I'll be late, she'll worry and then I'll feel guilty."

Most important, you can transform hindsight into foresight: mentalizing about problems in the past can enhance your ability to mentalize in the future. "I know I'm extremely sensitive to criticism and I get so defensive that I can't listen to her point of view. Next time, I'll try to think about where she's coming from, listen carefully to what she's saying, and avoid another blowup."

Just as you can mentalize about the present, past, or future, you can mentalize with a narrower or broader perspective. You can focus narrowly on a person's feelings at a given moment: "She looks irritated." In addition, you can be aware of the broader context of her mental state: "She thinks I lied to her." You can even take into account a broad swath of the person's history: "She's extremely sensitive to any sign of betrayal because of her father's recurrent untrustworthy behavior." Thus, expanding the scope of mentalizing may take into account a broader time frame as well as the wider network of interactions and relationships that influence an individual's mental states.

The same applies to your own mental states: self-understanding often requires you to consider the wider context beyond the present moment. You might wonder, "Why am I so upset that he didn't acknowledge how much work I did on this project?" Mentalizing, you might realize that you've been feeling unappreciated for a long time and that not having this particular project recognized was the last straw. You can take this line of thinking all the way back to your childhood, for example, connecting your current feelings with repeated disappointments in the past, when a parent routinely failed to attend school plays or sports events. Your feelings about the present invariably are colored by your past experiences, and mentalizing involves being aware of this coloring—the "baggage" from the past—so that you can see the present for what it is.

You can mentalize more or less consciously. Mentalizing *explicitly* is a conscious process in which you think deliberately about the reasons for actions—often when you are puzzled: "Why would she have said that?" "How could I have forgotten to do that when I knew it was so important to him?" You mentalize explicitly when you put your feelings into words, whether you're trying to make sense of yourself in your own mind or needing to express what you're feeling to someone else.

Most often, however, you don't have time to mentalize explicitly when you're interacting with others; you're mentalizing *implicitly*—that is, spontaneously and intuitively, without thinking about it. Mentalizing implicitly, you're guided by your gut feelings. When your friend tells you about a major disappointment, you automatically adopt an expression combining sadness and caring, leaning forward to make emotional contact. Thus the natural empathy you have for others is based on your ability to mentalize implicitly. You also mentalize implicitly when you engage in conversation, keeping the other person's perspective in mind and taking turns naturally without having to think about it. (You're likely to find conversations annoying when others fail to mentalize, mentioning names of people you don't know without taking into consideration that you have no idea who they're talking about.)

When all goes well, you can get by with mentalizing intuitively and implicitly. Using language naturally, you don't need to think about your choice of words until you're misunderstood. Similarly, you need to mentalize deliberately and explicitly when you hit a snag in a relationship. Much of your *explicit* mentalizing takes the form of *narrative*, through which you make your own and others' actions intelligible. You ceaselessly create stories involving thoughts and feelings. Think of a time when you had to justify your actions to someone, such as asking your boss for time off. Think about how you explain your emotional reactions to someone else's behavior. Think about how squabbling children behave when a parent confronts them. Each one comes up with a different story; then the parent needs to mentalize to sort it out and intervene appropriately.

You begin learning to mentalize early in life by creating stories to account for your actions. And you do this in your own mind. For better and at times for worse, you continually tell yourself stories about yourself, and these stories influence who you are. Self-critical stories, for example, can undermine your self-confidence. "Nothing I do ever turns out right, no matter how hard I try. I'm useless. If anything goes wrong, I'm always the one to be blamed. The story of my life…"

Ideally, mentalizing, like story telling more generally, is creative: mentalizing, you come up with fresh perspectives, seeing yourself and others from more than one point of view. Thus you're mentalizing when you wonder, "I'm really irked at him. What *else* might I be feeling? I guess he hurt my feelings." Similarly, you're mentalizing when, after you think, "What an idiot I am," you reconsider and think, "I made an understandable mistake; I was trying to do too much at once." Jeremy Holmes insightfully construed psychotherapy as a "story-making" and "story-breaking" process. Mentalizing, you move out of old ruts in the stories you create about yourself and others.

Conditions for Mentalizing

Children learn language best in a language-rich environment, by hearing speech, being spoken to, and being listened to and responded to when they are learning to speak. Similarly, children learn to mentalize best when their family members are sensitive to their states of mind, especially their emotions. Children learn to mentalize by *being mentalized*, that is, when others have their mind in mind. Mentalizing will not flourish in emotionally neglectful relationships. Rather, mentalizing develops best in trusting and safe relationships—what we call secure attachment relationships. Moreover, once children begin to acquire language, talking openly with them about their own and others' needs, feelings, fears, and reasons for actions gives mentalizing a great boost. As with all other skills, mentalizing is learned through practice, and learning continues throughout the lifetime.

Developing the ability to mentalize is one thing; *using* it consistently is another. Some conditions are more conducive to mentalizing than others. Your level of emotional arousal is a major factor in being able to mentalize at any given moment. Mentalizing goes best when your level of emotional arousal is neither too high nor too low. You need to feel relatively safe to mentalize. If you're feeling threatened—angry or frightened—you'll be more concerned with self-protection than with taking the time and effort to mentalize. In states of high emotional arousal, the instinctive fight-or-flight response takes over, and mentalizing falls by the wayside. You can feel so panicky or infuriated that you can't think straight, much less consider what someone else is thinking or feeling.

As we already indicated, you're generally likely to have most difficulty mentalizing in emotionally close attachment relationships when conflicts arise and feelings run high. Catch-22: *mentalizing is most difficult when you most need to do it*. That's why much of our mentalizing takes place after the fact; fortunately, you can translate hindsight into foresight and thereby turn your misunderstandings into understandings, much like you might do with your partner after a falling out. And you may need professional help in the form of individual or couples therapy so that you can learn to mentalize when you're experiencing conflict or feeling threatened in your attachment relationships. Mentalizing enables you to be aware of your feelings as well as those of your partner. To engage in constructive problem solving, each person needs to keep their own mind as well as the other's mind in mind. And the best way to engage another person in mentalizing is to be doing it yourself.

Either too much or too little emotional arousal can interfere with mentalizing. If you're too depressed or lethargic, you won't be inclined to mentalize. Mentalizing takes effort, and you must be motivated to do it. If you're indifferent to others' needs or feelings, you won't be inclined to mentalize.

Skillful Mentalizing

The two hallmarks of skillful mentalizing are *accuracy* and *richness*. Mentalizing accurately means seeing others for who they really are as well as seeing yourself for who you really are. Mentalizing requires imagination—for example, being able to project your own experience into others, putting yourself in their shoes, and imagining how you might feel if you were in their situation. But projecting from your own experience can be a slippery slope; your imagination can lead to distorted mentalizing. For example, feeling ashamed and inadequate or being excessively self-critical, you might wrongly imagine that others look down on you or judge you harshly. In so doing, you would be mentalizing, but you would be mentalizing inaccurately.

We are often asked, "Can you mentalize too much?" Frequently, this question reveals ineffective or inaccurate mentalizing such as obsessing or worrying about what someone else is thinking or ruminating about your past failures and deficiencies. Skillful mentalizing, on the contrary, is flexible and exploratory; you're not stuck in a rut. Of course, as with all else, health lies in balance; there's more to life than mentalizing.

As problems with worrying and ruminating illustrate, mentalizing accurately means *grounding your imagination in reality*; you might do this by asking others what they think and feel instead of relying solely on your assumptions or projections. If you think someone is put out with you or critical of what you've done but you're not sure, you can ask. If you're unsure of your interpretation of a situation, you can check out how others saw it. Often, different people interpret the same situation in different ways. This brings us to the essence of mentalizing: recognizing that there are many mental perspectives on the same outer reality. That's *mental* reality.

Richness in mentalizing refers to the process of *mental elaboration*—making the effort to use your imagination and think beyond the surface. A father is failing to mentalize when he dismisses his son's tears as showing that "he's just a spoiled brat" rather than considering the basis of his son's disappointment or frustration. Similarly, thinking that a co-worker is "just a jerk" is a non-mentalizing view. You might think of yourself in the same non-mentalizing way: "I'm just lazy" or "I'm just impulsive." The word "just" is a tip-off to non-mentalizing; it closes off thoughtful exploration of the potential multitude of reasons for behavior.

In her book *The Sovereignty of Good*, novelist and philosopher Iris Murdoch provided a now-celebrated example of a mother-in-law's shift in perspective regarding her daughter-in-law, a shift in viewpoint that illustrates a transformation from inaccurate to accurate mentalizing. Initially, the mother-in-law found her daughter-in-law to be crude, unrefined, and juvenile; she thought her son had married beneath him. Outwardly, she treated her daughter-in-law with impeccable kindness, but, inwardly, she felt scorn. Yet the mother-in-law was uncomfortable with her attitude and wondered if she was being snobbish. She put her mind to seeing her daughter-in-law accurately, justly, and lovingly. She was determined to see her daughter-in-law for who she really was. Through a concerted effort of attention and imagination, she came to see her daughter-in-law not as vulgar but rather as refreshingly simple, spontaneous, and delightfully youthful—a dramatic shift of perspective.

Because mentalizing is inherently open-ended, allowing for multiple perspectives, you know you've stopped mentalizing whenever you have a sense of certainty. You've stopped mentalizing when you declare, "I *know* you really don't want me here!" You've shifted into mentalizing when you say, "I'm *thinking* you really don't want me here—is that so?"

The Benefits of Mentalizing

The most obvious benefit of mentalizing is *engaging in fulfilling relationships with others,* particularly those to whom you are emotionally attached. Mentalizing—each person having the other's mind in mind—lies at the heart of intimacy. Mentalizing skillfully also enables you to influence others effectively, taking their point of view into account while respecting their individuality. When you fail to mentalize, you tend to *impose* your point of view and your will on others, trying to force them to comply with your wishes, needs, or beliefs. Conflict, antagonism, and resentment are bound to ensue. And mentalizing not only allows you to influence others but also opens you up to *being influenced* by others. You could not learn from others by seeing things from their perspective if you were unable to have their mind in your mind. Healthy relationships depend on it.

Ironically, while mentalizing develops best in secure attachment relationships in childhood, one advantage of secure attachments is that you typically don't have to put too much conscious effort into mentalizing as long as things are going smoothly. You will need to put effort into mentalizing, however, when you are in competitive relationships as well as when you are not sure of another person's trustworthiness. If you are naively trusting—not making the effort to discern the other person's true intentions or motives—you can put yourself in danger. Thus, in a new relationship, cautious appraisal as well as being attuned to your gut reactions is essential. Failing to mentalize can be even more calamitous if the other person senses your naiveté through his or her own mentalizing but then exploits your innocence for personal gain. Such misuse of mentalizing becomes a way of gratifying oneself or furthering one's own interests rather than a self-reflective process or joint project of mutual understanding. Of course, some leaders of organizations climb the competitive ladder in this way, and con men also must understand others' minds if they are to be successful. Like any other skill, mentalizing can be misused.

Mentalizing not only is essential to good relationships with others but also to *your relationship with yourself.* Just as you need to influence others, you need to be able to influence yourself—for example, when you want to change your feelings, attitudes, thought patterns, or behavior. To influence yourself, you must know yourself and be attuned to yourself, keeping your own mind in mind. If you're struggling with an addiction, for example, you need to anticipate situations that will tempt you and then steer clear of them.

Mentalizing your emotions is most important and most difficult. You can be immersed in an emotional state without mentalizing. You can be emotionally agitated and appear tense and edgy to others without being aware of your feelings. Or you may be dimly aware of feeling "out of sorts" but not be clear about just what you are feeling or why. Mentalizing emotion requires *feeling* and *thinking about feeling* at the same time, clarifying your feelings and their basis. Your feelings are your gut-level guide to your needs and to how your relationships are going. You feel annoyed when someone invades your space, and your annoyance prompts you to stand up for yourself. When you're aware of your feelings through mentalizing, you're in the best position to get your needs met effectively. You can express your feelings to others accordingly and thus solve the problems that your feelings are signaling: "I don't like it when you just barge in without knocking." Even when it's not a good idea to express your feelings outwardly to others, you can at least express them inwardly to yourself. Ideally, you can take an understanding and compassionate attitude toward your feelings, just as you would wish others to do. You might not want to tell your boss how angry you are about his being unreasonable, but you might say to yourself, "I can't believe how aggravating this is—no wonder I was anxious about asking him for time off!" And you might express your feelings later to a trusted friend as well.

Mentalizing your emotions also enables you to refrain from impulsive and self-defeating behavior—storming out of your boss's office. Mentalizing is like pushing a *pause button*—not merely "counting to ten" but also giving yourself time to think about your needs and feelings and the best way to manage them rather than employing desperate measures to quell them. For example, mentalizing enables you to recognize, tolerate, regulate, and express your feelings of frustration rather than having to drink to the point of intoxication to get rid of them.

A Mentalizing Stance

To repeat, mentalizing is like language: short of rare genetic abnormalities or extreme deprivation, we all learn to talk and we all learn to mentalize. Yet all of us can learn to speak and write more articulately, and all of us can learn to mentalize more effectively and consistently. The most frequent problem with mentalizing is not lacking the basic ability but rather failing to cultivate it and put it to use. When you're having trouble in close relationships or difficulty managing your own emotional states, you'll need to pay more attention to mentalizing and put more effort into it. You may need professional help. We've said that the best way to influence another person to mentalize is to do it yourself; mentalizing begets mentalizing. This is what we therapists aspire to do: by mentalizing, we help our patients to mentalize. In fact, we believe that the success of all forms of therapy rests on mentalizing on the part of therapists and their patients.

As therapists, we wrote this description to inspire what we call a *mentalizing stance:* an attitude of openness, inquisitiveness, and curiosity about what's going on in others' minds and in your own. This mentalizing stance requires tolerance for ambiguity—that is, comfort with not knowing. Mentalizing involves exploring possibilities with an open-minded attitude, a sense that there's always more to the story. Accordingly, this brief account is a mere introduction.

Chapter 11

Social Systems

Inasmuch as attachment relationships are the crucible for mentalizing, we have followed Bowlby's (1988) lead in extrapolating from the mother-child relationship to the individual psychotherapy relationship: we strive to provide belated developmental help through a relationship that exploits the synergy between secure attachment and mentalizing. Yet, building on Fraiberg and colleagues' (1975) pioneering work, we have gone beyond dyadic attachment relationships to consider how the therapist-parent relationship can be employed to promote mentalizing in the parent-infant relationship. In addition, we have described how therapists can promote mentalizing at a family system level. We also recognize, however, that influences on mentalizing extend beyond attachment relationships and the family: not only peer relationships but also the wider environment influences the refinement and use of whatever mentalizing capacities the individual has developed. Accordingly, there is a potential role for mentalizing interventions to extend beyond the individual and family to the wider social community.

As we describe in this chapter, our interest in mentalizing at the level of the community evolved in conjunction with the pervasive problem of community violence. To a considerable degree, violence and trauma are the flip sides of one coin: violence—psychological as well as physical—is traumatizing behavior. Correspondingly, as we explicate in this chapter, not only being traumatized but also inflicting trauma is associated with impaired mentalizing capacity. It was the potentially unending intergenerational cycles of violence and trauma that Fraiberg and colleagues' (1975) interventions were designed to interrupt.

We begin this chapter by highlighting the role of mentalizing failures in violence. Then we describe mentalizing-promoting interventions in schools. Taking a bold leap, we conclude the chapter by drawing attention to the potential relevance of mentalizing failures to global conflicts.

Mentalizing and Violence

Notwithstanding the current course of world events, Freud's concept of the death instinct would find few contemporary adherents. Yet recent developmental research indicates that Freud (1929) was on the right track when he proposed that

> men are not gentle creatures who want to be loved, and who at the most can defend themselves if they are attacked; they are, on the contrary, creatures among whose instinctual endowments is to be reckoned a powerful share of aggressiveness. (p. 68)

As is well known, Freud believed that as a result of our inherent penchant for aggression, "civilized society is perpetually threatened with disintegration.... [hence] Civilization has to use its utmost efforts in order to set limits to man's aggressive instincts" (pp. 69–70).

Consistent with Freud's view, longitudinal studies of aggressiveness in children indicate that violence is *unlearned*, not learned: "Biological predisposition and social influence do not create destructiveness, but rather compromise the social processes that normally serve to regulate and tame it" (Fonagy 2004, p. 185). In the course of optimal development, physical aggression decreases with age, from early childhood to adulthood. Yet there are wide individual differences in the developmental trajectory of aggressiveness, and longitudinal studies have delineated distinct patterns that include subgroups whose aggression fails to abate or even increases over the course of development (Boidy et al. 2003; White et al. 2001).

A wide range of risk and protective factors relating to the development of aggression have been identified (Rutter et al. 1998); while recognizing this complexity, we focus on mentalizing capacity, a critical means by which civilization tames aggression. As described elsewhere (Fonagy 2004), the propensity for physical aggression ordinarily decreases over the course of development as mentalizing and the associated capacities for self-regulation become more solidly established. A core facet of mentalizing inhibits aggression: attunement and emotional responsiveness to the current mental state of the other individual. Conversely, although a host of risk factors come into play, the final common pathway for acts of violence is the momentary inhibition of mentalizing—temporary mindblindness. Hence it is difficult to hurt another person while maintaining prolonged eye contact, which is conducive to mentalizing, and it becomes progressively easier to do so as the physical and psychological distance increases. Thus it is most difficult to assault another person with one's hands and becomes progressively easier with a knife, a gun, or a bomb. Little wonder that despite its limited effectiveness, aerial bombing remains a preferred mode of waging war (Grayling 2006).

As reviewed elsewhere (Fonagy 2003b, 2004; Fonagy and Higgitt 2004), secure attachment relationships, by virtue of promoting mentalizing, serve as a buffer against the development of aggression. Conversely, non-mentalizing parental behavior—such as coercion, assertion of power, and rejection—abets children's aggression. Hence secure attachment is conducive to the *unlearning* of aggression over the course of development, whereas insecure attachment is conducive to its maintenance or escalation.

To reiterate, in this chapter we are reconsidering the intergenerational transmission of trauma from the perspective of violence. Abusive and violent behavior evoke frustration and anger while at the same time undermining mentalizing capacity; accordingly, violence not only produces trauma but also increases the risk that the victim will engage in traumatizing violence toward others. We note, however, that maltreatment and neglect, both of which interfere with the development of mentalizing, are not the only pathway to mindblind violence. As we described in Chapter 4 ("Neurobiology"), psychopathy, which entails a partial failure of mentalizing (i.e., mindreading without empathy), also is associated with aggression. More generally, a relatively fearless temperament is associated with aggressiveness insofar as fearless children are less inclined to rely on the secure base of attachment, and thus they miss out on the opportunity to develop a robust capacity to mentalize (Fonagy 2004).

We have discussed the role of promoting mentalizing in healing from trauma in Chapter 7 ("Treating Attachment Trauma"); next we illustrate two efforts to promote mentalizing in the community for the purpose of stemming aggressive and potentially traumatizing behavior.

Violence Prevention in Schools

We present two school-based programs related to community violence, one primarily intended to prevent exposure to potentially traumatizing violence in high school students and another designed to prevent violent behavior among elementary school students. The first program, although conducted in the community, was directed primarily at influencing individual adolescents through psychoeducation. The primary target of the second program was the children's school community.

Trauma Psychoeducation

The senior author developed an interest in violence prevention in schools as an unanticipated spinoff from having extended an adult psychoeducational program on trauma (Allen 2005) to hospitalized adolescents. Initiated by our social worker colleague AnnMarie Glodich, what began as an intervention designed to facilitate coping with *past* trauma evolved into an intervention designed to promote mentalizing with the primary intention of helping traumatized adolescents avoid exposure to *future* traumatizing violence in the community.

When we began discussing ways of coping with the impact of previous exposure to traumatic stress with adolescents, we quickly became aware that we were rowing upstream: they spontaneously talked about ongoing exposure to violence along with their proclivity to engage in high-risk behavior that continually put them at risk for more of the same. Substance abuse loomed large as a factor that is notoriously associated with a high risk of exposure to potentially traumatizing events, such as assault, rape, automobile crashes, and altercations with law enforcement officers (Allen 2001). Accordingly, while not giving up our interest in trauma education, we focused the intervention rather single-mindedly on preventing reenactment of past trauma by means of promoting mentalizing (Glodich et al. 2001).

As the trauma psychoeducation group became established, we began including outpatients along with those in hospital and residential treatment; then we extended the intervention into the community, taking advantage of an opportunity to work with counselors in a local public high school. Although there is no dearth of challenges, there are many advantages to school-based mental health interventions for high-risk populations (Allen-Meares et al. 1996; Lightburn and Sessions 2006). Moreover, the school setting, where students are accustomed to classes and learning, was especially compatible with our psychoeducational format.

As in our psychoeducational approach to mentalizing, the school-based trauma psychoeducation groups included a combination of discussion and experiential exercises. Although we did not discuss "mentalizing" explicitly, we promoted it implicitly. That is, we endeavored to provide participants with a conceptual framework for understanding the relation between past exposure to traumatic events and their proclivity for ongoing traumatic reenactments. As in the adult psychoeducational program, we promoted awareness of various emotional responses to traumatic events as well as constructive means of emotion regulation. Yet, with an eye toward reenactment, we focused on power dynamics in trauma, employing the paradigmatic roles of persecutor, victim, witnessing bystander, and rescuer (Davies and Frawley 1994; Twemlow et al. 1996); at the same time, we emphasized participants' inclination to alternate among these roles in reenactments that perpetuate trauma. We based this intervention on the assumption that coercive power dynamics manifested in violent relationships and social systems tend to drive individuals out of the mentalizing mode and into enacting these trauma-related roles (Twemlow et al. 2005a). Conversely, individuals with well established mentalizing capacities are more likely to resist such coercive influence—although few of us are entirely immune to it.

In addition to highlighting these adolescents' exposure to violence in the community, our experience with the adolescent group underscored the potential for further transgenerational reenactments in their family systems. We engaged participants in creating a future family diagram, in which they created a genogram (Bowen 1980) to depict their relationships with their (future) romantic partner and children. After they had diagrammed the structure of their future family, they described their own imagined functioning in the future, their relationship with their partner and children, and their children's functioning. Routinely, we were chagrined by the extent to which maltreatment, substance abuse, and violence pervaded their imagined families of the future in a way that seemed entirely ego-syntonic to the participants; they had experienced continual violence and trauma in the past and unreflectively anticipated that the future would bring more of the same.

We promoted mentalizing in action through role-playing, using the perpetrator, victim, rescuer, and bystander roles. Videotaping these role-plays sensitized participants to the impact of their actions on others. We also engaged participants in role-playing behaviors that might defuse violence along with those that would incite violence; in so doing, we aimed to promote flexibility in responding that is compatible with mentalizing. To enhance generalization to behavior in the community, we engaged local law enforcement officers in the role-playing. The officers not only counseled participants regarding means of de-escalating violence but also talked about their own experience of interacting with violent adolescents; hence the officers, by virtue of drawing attention to their own vulnerabilities and frustrations, promoted perspective-taking responses consistent with mentalizing.

As clinicians accustomed to working with adolescent groups will appreciate readily, the group *process* bears as much relation to mentalizing as does the clinical content. The leaders quickly came to appreciate that the group members were far more interested in talking with each other than in listening to them. Moreover, the leaders soon adopted the primary goal of encouraging members to listen respectfully to one another—to mentalize vis-à-vis the other. This process orientation parallels interventions in family therapy intended to promote mentalizing through more attentive listening (Fearon et al. 2006a; see Chapter 8, "Parenting and Family Therapy").

This relatively small-scale clinical project included an evaluation component with a wait-list control (Glodich 1999). An initial study based on an 8-session intervention showed that the participants, despite reporting a history of substantial exposure to violence in the family and community, along with a high level of engagement in risk-taking behaviors in the community, reported relatively low levels of classic posttraumatic symptoms. Moreover, despite having acquired a high level of knowledge about trauma, participants in the intervention group did not differ from those in the control group in reported propensity to high-risk behavior at post-test. Yet across all participants, there was a positive correlation between knowledge about trauma and holding adaptive attitudes toward risk-taking behaviors. Furthermore, quite uniformly, participants reported highly positive attitudes toward the group. A replication of this initial study employed a somewhat more intensive 12-session intervention (Glodich et al. 2006); Table 11–1 presents an overview of this curriculum. Notwithstanding the incorporation of more refined psychometric measures, this replication likewise failed to demonstrate significant differences between intervention and control groups, notwithstanding that participants highly valued the group experience. The project was hampered, however, by high rates of attrition and sporadic attendance. Moreover, we had the impression that our adolescent participants were neither forthcoming nor careful in their responses to self-report questionnaires.

TABLE 11–1. ADOLESCENT TRAUMA PSYCHOEDUCATIONAL GROUP
CURRICULUM

Session 1: Participants discuss typical situations that entail exposure to
violence, with an emphasis on power differences among participants; group
members write down one personal experience of exposure to violence.

Session 2: Co-leaders review the fight-or-flight response, reexperiencing
trauma, reenactments, and risk-taking behavior; group members discuss the
capacity to make choices and the importance of compassion.

Session 3: Group discussion focuses on the impact of trauma on self-esteem
and ways of restoring self-esteem.

Session 4: Reenactments of traumatic relationships are explicated through the
roles of victim, abuser, rescuer, and bystander; co-leaders model by role-
playing.

Session 5: Group members engage in role playing the trauma-related roles,
and they practice alternatives to behaving in abusive, victimized, and
neglectful ways.

Session 6: Co-leaders videotape group members role-playing a stressful
interaction, followed by a second version of the role-play that illustrates ways
of averting reenactment of trauma.

Session 7: Group discusses the videotape made in Session 6; participants
identify the various trauma-related roles and consider ways of avoiding
traumatic reenactments.

Session 8: Local police officers join the group in street clothes to discuss high-
risk situations and ways of defusing violence; police officers engage in role-
playing with participants.

Session 9: Police officers come to the group in uniform, and group members
continue role-playing and discussing high-risk situations and coping
strategies.

Session 10: Group members discuss ways that feelings such as fear, anger, and
guilt, as well as externalizing blame, contribute to reenactments and violence;
participants receive help in identifying their own contributions to
interpersonal conflicts and in identifying self-deception in relationships.

Session 11: Group members discuss their future plans and goals centering
around imagining their future family; discussion highlights the potential for
intergenerational transmission of trauma in the future family and ways of
averting such reenactments.

Session 12: Participants rewrite the traumatic experience about which they
wrote in Session 1 and identify differences between the two narratives; group
members engage in a general discussion of what they have learned and
provide feedback to the co-leaders.

Having failed to demonstrate effectiveness with psychometric measures, we conducted a more clinically oriented qualitative study of the impact of the group. We engaged facilitators and the law enforcement officers in focus groups aiming to develop interview questions and procedures to explore the potential impact of the group on an individual basis. Qualitative analysis of a brief semistructured interview with each participant indicated several domains of direct benefit from the group, which we coded in several categories as listed in Table 11–2. Interviewers were trained to elicit specific examples from daily life as evidence of benefit. Although there was individual variation in the nature and extent of benefit, most participants gave anecdotal evidence of benefit in a number of the categories we had delineated (Glodich et al. 2006). For example, participants reported walking away from fights, employing self-regulation skills to calm their anger, improving antagonistic relationships with family members, and having greater awareness of the influence of past trauma on their current behavior. This shift in evaluation

---

TABLE 11–2.   CATEGORIES OF BENEFIT FROM THE PSYCHOEDUCATIONAL GROUP

Awareness and insight

- Self-awareness (e.g., the relation between trauma history and present behavior)
- Awareness of exercising one's will (e.g., thinking before acting)

Active coping

- Trauma avoidance (e.g., extricating oneself from conflicts and risky situations)
- Control of anger and aggression (e.g., avoiding arguments; cooperating with teachers' and administrators' requests)
- Positive coping skills (e.g., self-regulation skills such as ways of calming fear and anger)

Relationships

- Feeling of connection with others (e.g., empathy and compassion; universality)
- Trust (e.g., feeling safe and opening up to others)
- Relationship repair (e.g., negotiating and resolving conflicts with peers and parents)
- Seeking help (e.g., talking about problems and feelings with others)
- Giving help (e.g., offering support to others)

---

strategy from questionnaires to interviews sensitized us to the fact—now obvious in hindsight—that different individuals benefited in different ways.

In the course of moving the psychoeducational intervention from the clinic to the school, we were keenly aware of aspiring to influence not only the student participants but also some of the school personnel. Individual interviews of the group facilitators indicated that as a result of conducting the groups, facilitators felt less helpless and more effective in working with traumatized students. They gave numerous examples of applying what they learned in the psychoeducational group to their interactions with students in other contexts, and they also gave evidence of personal growth. Thus, as we had done with the adolescent participants, we aspired to cultivate a mentalizing stance among the facilitators, and in the process, we established a small network of advocates in the school and police department who learned about trauma-related violence and ways of averting it.

We have no illusions about the depth of the impact of this psycho-educational intervention; we were challenged to demonstrate a systematic short-term benefit, and we did not assess its long-range impact. We recognize that the enthusiasm for the intervention in the school system might reflect the pressing need to *do something* about pervasive violence and trauma and the relief at doing anything reasonable. The limitations of education alone as well as those of brief interventions for such entrenched social problems are all too apparent (Fonagy and Higgitt 2004). Thus we present this work primarily to illustrate a general theme of this book, namely, how a focus on enhancing mentalizing can provide a useful conceptual framework for developing psychosocial interventions. Next, we present a more ambitious and extensively researched intervention designed to prevent violence, an intervention pitched explicitly at the social-system level.

Peaceful Schools Project

Throughout this book we have focused on mentalizing impairments in individuals, although we have viewed the family group as the crucible for mentalizing. We find it useful, however, to go beyond the individual and family to consider that social groups and communities can be more or less inclined to mentalize or supportive of mentalizing. At worst, "Mentalizing is a key psychological skill absent from violent individuals and communities" (Twemlow et al. 2005a, p. 265). Our approach to promoting mentalizing in school systems was instigated by an incident in which several second-grade boys participated in the attempted sexual assault of a second-grade girl. Although this was a shocking and atypical event, it occurred in the context of a Midwestern city school with the highest out-of-school suspension rate and the lowest performance on standardized achievement tests in the entire school district. The assault was atypical, but the problems with interpersonal violence and bullying were not. Here we summarize briefly a program that has evolved over more than a decade and continues to do so (Twemlow and Fonagy 2006; Twemlow et al. 2005b).

The traditional approach to violent behavior entails intervening at the level of individuals (e.g., placement in special classrooms or schools) and, sometimes, families (e.g., family counseling or therapy). Such approaches are liable to be limited in effectiveness to the extent that the community itself is conducive to non-mentalizing violent behavior. Hence the Peaceful Schools Project was developed to cultivate a mentalizing social system, that is, a community with a social climate conducive to awareness of one's own and others' mental states in conjunction with compassion for others' suffering.

Central to the social-systems perspective is the view that *all* persons in the community play a significant part in bullying and violence. Hence, from the standpoint that bullying is a triadic rather than a dyadic problem, students are taught that three roles always must be taken into consideration: bully, victim, and bystander. Although only a subgroup of students are likely to be actively involved as bullies and victims, the remainder perforce will be involved as bystanders (Twemlow et al. 2004, 2005b). Aggressive bystanders encourage bullying (e.g., by laughing or egging on the aggressors). Less obviously, sheer passivity in the bystander role—doing nothing—can abet aggression. Thus a major goal of the Peaceful Schools program is to engage bystanders in actively helping to identify and curb bullying—collectively, as a community.

Although the intervention is addressed explicitly to bullying and interpersonal violence among students, the Peaceful Schools program also is designed to promote mentalizing among teachers and other school personnel. To reiterate, the entire community must be engaged in mentalizing—promoting curiosity, understanding, and compassion. Sadly, teachers are an important part of the problem, not only as bystanders and victims but also as bullies. A systematic study revealed that a substantial proportion of elementary school teachers observe other teachers bullying students, and in one sample, 45% of teachers acknowledged bullying students at least on occasion (Twemlow and Fonagy 2005; Twemlow et al. 2006). Attesting to the intergenerational nature of the problem, teachers who bullied were more likely to report a history of having been bullied as students. Furthermore, high rates of bullying by teachers were observed in schools with high rates of suspension, suggesting that teachers disposed to bullying may either assimilate to the violent culture or drift toward more violent institutions and remain in them—or both. Given their direct or indirect involvement in the problem, engaging teachers in promoting mentalizing among students and embracing the associated values is an optimal way of encouraging them to use their own mentalizing capacities more consistently. The multifaceted Peaceful Schools intervention includes several components summarized in Table 11–3.

Compared with two control conditions, psychiatric consultation and treatment as usual, the Peaceful Schools intervention was effective

---

TABLE 11–3. CORE COMPONENTS OF PEACEFUL SCHOOLS

The positive climate campaign aspires to raise awareness of bullying, victimization, and bystander behavior at the time these behaviors are occurring as well as to foster a shift in attitudes toward bullying. This consciousness raising is done by means of counselor-led discussions, posters, magnets, and bookmarks.

Classroom management strategies and discipline plans include attention to bullying when it is occurring; this process involves identifying those occupying the bully, victim, and bystander roles. The whole classroom participates in the identification of the problem, and the class as a whole takes responsibility for the conduct of its members. Repeated offenses are dealt with by a power-referral chart, filled out collectively, which can result in a more concerted effort at understanding that might involve the school counselor or social worker as well as the family. This intervention is intended to maintain a mentalizing stance rather than a punitive orientation.

Mentors—typically, relaxed and noncompetitive older men—serve as mentalizing role models who help children negotiate and resolve conflicts, for example, on the playground. The mentor's intervention in antagonistic interactions brings in a third perspective and thereby helps antagonists with perspective taking.

The Gentle Warrior physical education program incorporates role-playing and relaxation exercises along with defensive martial arts techniques. Non-aggressive, cognitive strategies are learned as alternatives to fighting. Increasing physical and interpersonal self-confidence decreases fearfulness and thereby enhances a sense of safety that is conducive to mentalizing.

Ten minutes of class reflection time is built into the end of each day. During this time, the class reflects on bullying, victimization, and bystander behavior; then the class makes a collective decision about whether to display a banner outside the classroom proclaiming that the class has had a good day.

---

in decreasing peer-reported victimization, aggression, and aggressive bystander behavior (Twemlow and Fonagy 2006; Twemlow et al. 2005b; P. Fonagy, S.W. Twemlow, E. Vernberg, et al.: "A Randomized Controlled Trial of a Child-Focused Psychiatric Consultation and a School Systems-Focused Intervention to Reduce Aggression," submitted for publication). Moreover, these beneficial changes were maintained at one-year follow-up. Further strengthening these findings, research ratings of extent of individual teacher adherence to the Peaceful Schools philosophy showed the most beneficial effects for those teachers who followed the protocol more closely.

Concomitant with its impact on aggression, exposure to two consecutive years of the Peaceful Schools intervention led to pronounced improvements in achievement test scores in reading, language, and mathematics—on average, a gain of 8–10 percentile points (Fonagy et al. 2005). These gains are consistent with observed decreases in off-task and disruptive behavior in Peaceful Schools classrooms. It is likely that the increased sense of safety and associated decrease in anxiety promoted better concentration and task orientation among Peaceful Schools students. Notably, students who changed schools after only one year of the intervention showed a substantial decline in performance, attesting to the detrimental effects of moving from a protective, nonviolent environment to one in which no special effort is made to promote safety in a way that is conducive to learning.

With an eye toward prevention and early intervention, the Peaceful Schools program targeted several elementary schools. Albeit communities in themselves, these schools are merely part of a still larger community. As the size of the community under consideration grows, the sheer difficulty as well as the profound importance of promoting mentalizing only increases:

> The larger question of whether a community can reflect the mentalizing power-dynamics perspective in the way it organizes itself remains unanswered. We believe that for communities to reflect the high quality of life demanded by citizens in an open democracy, such changes in how the system as a whole operates must occur. (Twemlow and Fonagy 2006, pp. 304–305)

Global Conflicts

Plainly, the power struggles witnessed on elementary school playgrounds are merely a microcosm of exponentially more dangerous global conflicts that are brought to our attention on a daily basis with news of terrorist attacks, war, and genocide. Current events are dire enough, but it could become worse: more than 99.9% of species that ever existed on earth have become extinct (Mayr 1988), and we humans have been developing technologies that promise to hasten the seemingly inevitable—our own extinction. Even before the development of nuclear and biological weapons, Freud (1929) explicated this plight:

> Men have gained control over the forces of nature to such an extent that with their help they would have no difficulty in exterminating one another to the last man. They know this, and hence comes a large part of their current unrest, their unhappiness and their mood of anxiety. (p. 112)

Philosopher Hannah Arendt's (1963) controversial book *Eichmann in Jerusalem: A Report on the Banality of Evil* drew our attention to the potentially global scale of trauma wrought, in part, by failures of mentalizing (Allen 2007). What we construe as mindblindness fits precisely Arendt's (2003) psychologically perspicacious characterization of Eichmann as a man

> whose only personal distinction was perhaps *extraordinary shallowness.* However monstrous the deeds were, the doer was neither monstrous nor demonic, and the only specific characteristic one could detect in his past as well as in his behavior during the trial and the preceding police examination was something entirely negative: it was not stupidity but a curious, quite authentic *inability to think.* (p. 159, emphasis added)

Perhaps better than anyone else, Arendt apprehended the gravity of what we are calling mindblindness. Writing a few decades after Freud (1929), and no stranger to the phenomenon of reenactment, she was equally alarmed about the potential for global havoc:

> It is in the very nature of things human that every act that has once made its appearance and has been recorded in the history of mankind stays with mankind as a potentiality long after its actuality has become a thing of the past. No punishment has ever possessed enough power of deterrence to prevent the commission of crimes. On the contrary, whatever the punishment, once a specific crime has appeared for the first time, its reappearance is more likely than its initial emergence could ever have been. The particular reasons that speak for the possibility of a repetition of the crimes committed by the Nazis are even more plausible. The frightening coincidence of the modern population explosion with the discovery of technical devices that, through automation, will make large sections of the population "superfluous" even in terms of labor, and that, through nuclear energy, make it possible to deal with this twofold threat by the use of instruments beside which Hitler's gassing installations look like an evil child's fumbling toys, should be enough to make us tremble. (Arendt 1963, p. 273)

This vision of automated evildoing brings us back to what Arendt saw as Eichmann's "inability to think." Of course, "thinking" encompasses far more than mentalizing. Yet mentalizing was precisely the *domain* of thinking that Arendt perceived Eichmann to be lacking. In embracing the Nazi ideology, he dehumanized those whose slaughter he engineered in a mindless bureaucratic machine of "industrialized murder" (Arendt 2003, p. xii). Many of Arendt's readers took umbrage at her provocative thesis: "The trouble with Eichmann was precisely that so many were like him, and that so many were neither perverted nor sadistic, that they were, and still are, terribly and terrifyingly normal" (Arendt 1963, p. 276). Arendt quoted one psychiatrist as declaring Eichmann as "More normal, at any rate, than I am after having examined him" (Arendt 1963, p. 25). The banal point: normal persons can do incalculable damage by the mundane act of failing to mentalize—behaving mindblindly. And mentalizing failures are ubiquitous; as Arendt (1971) maintained, "inability to think is not a failing of the many who lack brain power but an ever-present possibility for everybody—scientists, scholars, and other specialists in mental enterprises not excluded" (p. 191).

On the basis of his examinations of violent offenders, Baumeister (1997) came to a conclusion similar to Arendt's; his most unwelcome inference: "Understanding evil begins with the realization that we ourselves are capable of doing many of these [evil] things" (p. 5). In using the term "evil" we do not imply any supernatural phenomenon, nor are we adopting any religious perspective. Rather, we adhere to Card's (2002) secular conception of evil: *culpable wrongdoing that results in intolerable harms.* While we might seem to be going off the deep end in bringing "evil" into the discussion of mentalizing, many traumatized persons wrestle explicitly with concerns about good and evil (Allen 2005), and their concerns have been a mainstay of centuries of philosophy (Neiman 2002) and theology (Taliaferro 2005). Now, references to "evil" routinely punctuate political dialogue.

Encompassing mindblindness, Card's view of culpability includes negligence and recklessness as well as malicious intent. As Arendt grasped, relatively few persons who commit evil acts are motivated by conscious sadism. Numerous motives for evildoing are more common than sheer malice: desire for material gain, narcissistic threats, pursuit of ideological aims, ambition, honor, envy, and boredom (Baumeister 1997; Kekes 2005). Coupled with mindblindness, such ubiquitous motives and affects can be profoundly dangerous. Of course, sometimes the level of mindblindness and aggression goes far beyond the ordinary, as some of Baumeister's (1997) examples attest: Spree killer Frederick Tresh stated, "Other than the two we killed, the two we wounded, the woman we pistol-whipped, and the light bulbs we stuck in people's mouths, we didn't really hurt anybody" (p. 6). A man who captured five different women at gunpoint, raped them, and stabbed them to death "said he had always made sure to be 'kind and gentle' with them, at least 'until I started to kill them'" (p. 41).

Prompted by her disquieting insights about Eichmann, Arendt (1971) became captivated by the process and significance of *thinking*, and her thinking about thinking not only underscores the potentially dire social consequences of mindblindness but also brilliantly illuminates the spirit of what we have come to call the mentalizing *stance*—an exploratory attitude of inquisitiveness and curiosity. Arendt (1971) was taken by what Kant had called the scandal of reason—in Arendt's words, "the fact that our mind is not capable of certain and verifiable knowledge regarding matters and questions that it nevertheless cannot help thinking about" (p. 14). Elaborating this point, she stated that "man's need to reflect encompasses nearly everything that happens to him, things he knows as well as things he can never know" (p. 14). She made use of Kant's distinction between knowing and thinking: knowing entails the search for *truth*, whereas thinking entails a quest for *meaning*. Pertinent to our clinical concerns, this distinction marks the difference between scientific inquiry and psychotherapeutic exploration (Strenger 1991). Pressing her point, Arendt formulated an inevitable conflict between the relentless need to think and the desire to know: "To expect truth to come from thinking signifies that we mistake the need to think with the urge to know" (Arendt 1971, p. 61). We must be able to continue thinking without being able to know. Accordingly, in focusing on our potentially ever-present inclination to find meaning, Arendt captured what we construe as the not-knowing stance of mentalizing: we explore multilayered meanings without aspiring to a sense of certainty that would bring mentalizing to an abrupt halt.

As her work on Eichmann reveals, Arendt was concerned with the interpersonal, social, and moral implications of thinking—and *not* thinking. As we noted in Chapter 5 ("The Art of Mentalizing"), mentalizing has an inescapable ethical texture. To put this point more forcefully, moral development requires mentalizing. Arendt construed the activity of thinking as essential to preventing evildoing, and she also viewed thinking as the basis of judging right from wrong. Inasmuch as morality is fundamentally about how we treat each other (Scanlon 1998), these judgments of right and wrong are founded in mentalizing. Moreover, the reflective aspect of mentalizing is essential for the highest level of moral development, as philosopher Christine Korsgaard's (2006) understanding of the uniquely human capacity for morality attests:

a nonhuman agent may be conscious of the object of his fear or desire, and conscious of it as *fearful* or *desirable*, and so as something to be avoided or to be sought. That is the ground of his action. But a rational animal is, in addition, conscious *that* she fears or desires the object, and *that* she is inclined to act in a certain way as a result.... Once you are aware that you are being moved in a certain way, you have a certain reflective distance from the motive, and you are in a position to ask yourself "but should I be moved in that way? Wanting that end inclines me to do that act, but does it really give me a reason to do that act?" You are now in a position to raise a normative question about what you *ought* to do. (p. 113; emphasis in original)

This self-reflective aspect of morality also is consistent with the relational development of mentalizing. Arendt construed thinking as an interpersonal process, a dialogue—albeit with oneself. With great insight, she reasoned that the capacity to think freely—and morality along with it—depends on the quality of one's relationship with oneself. A passage we quoted earlier bears repeating in this context: "if you want to think, you must see to it that the two who carry on the dialogue be in good shape, that the partners be *friends*" (Arendt 1971, pp. 187–188; emphasis in original). Hence, with evildoing in mind, she averred that "the self we all are must take care not to do anything that would make it impossible for the two-in-one to be friends and live in harmony" (p. 191). Alternatively, one can do evil and live comfortably with oneself only by *not* thinking, that is, remaining mindblind. Arendt's (1971) conclusion:

The manifestation of the wind of thought is not knowledge; it is the ability to tell right from wrong, beautiful from ugly. And this, at the rare moments when the stakes are on the table, may indeed prevent catastrophes, at least for the self. (p. 193)

It would be simplistic to imply that mentalizing failures are the root of all evil; the psychological and social factors that contribute to evildoing on small and large scales are extremely complex and, as always, individual differences loom large (Kekes 2005). And we would be extraordinarily naïve to imply that preventing violence by promoting greater mentalizing on a grand scale would be easy, possible, or a panacea. It is a long way from positively influencing a small number of elementary schools to resolving global conflicts. Moreover, even at the elementary school level, some classrooms were more amenable to influence than others.

Even on the smaller scale, effective prevention of adverse developmental outcomes of the kind we have been considering requires intensive and costly interventions. More specifically, as Fonagy and Higgitt (2004) delineated, interventions that are effective in promoting mental health share the following features: 1) comprehensiveness; 2) a system orientation; 3) relatively high intensity over a long duration; 4) a structured curriculum; 5) commencement early in development, for example, during pregnancy; 6) specificity with respect to particular risk factors; and 7) specific training. Accordingly, "the easiest interventions are usually the least effective" (p. 292). Even in small communities—or many families, for that matter—enduring peace is not easily achieved.

Recapitulation

We introduced this book by making a grand leap from previous applications of mentalizing to autism, developmental psychopathology, and borderline personality disorder to construing mentalizing as the most fundamental common factor in all psychotherapeutic interventions for a range of psychiatric conditions. We have ended the book by making an even grander leap into global social problems. Yet our grandiosity has limits; we endeavor merely to continue gradually expanding the purview of mentalizing and exploring its potential applications. Nonetheless, we hope that our foray into the realm of global conflicts has served to underscore what we consider to be the profound importance of mentalizing and the potentially grave implications of mindblindness.

As this book aspires to show, we have some basis for hope in our accruing knowledge about relationship conditions and associated clinical interventions that enhance mentalizing. We are heartened by the burgeoning international interest in mentalizing, especially considering that the term began to take hold in the English professional literature less than two decades ago and the word still does not appear in most dictionaries. Yet the concept has broad and deep roots in psychoanalysis, attachment theory, and developmental psychology as well as in philosophy; now its underpinnings are substantially bolstered by rapidly proliferating connections to social-cognitive neuroscience. Accordingly, while we have been mentalizing since we became a species, we now understand this essence of our human nature better than ever before. But we have no reason to be sanguine about our newfound self-understanding: as we have glimpsed in this chapter, the need to enlarge our sphere of mentalizing never has been more urgent.

Key Clinical Points

- *Mentalizing and aggression:* Aggression is normally unlearned over the course of development through the establishment of secure attachment relationships that promote mentalizing, which provides a buffer against aggression.

- *Influence of social setting:* In non-mentalizing social environments, social influence is teleological, via actions rather than verbal communication, limiting the creative potential of such social settings. Reactive, non-mentalizing interventions aggravate rather than alleviate the problems they endeavor to address.

- *Influence of schools:* School systems provide a natural arena for violence prevention interventions in the community. Illustratively, a mentalizing-focused intervention in elementary schools designed to enhance awareness of bully-victim-bystander roles not only decreased aggression but also enhanced academic performance.

- *Societal importance of mentalizing:* The concept of mindblindness —the antithesis of mentalizing—can be applied to traumatizing behavior on different scales ranging from the family to the local and global communities; the Holocaust is merely one of innumerable horrific examples of grand-scale trauma in which mindblindness can be implicated. As attachment relationships exemplify, clinical and social perspectives are inextricable; taking the broadest view, the moral and ethical fabric of society depends on mentalizing.

Epilogue

This scholarly volume persuasively presents the concept of mentalizing as a central organizing construct to help us understand the successes and failures of interpersonal human behavior. Much previous work has been done and published, by the authors of this volume and their colleagues, on mentalizing and its emergence in normal human development, contingent on the establishment of secure attachment early in life. This book reviews and consolidates that earlier work. With clarity and, if you will, mentalizing attention to the mind of the reader, the authors elucidate contributions of others and lines of thought that constitute precursors to the more encompassing notion called mentalizing. At each step, after presenting an area or body of work in detail, they pause to recapitulate the main points being made and to provide a summary—a format helpful both to the newcomer to this material and the veteran. The reader is then well equipped to move into the second half of the book, the application of a mentalizing approach in treatment—the main goal of the book, as its title implies.

I have been asked to write a brief epilogue to this volume, a challenge indeed, since the elegant and comprehensive words of the authors themselves leave very little room for additional comment. But I shall try!

The Concept of Mentalizing

Mentalizing can be viewed as a fundamental characteristic of mature mental and emotional health, of particular value in facilitating and enhancing effective interpersonal relationships and transactions. A well established, mature capacity to mentalize implies a sturdy sense of self, or identity, or *agency*, perhaps intuitively recognized by others as solid self-directedness and goal-directedness. But as the authors emphasize, it also implies an ability to recognize or "tune in to" one's own thoughts and feelings, and to have the capacity to read the emotional language of others, that is, to put oneself in others' shoes. I would extend these descriptions a bit to suggest that successful mentalizing implies an ability to care for and to forgive—which applies both to oneself and to others, and which makes a difference in the vast daily menu of decisions, both deliberate and subliminal, that we make every day about what we say and what we do.

After identifying secure attachment as the developmental platform on which the capacity to mentalize is built, Allen and colleagues review the latest neurobiological findings relevant to attachment and mentalizing, for example, the exciting recent work on mirror neurons. Brain imaging techniques are becoming increasingly sophisticated, enabling us to know more and more about neural circuitry and the capacity and plasticity of the brain. This awesome executive organ, the biological hard drive we call the brain, stands at the ready to be booted up to implement our commands. Part of our challenge is to learn how and when the hardwired circuits become underdeveloped or overdeveloped, what makes them misfire, how much of the brain constitutes software that can be reprogrammed, and how to identify resilience and risk factors at the level of the individual patient.

Mentalizing and Psychopathology

The authors' enthusiasm and excitement about the value of a mentalizing approach in clinical practice are engaging and well justified. They describe the relationship between mentalizing and psychopathology in the context of the two dominant arenas pertinent to all psychopathology: development and neurobiology. Regarding neurobiology, the authors emphasize brain imaging research—where indeed great progress is being made, particularly shedding light on the critical role of the limbic system in regulating affect and of the prefrontal cortex in reining in impulsivity and implementing reasoned decision making and judgment. Other broad areas of research are increasingly important in our

understanding of psychopathology, such as key heritable endophenotypes that are predisposing to future pathology—especially if combined with developmental neglect or trauma, or even with sustained
stress later in life. Knowledge in the field of genomics is accelerating
rapidly, filling in critical gaps in the stress/vulnerability model of disease. Each of us, after all, carries unknown amounts of heritable risk for
a range of conditions from hypertension to diabetes to depression to
schizophrenia, and many more—the list is long. The challenge ahead is
to better understand and identify these genetic risk factors and their relationship to developmental experience as critical elements influencing
the eventual structure and functioning of the adult brain.

The authors have done a masterful job of condensing what could
otherwise be an encyclopedia of information into critical selected elements of development and neurobiology. What is not always clear is
whether the authors have "modal" or typical patients in mind as they
describe this research and its importance to the concept of mentalizing.
In familiar clinical terminology, are we referring to patients with, for example, severe personality disorders, major depressive disorder, bipolar
disorder, substance use disorders, or all of the above and more? The focus of the material is, by design, on the development of the capacity (or
the lack of it) to mentalize. One population singled out is that of psychopathy, and this enlightening focus is pertinent, since this trait is a
highly disabling subtype of personality pathology, and it is also a pervasive and clinically challenging component of many other conditions,
such as borderline personality disorder. Similarly, the authors drill
down to focus on borderline personality disorder itself, as well as on
trauma; these sections of the book are extremely valuable, since patients
with these conditions are common in treatment populations. Although
the authors do not emphasize the diagnostic language of mainstream
psychiatry, systematic consideration in future work of the role of mentalizing in patients in other specified diagnostic categories would be
welcome.

Mentalizing and Treatment

The capacity to mentalize is logically a prerequisite to becoming a
skilled and effective psychotherapist, regardless of the specific type of
therapy employed. We sometimes refer to "psychodynamically informed" psychotherapy, to underscore the importance of a psychodynamic framework to help us understand the way our patients think,
feel, and behave, but not necessarily to indicate a specific type of treatment. In the same way, as the authors make clear, one can choose to

learn and practice Mentalization-Based Therapy, or not, but in either case the concept of mentalizing can be an invaluable touchstone for assessing our own mental state as we work with patients, and for understanding our patients themselves.

It is important to recognize that this book is not intended to be a comprehensive source (nor could it be) of the entire scope of the concept of mentalizing and its application in clinical work. References to treatment in this work refer to psychotherapy, though it is not systematically specified if this occurs in an inpatient, partial hospital, outpatient, or other settings. The authors have written a separate treatment manual (Bateman and Fonagy 2006), a valuable companion to the present volume, that provides more detailed guidance to practitioners wishing to learn Mentalization-Based Therapy.

Future Directions and Research

Reading this book taught me a great deal. One of its many merits is its translational utility, since the authors take pains to correlate the new (for many) language of mentalizing with terms perhaps more familiar to some. Terms such as *mentalizing* itself, agency, mind-mindedness, quarantine failure, switching off mentalizing, and many others are compared and contrasted to traditional psychodynamic terms such as psychological mindedness, transference, countertransference, identity, defense mechanisms, and the dynamic unconscious. Still other parallels are drawn, such as explicit and implicit mentalizing, correlated with declarative and procedural memory. There are many other languages of our field, some of which are incorporated into treatment strategies, and psychotherapy is anything but a "one size fits all" world. From time to time, when making professional presentations about personality disorders, I have been asked "Are you a Kohutian or a Kernbergian?" (And I now may be at risk of being asked whether I am an Allenian, a Fonagian, or a Batemanian!) My invariable answer is that such a question is the wrong question. First one needs to know all about the individual patient, and then one can think about the best treatment approach for that patient. What impresses me more and more are the many areas that presumably different psychotherapies have in common. Plakun and others have described a theoretical model they call the "Y" model of psychotherapy, where the lower stem of the Y represents the common features many types of psychotherapy share and the upper arms of the Y represent specific unique aspects that differentiate one therapy from another. One could persuasively argue, it seems to me, that the framework of mentalizing could constitute the common basis for psychotherapeutic work, supporting on its shoulders a valuable array of special techniques tailored for specific patient groups and always molded to the needs of each individual patient.

In spite of great progress and the hugely important contributions made by the authors of this book and by many others, we must acknowledge that we still have much to learn. We *do* need more psychotherapy research. Randomized controlled psychotherapy trials have usually focused on brief therapy utilizing cognitive-behavioral approaches. These studies are extremely valuable. But we must remember that absence of data is not the same thing as negative data, and there are very few head-to-head studies comparing different forms of long-term psychotherapy. Thankfully, these difficult studies are now being done, and we are grateful to the authors of this book for their pioneering work in this regard.

Closing Thoughts

Many years ago, I had the privilege to hear a presentation at the New York Psychoanalytic Society by D.W. Winnicott entitled "The Use of an Object," which later became one of his published works. In the language of the time, but with his usual prescience, Winnicott argued the importance of sensitively helping patients relinquish their fiercely defended fantasy of the object (the analyst) and replacing it with recognition of the analyst as a real, separate person, there to be used for their help. He illustrated his thesis by describing one of his patients, a young man whose development had been derailed by severe neglect and who had no sense of secure footing in the world, no sense of basic trust. Winnicott reviewed the course of his psychoanalytic work with this patient, a stormy and challenging process that revolved around the patient's mistrust of the analyst—a mistrust that painfully but steadfastly was transformed into the patient's recognition of the analyst's trustworthiness and of the analyst's genuine respect and regard for the patient. Winnicott's poignant concluding sentence, which has remained vivid in my memory, was: "For this patient, an object now exists in the world, and the world can begin." In the language of this book, I believe it would be fair to say that Winnicott's patient had achieved the capacity to mentalize, a capacity that truly does invite membership in the interpersonal world. Such membership does not imply sustained bliss or freedom from pain, but rather the capacity to "connect" to others, to understand and share their joys and sorrows, and to allow them to understand and share one's own. By citing this example from the work of a master clinician, I am reiterating that mentalizing, even if not always explicit in our language, is implicit in many forms of psychotherapy and is an invaluable conceptual beacon to guide us in our work. Allen and colleagues, of course, have already said this, when they suggest: "You're already doing it." And indeed we are, if we're doing our job.

John M. Oldham, M.D., M.S.
The Menninger Clinic
and Baylor College of Medicine

Glossary

attachment trauma   trauma in attachment relationships, mediated in part by mentalizing failures in the caregiver that undermine the development of mentalizing in the child

contingent responsiveness   a high, but imperfect, level of caregiver responsiveness to infant behavior that facilitates the infant's attention to the caregiver's mental states and thereby lays the developmental foundation for mentalizing

egocentrism   the default mentalizing mode of equating others' mental states with one's own

emotional intelligence   a multifaceted assessment pertinent to mentalizing emotion; includes competence in perception and expression of emotion as well as emotion understanding and emotion regulation

empathy   as Simon Baron-Cohen defines it, identifying others' emotional responses and responding with appropriate emotion; broadly conceived, mentalizing is more inclusive than empathizing, encompassing empathy for the self as well as others

intentionality   the distinguishing feature of mental states, namely, that these states are representational or about something

intergenerational transmission   the interactive process whereby patterns of behavior are learned and reenacted across generations; for example, as the intergenerational transmission of trauma is perpetuated by mentalizing failures that cascade across generations

joint attention   occurs in interactions in which infant and caregiver jointly attend to a third object; a significant contributor to the development of mentalizing in cultivating the sense of multiple perspectives, including another person's perspective on the self when the infant is the object of attention

marked emotion   a characterization of emotional mirroring that denotes the caregiver's modified expression of the infant's emotion back to the infant, for example, alloying the reflection of the infant's distress with an expression of concern; promotes the infant's capacity to develop self-representations of emotional states

mentalizing   imaginatively perceiving and interpreting behavior of oneself and others as conjoined with intentional mental states, shorthand for which is *holding mind in mind*

mentalizing emotion   includes identifying emotional states and their meaning, modulating the intensity of emotion, and expressing emotion outwardly and inwardly; crucial for emotion-regulation, mentalizing emotion includes mentalizing while remaining in the emotional state

mentalizing region   an area in the medial prefrontal cortex overlapping the anterior cingulate that consistently shows activation in neuroimaging studies when participants are engaged in mentalizing tasks

mentalizing stance   an exploratory attitude of inquisitiveness and curiosity about mental states that mentalizing interventions aspire to promote

metacognition   a facet of mentalizing, namely, thinking about thinking; serves the function of monitoring and regulating cognitive processes

mindblindness   Simon Baron-Cohen's term for the absence of mentalizing in autism; the term can be extended to more transient and dynamic mentalizing failures, as evident, for example, when one experiences threats to attachment relationships

mindfulness   a Buddhist concept referring to attentiveness to the present; mentalizing entails mindfulness of mind in particular

mind-mindedness   a term employed by Elizabeth Meins and colleagues to refer to caregivers' recognition of their children as a mental agents and their proclivity to refer to their children's mental states in their speech

mindreading   a term widely employed in the theory-of-mind literature to refer to interpreting others' mental states; sometimes used synonymously with mentalizing

mirror neurons neurons activated by observing an action or emotion as well as when performing an action or experiencing an emotion; a potential neurobiological substrate of empathy

moments of meeting as characterized by Daniel Stern and colleagues, poignant moments of intersubjective contact in psychotherapy that have a potentially powerful therapeutic impact; in their spontaneity, moments of meeting exemplify the artful nature of mentalizing

not-knowing stance an aspect of the mentalizing stance that respects the opaqueness of the patient's mental states, as contrasted with making unwarranted assumptions and interpretations

parental meta-emotion philosophy a term employed by John Gottman and colleagues to refer to parents' awareness of their children's emotional states and an interest in cultivating children's emotional awareness; consistent with a parental mentalizing stance

pedagogy a term employed by George Gergely and colleagues to refer to the uniquely human capacity to teach and learn cultural information, including information about mental states; a foundation for mentalizing and, through marked emotion, a means of learning about one's own emotional states in particular

prementalizing modes ways of thinking and interacting that are developmental precursors to mentalizing, including the psychic equivalence, pretend, and teleological modes

pretend mode one of the prementalizing modes of thinking in which, unlike psychic equivalence, mental states are decoupled from reality yet, unlike in mentalizing, not flexibly linked to reality; in psychotherapy, evident in pseudo-mentalizing, intellectualizing, or (to use philosopher Harry Frankfurt's term of art) bullshitting

psychic equivalence mode one of the prementalizing modes of thinking in which reality is equated with mental states and the sense of representingness of mental states is absent; examples are dreams, posttraumatic flashbacks, and paranoid delusions

psychological unavailability a term for emotional neglect, referring to a lack of attunement to the child's mental states; exemplifies a critical mentalizing failure

reenactment unwittingly repeating past traumatic relationship patterns in current relationships; a mentalizing failure that entails retraumatization and puts patients at risk for posttraumatic symptoms

reflective functioning   Peter Fonagy and colleagues' operationalization of mentalizing capacity, as exemplified by their reflective functioning scale employed in research; used synonymously with mentalizing in some research and clinical literature

representingness   a term employed by Radu Bogdan to capture the sense one has of mental states as representing something in a particular way; the sense of representingness of mental states is lost in the psychic-equivalence mode—for example, when the depressed patient cannot appreciate that self-condemnation is a reflection of depressed mood rather than indicative of objective reality

secure base   a facet of secure attachment in which the attachment relationship serves as a platform for exploration; a secure base in attachment promotes exploration of mental reality as well as external reality and thus is conducive to mentalizing

social cognition   an extensive domain of research pertaining to mental processes that mediate social relationships and, accordingly, a large body of knowledge pertinent to mentalizing

systemizing   as defined by Simon Baron-Cohen, the antithesis of empathizing, namely, a rule-based way of understanding and predicting the behavior of a system; some persons with autism exemplify exceptional systemizing ability coupled with profoundly impaired empathizing

teleological mode   one of the prementalizing modes in which mental states are expressed in goal-directed actions instead of explicit mental representations such as words; for example, when self-cutting is employed as a way of communicating extreme emotional pain

theory of mind   a domain of extensive research bearing on the individual's development of an understanding of the representational nature of mind, as exemplified explicitly in the ability to interpret behavior as stemming from false beliefs; prominent theories to explain theory-of-mind development include the theory-theory, simulation theory, and modularity theory

References

Adam KS, Sheldon Keller AE, West M: Attachment organization and vulnerability to loss, separation and abuse in disturbed adolescents, in Attachment Theory: Social, Developmental and Clinical Perspectives. Edited by Goldberg S, Muir R, Kerr J. Hillsdale NJ Analytic Press, 1995, pp 309–341

Adolphs R: Cognitive neuroscience of human social behavior. Nat Rev Neurosci 4:165–178, 2003

Adolphs R, Gosselin F, Buchanan TW, et al: A mechanism for fear recognition after amygdala damage. Nature 433:68–72, 2005

Aggleton JP, Young AW: The enigma of the amygdala: on its contribution to human emotion, in Cognitive Neuroscience of Emotion. Edited by Lane RD, Nadel L. New York, Oxford University Press, 2000, pp 106–128

Ainsworth MDS, Blehar MC, Waters E, et al: Patterns of Attachment: A Psychological Study of the Strange Situation. Hillsdale, NJ, Erlbaum, 1978

Akhtar S: Broken Structures: Severe Personality Disorders and their Treatment. Northvale, NJ, Aronson, 1992

Alexander RD: Evolution of the human psyche, in The Human Revolution: Behavioral and Biological Perspectives on the Origins of Modern Humans. Edited by Mellars P, Stringer C. Princeton, NJ, Princeton University Press, 1989, pp 455–513

Allen JG: The spectrum of accuracy in memories of childhood trauma. Harv Rev Psychiatry 3:84–95, 1995

Allen JG: Loosening traumatic bonds. Renfrew Perspective 22:7–8, 1996

Allen JG: Traumatic Relationships and Serious Mental Disorders. Chichester, UK, Wiley, 2001

Allen JG: Mentalizing. Bull Menninger Clin 67:87–108, 2003

Allen JG: Coping With Trauma: Hope Through Understanding, 2nd Edition. Washington, DC, American Psychiatric Publishing, 2005

Allen JG: Coping With Depression: From Catch-22 to Hope. Washington DC, American Psychiatric Publishing, 2006a

Allen JG: Mentalizing in practice, in Handbook of Mentalization-Based Treatment. Edited by Allen JG, Fonagy, P. Chichester, UK, Wiley, 2006b, pp 3–30

Allen JG: Evil, mindblindness and trauma: challenges to hope. Smith Coll Stud Soc Work 77:9–31, 2007

Allen JG: Psychotherapy: the artful use of science. Smith Coll Stud Soc Work (in press)

Allen JG, Fonagy P (eds): Handbook of Mentalization-Based Treatment. Chichester, UK, Wiley, 2006a

Allen JG, Fonagy P: Preface, in Handbook of Mentalization-Based Treatment. Edited by Allen JG, Fonagy P. Chichester, UK, Wiley, 2006b, pp ix–xxi

Allen JG, Munich RL: The j-word. Menninger Perspect 36:5, 2006

Allen JG, Huntoon J, Fultz J, et al: A model for brief assessment of attachment and its application to women in inpatient treatment for trauma-related psychiatric disorders. J Pers Assess 76:420–446, 2001

Allen JG, Bleiberg E, Haslam-Hopwood GTG: Mentalizing as a Compass for Treatment. Houston, TX, The Menninger Clinic, 2003

Allen-Meares P, Washington R, Welsch B: Social Work Services in Schools. Boston, MA, Allyn & Bacon, 1996

American Psychiatric Association: Diagnostic and Statistical Manual of Mental Disorders, 4th Edition, Text Revision. Washington, DC, American Psychiatric Association, 2000

Ames DR: Everyday solutions to the problem of other minds: which tools are used when? in Other Minds: How Humans Bridge the Divide between Self and Others. Edited by Malle BF, Hodges SD. New York, Guilford, 2005, pp 158–173

Antonaccio M: Picturing the Human: The Moral Thought of Iris Murdoch. New York, Oxford University Press, 2000

Appelbaum SA: Psychological-mindedness: word, concept and essence. Int J Psychoanal 54:35–46, 1973

Ards S, Harrell A: Reporting of child maltreatment: a secondary analysis of the national incidence surveys. Child Abuse Negl 17:337–344, 1993

Arendt H: Eichmann in Jerusalem: A Report on the Banality of Evil (1963). New York, Penguin, 1994

Arendt H: The Life of the Mind, I. Thinking. New York, Harcourt, 1971

Arendt H: Responsibility and Judgment. New York, Schocken, 2003

Armony JL, LeDoux JE: How the brain processes emotional information, in Psychobiology of Posttraumatic Stress Disorder, Vol 821. Edited by Yehuda R, MacFarlane AC. New York, New York Academy of Sciences, 1997, pp 259–270

Arnott B, Meins E: Links between antenatal attachment representations, postnatal mind-mindedness and infant attachment security: a preliminary study of mothers and fathers. Bull Menninger Clin 71:132–149, 2007

Arnsten AFT: The biology of being frazzled. Science 280:1711–1712, 1998

Arnsten AFT, Goldman-Rakic PS: Noise stress impairs prefrontal cortical cognitive function in monkeys. Arch Gen Psychiatry 55:362–368, 1998

Arnsten AFT, Mathew R, Ubriani R, et al: Alpha-1 noradrenergic receptor stimulation impairs prefrontal cortical cognitive function. Biol Psychiatry 45:26–31, 1999

Aron A: Reward motivation and emotion systems associated with early stage intense romantic love. J Neurophysiol 94:327–337, 2005

Astington JW: What is theoretical about the child's theory of mind? A Vygotskian view of its development, in Theories of Theories of Mind. Edited by Carruthers P, Smith PK. Cambridge, UK, Cambridge University Press, 1996, pp 184–199

Astington JW, Filippova E: Language as the route into other minds, in Other Minds: How Humans Bridge the Divide between Self and Others. Edited by Malle BF, Hodges SD. New York, Guilford, 2005, pp 209–222

Aviram RB, Brodsky BS, Stanley B: Borderline personality disorder: stigma and treatment implications. Harv Rev Psychiatry 14:249–256, 2006

Baars BJ: A Cognitive Theory of Consciousness. New York, Cambridge University Press, 1988

Bahrick LE, Watson JS: Detection of intermodal proprioceptive-visual contingency as a potential basis of self-perception in infancy. Dev Psychol 21:963–973, 1985

Baird AA, Veague HB, Rabbitt CE: Developmental precipitants of borderline personality disorder. Dev Psychopathol 17:1031–1049, 2005

Baker L, Silk KR, Westen D, et al: Malevolence, splitting and parental ratings by borderlines. J Nerv Ment Dis 180:258–264, 1992

Barker M, Givon T: Representation of the interlocutor's mind during conversation, in Other Minds: How Humans Bridge the Divide between Self and Others. Edited by Malle BF, Hodges SD. New York, Guilford, 2005, pp 223–238

Barnett D, Manly JT, Cicchetti D: Defining child maltreatment: the interface between policy and research, in Child Abuse, Child Development and Social Policy: Advances in Applied Developmental Psychology, Vol 8. Edited by Cicchetti D, Toth SL. Norwood, NJ, Ablex, 1993, pp 7–73

Baron-Cohen S: Mindblindness: An Essay on Autism and Theory of Mind. Cambridge, MA, MIT Press, 1995

Baron-Cohen S: Theory of mind and autism: a fifteen year review, in Understanding Other Minds: Perspectives from Developmental Cognitive Neuroscience, 2nd Edition. Edited by Baron-Cohen S, Tager-Flusberg H, Cohen DJ. New York, Oxford University Press, 2000, pp 3–20

Baron-Cohen S: The Essential Difference: Male and Female Brains and the Truth about Autism. New York, Basic Books, 2003

Baron-Cohen S: The empathizing system: a revision of the 1994 model of the mindreading system, in Origins of the Social Mind: Evolutionary Psychology and Child Development. Edited by Ellis BJ, Bjorklund DF. New York, Guilford, 2005, pp 468–492

Baron-Cohen S, Swettenham J: The relationship between SAM and ToMM: two hypotheses, in Theories of Theories of Mind. Edited by Carruthers P, Smith PK. Cambridge, UK, Cambridge University Press, 1996, pp 158–168

Baron-Cohen S, Tager-Flusberg H, Cohen DJ (eds): Understanding Other Minds: Perspectives from Developmental Cognitive Neuroscience, 2nd Edition. New York, Oxford University Press, 2000

Baron-Cohen S, Wheelwright S, Hill J, et al: The "Reading the Mind in the Eyes" Test, Revised Version: a study with normal adults and adults with Asperger syndrome or high-functioning autism. J Child Psychol Psychiatry 42:241–251, 2001

Baron-Cohen S, Wheelwright S, Lawson J, et al: Empathizing and systemizing in autism spectrum conditions, in Handbook of Autism and Pervasive Developmental Disorders, 3rd edition. Edited by Volkmar F, Klinkman MS, Paul R. New York, Wiley, 2005, pp 628–639

Barr DJ, Keysar B: Mindreading in an exotic case: the normal adult human, in Other Minds: How Humans Bridge the Divide between Self and Others. Edited by Malle BF, Hodges SD. New York, Guilford, 2005, pp 271–283

Barrett LF, Salovey P (eds): The Wisdom in Feeling: Psychological Processes in Emotional Intelligence. New York, Guilford, 2002

Bartles A, Zeki S: The neural basis of romantic love. Neuroreport 11:3829–3834, 2000

Bartles A, Zeki S: The neural correlates of maternal and romantic love. Neuroimage 21:1155–1166, 2004

Bateman AW, Fonagy P: Effectiveness of partial hospitalization in the treatment of borderline personality disorder: a randomized controlled trial. Am J Psychiatry 156:1563–1569, 1999

Bateman AW, Fonagy P: Treatment of borderline personality disorder with psychoanalytically oriented partial hospitalization: an 18-month follow-up. Am J Psychiatry 158:36–42, 2001

Bateman AW, Fonagy P: Health service utilization costs for borderline personality disorder patients treated with psychoanalytically oriented partial hospitalization versus general psychiatric care. Am J Psychiatry 160:169–171, 2003

Bateman AW, Fonagy P: Psychotherapy for Borderline Personality Disorder: Mentalization-Based Treatment. New York, Oxford University Press, 2004

Bateman AW, Fonagy P: Mentalization-Based Treatment for Borderline Personality Disorder: A Practical Guide. New York, Oxford University Press, 2006

Battle CL, Shea MT, Johnson DM, et al: Childhood maltreatment associated with adult personality disorders: findings from the Collaborative Longitudinal Personality Disorders Study. J Pers Disord 18:193–211, 2004

Baumeister RF: Evil: Inside Human Violence and Cruelty. New York, Freeman, 1997

Baumrind D: Parenting styles and adolescent development, in The Encyclopedia on Adolescence. Edited by Brooks-Gunn R, Lerner R, Peterson AC. New York, Guilford, 1991, pp 746–758

Beck AT, Rush AJ, Shaw BF, et al: Cognitive Therapy of Depression. New York, Guilford, 1979

Beitel M, Cecero JJ: Predicting psychological mindedness from personality style and attachment security. J Clin Psychol 59:163–172, 2003

Beitel M, Ferrer E, Cecero JJ: Psychological mindedness and cognitive style. J Clin Psychol 60:567–582, 2004

Beitel M, Ferrer E, Cecero JJ: Psychological mindedness and awareness of self and others. J Clin Psychol 61:739–750, 2005

Belbo T, Driessen M, Mertens M, et al: Functional MRI correlates of the recall of unresolved life events in borderline personality disorder. Psychol Med 36:845–856, 2006

Belsky J, Fearon P: Infant-mother attachment security, contextual risk and early development: a moderational analysis. Dev Psychopathol 14:293–310, 2002

Bender DS, Skodol AE, Pagano ME, et al: Prospective assessment of treatment use by patients with personality disorders. Psychiatr Serv 57:254–257, 2006

Benoit D, Parker KCH: Stability and transmission of attachment across generations. Child Dev 65:1444–1456, 1994

Berger M: A model of preverbal social development and its application to social dysfunctions in autism. J Child Psychol Psychiatry 47:338–371, 2006

Bezirganian S, Cohen P, Brook JS: The impact of mother-child interaction on the development of borderline personality disorder. Am J Psychiatry 150:1836–1842, 1993

Bifulco A, Moran P: Wednesday's Child: Research into Women's Experience of Neglect and Abuse in Childhood, and Adult Depression. London, Routledge, 1998

Bifulco A, Brown GW, Harris TO: Childhood Experience of Care and Abuse (CECA): a retrospective interview measure. J Child Psychol Psychiatry 35:1419–1435, 1994a

Bifulco A, Brown GW, Neubauer A, et al: Childhood Experience of Care and Abuse (CECA) training manual. London, Royal Holloway, University of London, 1994b

Bifulco A, Moran PM, Baines R, et al: Exploring psychological abuse in childhood, II: association with other abuse and adult clinical depression. Bull Menninger Clin 66:241–258, 2002

Binder J, McNiel DE, Goldstone RL: Is adaptive coping possible for adult survivors of childhood sexual abuse? Psychiatr Serv 47:186–188, 1996

Binder JL: Issues in teaching and learning time-limited psychodynamic psychotherapy. Clin Psychol Rev 19:705–719, 1999

Bion WR: Learning from Experience. London, Heinemann, 1962a

Bion WR: The psycho-analytic study of thinking, II: a theory of thinking. Int J Psychoanal 43:306–310, 1962b

Björgvinsson T, Hart J: Cognitive behavioral therapy promotes mentalizing, in Handbook of Mentalization-Based Treatment. Edited by Allen JG, Fonagy P. Chichester, UK, Wiley, 2006, pp 157–170

Blair RJR: Facial expressions, their communicatory functions and neuro-cognitive substrates. Philos Trans R Soc Lond B Biol Sci 358:561–572, 2003

Blair RJR: The roles of orbital frontal cortex in the modulation of antisocial behavior. Brain Cogn 55:198–208, 2004

Blair RJR, Jones L, Clark F, et al: The psychopathic individual: a lack of responsiveness to distress cues? Psychophysiology 34:192–198, 1997

Blair RJR, Mitchell D, Blair K: The Psychopath: Emotion and the Brain. Oxford, UK, Blackwell, 2005

Blair RJR, Peschardt KS, Budhani S, et al: The development of psychopathy. J Child Psychol Psychiatry 47:262–275, 2006

Bland AR, Williams CA, Scharer K, et al: Emotion processing in borderline personality disorders. Issues Ment Health Nurs 25:655–672, 2004

Bleiberg E: Treating professionals in crisis: a mentalization-based specialized inpatient program, in Handbook of Mentalization-Based Treatment. Edited by Allen JG, Fonagy P. Chichester, UK, Wiley, 2006, pp 233–247

Bogdan RJ: Interpreting Minds: The Evolution of a Practice. Cambridge, MA, MIT Press, 1997

Bogdan RJ: Why self-ascriptions are difficult and develop late, in Other Minds: How Humans Bridge the Divide between Self and Others. Edited by Malle BF, Hodges SD. New York, Guilford, 2005, pp 190–206

Boidy LM, Nagin DS, Tremblay RE, et al: Developmental trajectories of childhood disruptive behaviors and adolescent delinquency: a six-site, cross-national study. Dev Psychol 39:222–245, 2003

Bokhorst CL, Bakermans-Kranenburg MJ, Fearon RM, et al: The importance of shared environment in mother-infant attachment security: a behavioral genetic study. Child Dev 74:1769–1782, 2003

Bonda E, Petrides M, Ostry D, et al: Specific involvement of human parietal systems and the amygdala in the perception of biological motion. J Neurosci 16:3737–3744, 1996

Bordin ES: The generalizability of the psychoanalytic concept of the working alliance. Psychotherapy: Theory Research and Practice 16:252–260, 1979

Botvinick MM, Nystrom LE, Fissell K, et al: Conflict monitoring versus selection-for-action in anterior cingulate cortex. Nature 402:179–181, 1999

Bowen M: Key to the use of the genogram family diagram, in The Family Life Cycle: A Framework for Family Therapy. Edited by Carter EA, McGoldrick M. New York, Gardner Press, 1980, p xxiii

Bowlby J: Attachment and Loss, Vol II: Separation. New York, Basic Books, 1973

Bowlby J: Attachment and Loss, Vol I: Attachment, 2nd Edition. New York, Basic Books, 1982

Bowlby J: A Secure Base: Parent-Child Attachment and Healthy Human Development. New York, Basic Books, 1988

Bradley R, Westen D: The psychodynamics of borderline personality disorder: a view from developmental psychopathology. Dev Psychopathol 17:927–957, 2005

Bradley R, Jenei J, Westen D: Etiology of borderline personality disorder: disentangling the contributions of intercorrelated antecedents. J Nerv Ment Dis 193:24–31, 2005

Bray S, Barrowclough C, Lobban F: The social problem-solving abilities of people with borderline personality disorder. Behav Res Ther 45:1409–1417, 2007

Brennan KA, Shaver PR: Attachment styles and personality disorders: their connections to each other and to parental divorce, parental death and perceptions of parental caregiving. J Pers 66:835–878, 1998

Brewin CR, Andrews B: Recovered memories of trauma: phenomenology and cognitive mechanisms. Clin Psychol Rev 18:949–970, 1998

Brewin CR, Dalgleish T, Joseph S: A dual representation theory of posttraumatic stress disorder. Psychol Rev 103:670–686, 1996

Brodsky BS, Groves SA, Oquendo MA, et al: Interpersonal precipitants and suicide attempts in borderline personality disorder. Suicide Life Threat Behav 36:313–322, 2006

Brothers L: Friday's Footprint: How Society Shapes the Human Mind. New York, Oxford University Press, 1997

Brown D, Scheflin AW, Hammond DC: Memory, Trauma Treatment and the Law. New York, WW Norton, 1998

Brown JR, Donelan-McCall N, Dunn J: Why talk about mental states? The significance of children's conversations with friends, siblings and mothers. Child Dev 67:836–849, 1996

Brown KW, Ryan RM: The benefits of being present: mindfulness and its role in psychological well-being. J Pers Soc Psychol 84:822–848, 2003

Brown MZ, Comptois KA, Linehan MM: Reasons for suicide attempts and non-suicidal self-injury in women with borderline personality disorder. J Abnorm Psychol 111:198–202, 2002

Bruner J: Acts of Meaning. Cambridge, MA, Harvard University Press, 1990

Bruschweiler-Stern N: A multifocal neonatal intervention, in Treating Parent-Infant Relationship Problems: Strategies for Intervention. Edited by Sameroff AJ, McDonough SC, Rosenblum KL. New York, Guilford, 2004, pp 188–212

Buccino G, Vogt S, Ritzl A, et al: Neural circuits underlying imitation learning of hand actions: an event-related fMRI study. Neuron 42:323–334, 2004

Bush G, Luu P, Posner MI: Cognitive and emotional influences in anterior cingulate cortex. Trends Cogn Sci 4:215–222, 2000

Byrne RW, Whiten A (eds): Machiavellian Intelligence: Social Expertise and the Evolution of Intellect in Monkeys, Apes and Humans. New York, Oxford University Press, 1988

Cahill SP, Carrigan MH, Frueh BC: Does EMDR work? And if so, why? A critical review of controlled outcome and dismantling research. J Anxiety Disord 13:5–33, 1999

Calhoun KS, Resick PA: Post-traumatic stress disorder, in Clinical Handbook of Psychological Disorders: A Step-by-Step Treatment Manual. Edited by Barlow DH. New York, Guilford, 1993, pp 48–98

Cannon WB: Bodily Changes in Pain, Hunger, Fear and Rage: An Account of Recent Researches into the Function of Emotional Excitement. Boston, MA, Charles T Branford, 1953

Card C: The Atrocity Paradigm: A Theory of Evil. New York, Oxford University Press, 2002

Carey S: Conceptual Change in Childhood. Cambridge, MA, MIT Press, 1985

Carr L, Iacoboni M, Dutton DG, et al: Neural mechanisms of empathy in humans: a relay from neural systems for imitation to limbic areas. Proc Natl Acad Sci USA 100:5497–5502, 2003

Carruthers P: Simulation and self-knowledge: a defence of theory-theory, in Theories of Theories of Mind. Edited by Carruthers P, Smith PK. Cambridge, UK, Cambridge University Press, 1996, pp 22–38

Carruthers P, Smith PK (eds): Theories of Theories of Mind. Cambridge, UK, Cambridge University Press, 1996

Carter CS, Braver TS, Barch D, et al: Anterior cingulate cortex error detection and the online monitoring of performance. Science 280:747–749, 1998

Child and Family Program: Short-Term Mentalization and Relational Therapy (SMART): A Mentalization-Based Therapy Manual for Children and Families, Version 1.7. Houston, TX, Menninger Department of Psychiatry and Behavioral Sciences, Baylor College of Medicine, 2005

Chirkov V, Ryan RM: Parent and teacher autonomy-support in Russian and US adolescents: common effects on well-being and academic motivation. J Cross Cult Psychol 32:618–635, 2001

Chu JA: Dissociative symptomatology in adult patients with histories of childhood physical and sexual abuse, in Trauma, Memory and Dissociation. Edited by Bremner JD, Marmar CR. Washington, DC, American Psychiatric Press, 1998, pp 179–203

Chugani HT, Behen ME, Muzik O, et al: Local brain functional activity following early deprivation: a study of postinstitutionalized Romanian orphans. Neuroimage 14:1290–1301, 2001

Cicchetti D, Rogosch FA: A developmental psychopathology perspective on adolescence. J Consult Clin Psychol 70:6–20, 2002

Cicchetti D, Rogosch FA, Maughan A, et al: False belief understanding in maltreated children. Dev Psychopathol 15:1067–1091, 2003

Clarkin JF, Yeomans F, Kernberg OF: Transference-Focused Psychodynamic Therapy for Borderline Personality Disorder Patients. New York, Wiley, 1999

Claussen AH, Mundy PC, Mallik SA, et al: Joint attention and disorganized attachment status in infants at risk. Dev Psychopathol 14:279–291, 2002

Cleckley H: The Mask of Sanity. St Louis, MO, Mosby, 1976

Cloitre M: Sexual revictimization: risk factors and prevention, in Cognitive-Behavioral Therapies for Trauma. Edited by Follette VM, Ruzek JI, Abueg FR. New York, Guilford, 1998, pp 278–304

Cloitre M, Tardiff K, Marzuk PM, et al: Childhood abuse and subsequent sexual assault among female inpatients. J Trauma Stress 9:473–482, 1996

Cloninger CR, Svrakic DM, Przybeck TR: A psychobiological model of temperament and character. Arch Gen Psychiatry 50:975–990, 1993

Coates SW: Introduction: Trauma and human bonds, in September 11: Trauma and Human Bonds. Edited by Coates SW, Rosenthal JL, Schechter DS. New York, Guilford, 2003, pp 1–14

Coates SW, Rosenthal JL, Schechter DS (eds): September 11: Trauma and Human Bonds. Hillsdale, NJ, Analytic Press, 2003a

Coates SW, Schechter DS, First E: Brief interventions with traumatized children and families after September 11, in September 11: Trauma and Human Bonds. Edited by Coates SW, Rosenthal JL, Schechter DS. Hillsdale, NJ, Analytic Press, 2003b, pp 23–49

Cohen P, Crawford TN, Johnson JG, et al: The children in the Community Study of developmental course of personality disorder. J Pers Disord 19:466–486, 2006

Comte-Sponville A: A Small Treatise on the Great Virtues: The Uses of Philosophy in Everyday Life. Translated by Temerson C. New York, Holt, 2001

Conklin CZ, Bradley R, Westen D: Affect regulation in borderline personality disorder. J Nerv Ment Dis 194:69–77, 2006

Conradi PJ: Iris Murdoch: A Life. New York, WW Norton, 2001

Conte HR, Ratto R, Karasu TB: The Psychological Mindedness Scale: factor structure and relationship to outcome of psychotherapy. J Psychother Pract Res 5:250–259, 1996

Cooke DJ, Michie C, Hart SD, et al: Reconstructing psychopathy: clarifying the significance of antisocial and socially deviant behavior in the diagnosis of psychopathic personality disorder. J Pers Disord 18:337–357, 2004

Corballis MC: From Hand to Mouth: The Origins of Language. Princeton, NJ, Princeton University Press, 2002

Craig JL: Survival skills workshops: support for families. Menninger Persp 2:21–23, 1985

Cramer V, Torgersen S, Kringlen E: Personality disorders and quality of life: a population study. Compr Psychiatry 47:178–184, 2006

Crandell LE, Patrick MPH, Hobson RP: "Still-face" interactions between mothers with borderline personality disorder and their 2-month old infants. Br J Psychiatry 183:239–247, 2003

Crick NR, Murray-Close D, Woods K: Borderline personality features in childhood: a short-term longitudinal study. Dev Psychopathol 17:1051–1070, 2005

Csibra G, Gergely G: The teleological origins of mentalistic action explanations: a developmental hypothesis. Dev Sci 1:255–259, 1998

Csibra G, Gergely G: Social learning and social cognition: the case for pedagogy, in Processes of Change in Brain and Cognitive Development: Attention and Performance. Edited by Johnson MH, Munakata Y. New York, Oxford University Press, 2005, pp 249–274

Cutting AL, Dunn J: Theory of mind, emotion understanding, language and family background: individual differences and interrelations. Child Dev 70:853–865, 1999

Damasio AR: Descartes' Error: Emotion, Reason and the Human Brain. New York, Avon, 1994

Damasio A: The Feeling of What Happens: Body and Emotion in the Making of Consciousness. New York, Harcourt Brace, 1999

Damasio A, Adolphs R, Damasio H: The contributions of the lesion method to the functional neuroanatomy of emotion, in Handbook of Affective Sciences. Edited by Davidson RJ, Scherer KR, Goldsmith HH. New York, Oxford University Press, 2003, pp 66–92

Danon G, Graignic R: Borderline personality disorder and mother-infant interaction. Paper presented at the Society for Child Development, Atlanta, GA, 2003

Dapretto M, Davies MS, Pfeifer JH: Understanding emotions in others: mirror neuron dysfunction in children with autism spectrum disorders. Nat Neurosci 9:28–30, 2005

Darwin C: The Expression of Emotion in Man and Animals (1872). Chicago, IL, University of Chicago Press, 1965

Davidson D: Subjective, Intersubjective, Objective. New York, Oxford University Press, 2001

Davidson RJ: Affective style, psychopathology and resilience: brain mechanisms and plasticity. Am Psychol 55:1196–1214, 2000

Davidson RJ, Jackson DC, Kalin NH: Emotion, plasticity, context and regulation: perspectives from affective neuroscience. Psychol Bull 126:890–909, 2000

Davidson RJ, Pizzagalli D, Nitschke JB, et al: Parsing the subcomponents of emotion and disorders of emotion: perspectives from affective neuroscience, in Handbook of Affective Sciences. Edited by Davidson RJ, Scherer KR, Goldsmith HH. New York, Oxford University Press, 2003, pp 8–24

Davies JM, Frawley MG: Treating the Adult Survivor of Childhood Sexual Abuse. New York, Basic Books, 1994

de Villers J: Language and theory of mind: what are the developmental relationships? in Understanding Other Minds: Perspectives from Developmental Cognitive Neuroscience, 2nd Edition. Edited by Baron-Cohen S, Tager-Flusberg H, Cohen DJ. New York, Oxford University Press, 2000, pp 83–123

de Waal F: Peacemaking Among Primates. Cambridge, MA, Harvard University Press, 1989

de Waal F: Morally evolved: primate social instincts, human morality and the rise and fall of "veneer theory," in Primates and Philosophers: How Morality Evolved. Edited by Macedo S, Ober J. Princeton, NJ, Princeton University Press, 2006, pp 1–80

Decety J: Perspective taking as the royal road to empathy, in Other Minds: How Humans Bridge the Divide between Self and Others. Edited by Malle BF, Hodges SD. New York, Guilford, 2005, pp 143–157

Denham SA, Zoller D, Couchoud E: Socialization of preschoolers' emotion understanding. Dev Psychol 30:928–936, 1994

Dennett DC: Are we explaining consciousness yet? Cognition 79:221–237, 2001

Depue RA, Lenzenweger MF: A neurobehavioral dimensional model, in The Handbook of Personality Disorders. Edited by Livesley WJ. New York, Guilford, 2001, pp 136–176

Depue RA, Lenzenweger MF: A neurobehavioral dimensional model of personality disturbance, in Major Theories of Personality Disorder, Second edition. Edited by Lenzenweger MF, Depue RA. New York, Guilford, 2005, pp 391–453

Descartes R: Discourse on Method and the Meditations. New York, Penguin, 1968

Diamond D, Stovall-McClough C, Clarkin JF, et al: Patient-therapist attachment in the treatment of borderline personality disorder. Bull Menninger Clin 67:227–259, 2003

Dias MG, Harris PL: The influence of the imagination on reasoning by young children. Br J Dev Psychol 8:305–318, 1990

Dimaggio G, Semerari A, Carcione A, et al: Psychotherapy of Personality Disorders: Metacognition, States of Mind and Interpersonal Cycles. New York, Routledge, 2007

Dinn WM, Harris CL, Aycicegi A, et al: Neurocognitive function in borderline personality disorder. Prog Neuropsychopharmacol Biol Psychiatry 28:329–341, 2004

Domes G, Winter B, Schnell K, et al: The influence of emotions on inhibitory functioning in borderline personality disorder. Psychol Med 36:1163–1172, 2006

Domes G, Heinrichs M, Michel A, et al: Oxytocin improves "mind-reading" in humans. Biol Psychiatry 61:731–733, 2007

Donegan NH, Sanislow CA, Blumberg HP, et al: Amygdala hyperreactivity in borderline personality disorder. Biol Psychiatry 54:1284–1293, 2003

Doody GA, Gotz M, Johnstone EC, et al: Theory of mind and psychosis. Psychol Med 28:397–405, 1998

Dunn J: The Emanuel Miller Memorial Lecture 1995: Children's relationships: bridging the divide between cognitive and social development. J Child Psychol Psychiatry 37:507–518, 1996

Dunn J, Brown J: Relationships, talk about feelings, and the development of affect regulation in early childhood, in Affect Regulation and Dysregulation in Childhood. Edited by Garber J, Dodge K. Cambridge, UK, Cambridge University Press, 2001, pp 89–108

Dunn J, Cutting A: Understanding others and individual differences in friendship interactions in young children. Soc Dev 8:201–219, 1999

Dunn J, Brown J, Beardsall L: Family talk about feeling states and children's later understanding of others' emotions. Dev Psychol 27:448–455, 1991

Dutton D, Painter SL: Traumatic bonding: the development of emotional attachments in battered women and other relationships of intermittent abuse. Victimology 6:139–155, 1981

Edelman GM: The Remembered Present: A Biological Theory of Consciousness. New York, Basic Books, 1989

Egeland B: Mediators of the effects of child maltreatment on developmental adaptation in adolescence, in Developmental Perspectives on Trauma: Theory, Research and Intervention, Vol 8. Edited by Cicchetti D, Toth SL. Rochester, NY, University of Rochester Press, 1997, pp 403–434

Eichenbaum H: The Cognitive Neuroscience of Memory: An Introduction. New York, Oxford University Press, 2002

Eilan N: Joint attention, communication and mind, in Joint Attention: Communication and Other Minds. Edited by Eilan N, Hoerl C, McCormack T, et al. New York, Oxford University Press, 2005, pp 1–33

Eilan N, Hoerl C, McCormack T, et al. (eds): Joint Attention: Communication and Other Minds. New York, Oxford University Press, 2005

Ekman P: Emotions Revealed. New York, Holt, 2003

Ekman P, Davidson RJ: Voluntary smiling changes regional brain activity. Psychol Sci 4:342–345, 1993

Elliott R, Dolan RJ, Frith CD: Dissociable functions in the medial and lateral orbitofrontal cortex: evidence from human neuroimaging studies. Cereb Cortex 10:308–317, 2000

Ellsworth PC, Scherer KR: Appraisal processes in emotion, in Handbook of Affective Sciences. Edited by Davidson RJ, Scherer KR, Goldsmith HH. New York, Oxford University Press, 2003, pp 572–595

Elman JL, Bates EA, Johnson MH, et al: Rethinking Innateness: A Connectionist Perspective on Development. Cambridge, MA, MIT Press, 1996

Emde RN, Everhart KD, Wise BK: Therapeutic relationships in infant mental health and the concept of leverage, in Treating Parent-Infant Relationship Problems: Strategies for Intervention. Edited by Sameroff AJ, McDonough SC, Rosenblum KL. New York, Guilford, 2004, pp 267–292

Erickson MF, Egeland B: Child neglect, in The APSAC Handbook on Child Maltreatment. Edited by Briere J, Berliner L, Bulkley JA, et al. Thousand Oaks, CA, Sage, 1996, pp 4–20

Estes D, Wellman HM, Wolley JD: Children's understanding of mental phenomena, in Advances in Child Development and Behavior. Edited by Reese H. New York, Academic Press, 1989, pp 41–87

Eurlings-Bontekoe E, Verschuur M, Schreuder B: Personality, temperament and attachment style among offspring of World War II victims: an integration of descriptive and structural features of personality. Traumatology 9:106–122, 2003

Farber BA: The genesis, development and implications of psychological-mindedness in psychotherapists. Psychotherapy 22:170–177, 1985

Fearon P, Belsky J: Attachment and attention: protection in relation to gender and cumulative social-contextual adversity. Child Dev 75:1677–1693, 2004

Fearon P, Target M, Sargent J, et al: Short-Term Mentalization and Relational Therapy (SMART): an integrative family therapy for children and adolescents, in Handbook of Mentalization-Based Treatment. Edited by Allen JG, Fonagy P. Chichester, UK, Wiley, 2006a, pp 201–222

Fearon P, van IJzendoorn MH, Fonagy P, et al: In search of shared and non-shared environmental factors in security of attachment: a behavior-genetic study of the association between sensitivity and attachment security. Dev Psychol 42:1026–1040, 2006b

Feldman RB, Zelkowitz P, Weiss M, et al: A comparison of the families of mothers with borderline and nonborderline personality disorders. Compr Psychiatry 36:157–163, 1995

Fernandez-Duque D, Baird JA: Is there a "social brain"? Lessons from eye-gaze following, joint attention and autism, in Other Minds: How Humans Bridge the Divide between Self and Others. Edited by Malle BF, Hodges SD. New York, Guilford, 2005, pp 75–90

Fernandez-Duque D, Baird JA, Posner MI: Executive attention and metacognitive regulation. Conscious Cogn 9:288–307, 2000

Fertuck EA, Lenzenweger MF, Clarkin JF, et al: Executive neurocognition, memory systems and borderline personality disorder. Clin Psychol Rev 26:346–375, 2006

First MB, Gibbon M, Spitzer RL, et al: User's Guide for the Structured Clinical Interview for DSM-IV Axis II Personality Disorders: SCID-II. Washington, DC, American Psychiatric Press, 1997

Flavell JH: Cognitive development: children's knowledge about the mind. Annu Rev Psychol 50:21–45, 1999

Flavell JH, Flavell ER, Green FL: Young children's knowledge about the apparent-real and pretend-real distinction. Dev Psychol 23:816–822, 1987

Fletcher PC, Happe F, Frith U, et al: Other minds in the brain: a functional imaging study of "theory of mind" in story comprehension. Cognition 57:109–128, 1995

Foa EB: Psychological processes related to recovery from a trauma and effective treatment for PTSD, in Psychobiology of Posttraumatic Stress Disorder. Edited by Yehuda R, McFarlane AC. New York, New York Academy of Sciences, 1997, pp 410–424

Foa EB, Kozak MJ: Emotional processing of fear: exposure to corrective information. Psychol Bull 99:20–35, 1986

Foa EB, Kozak MJ: Emotional processing: theory, research and clinical implications for anxiety disorders, in Emotion, Psychotherapy and Change. Edited by Safran JD, Greenberg LS. New York, Guilford, 1991, pp 21–49

Foa EB, Rothbaum BO: Treating the Trauma of Rape: Cognitive-Behavioral Therapy for PTSD. New York, Guilford, 1998

Foa EB, Riggs DS, Massie ED, et al: The impact of fear activation and anger on the efficacy of exposure treatment for posttraumatic stress disorder. Behav Ther 26:487–499, 1995

Foa EB, Ehlers A, Clark DM, et al: The Posttraumatic Cognitions Inventory (PTCI): development and validation. Psychol Assess 11:303–314, 1999

Fodor J: Hume Variations. New York, Oxford University Press, 2003

Fonagy P: Thinking about thinking: some clinical and theoretical considerations in the treatment of a borderline patient. Int J Psychoanal 72:639–656, 1991

Fonagy P: Playing with reality: the development of psychic reality and its malfunction in borderline personalities. Int J Psychoanal 76:39–44, 1995

Fonagy P: The transgenerational transmission of holocaust trauma: lessons learned from the analysis of an adolescent with obsessive-compulsive disorder. Attach Hum Dev 1:92–114, 1999

Fonagy P: Attachment Theory and Psychoanalysis. New York, Other Press, 2001a

Fonagy P: The human genome and the interpersonal world: the role of early mother-infant interaction in creating an interpersonal interpretive mechanism. Bull Menninger Clin 65:427–448, 2001b

Fonagy P: Understanding of mental states, mother-infant interaction and the development of the self, in Infant and Toddler Mental Health: Models of Clinical Intervention With Infants and Their Families. Edited by Maldonado-Duran JM. Washington, DC, American Psychiatric Publishing, 2002, pp 57–74

Fonagy P: The development of psychopathology from infancy to adulthood: the mysterious unfolding of disturbance over time. Infant Ment Health J 24:212–239, 2003a

Fonagy P: Towards a developmental understanding of violence. Br J Psychiatry 183:190–192, 2003b

Fonagy P: Early life trauma and the psychogenesis and prevention of violence. Ann NY Acad Sci 1036:181–200, 2004

Fonagy P: The mentalization-focused approach to social development, in Handbook of Mentalization-Based Treatment. Edited by Allen JG, Fonagy P. Chichester, UK, Wiley, 2006, pp 53–99

Fonagy P, Bateman AW: Mechanisms of change in mentalization-based therapy of borderline personality disorder. J Clin Psychol 62:411–430, 2006a

Fonagy P, Bateman AW: Progress in the treatment of borderline personality disorder. Br J Psychiatry 188:1–3, 2006b

Fonagy P, Higgitt A: Early mental health intervention and prevention: the implications for government and the wider community, in Analysts in the Trenches. Edited by Sklarew B, Twemlow SW, Wilkinson SM. Hillsdale, NJ, Analytic Press, 2004, pp 257–309

Fonagy P, Target M: Attachment and reflective function: their role in self-organization. Dev Psychopathol 9:679–700, 1997a

Fonagy P, Target M: Perspectives on the recovered memories debate, in Recovered Memories of Abuse: True or False? Edited by Sandler J, Fonagy P. Madison, CT, International Universities Press, 1997b, pp 183–237

Fonagy P, Target M: Early intervention and the development of self-regulation. Psychoanalytic Inquiry 22:307–335, 2002

Fonagy P, Steele H, Steele M: Maternal representations of attachment during pregnancy predict the organization of infant-mother attachment at one year of age. Child Dev 62:891–905, 1991a

Fonagy P, Steele M, Steele H, et al: The capacity for understanding mental states: the reflective self in parent and child and its significance for security of attachment. Infant Ment Health J 12:201–218, 1991b

Fonagy P, Moran GS, Edgcumbe R, et al: The roles of mental representations and mental processes in therapeutic action. Psychoanal Study Child 48:9–48, 1993

Fonagy P, Steele M, Steele H, et al: The Emmanuel Miller Memorial Lecture 1992: the theory and practice of resilience. J Child Psychol Psychiatry 35:231–257, 1994

Fonagy P, Steele M, Steele H, et al: Attachment, the reflective self and borderline states: the predictive specificity of the Adult Attachment Interview and pathological emotional development, in Attachment Theory: Social, Developmental and Clinical Perspectives. Edited by Goldberg S, Muir R, Kerr J. New York, Analytic Press, 1995, pp 233–278

Fonagy P, Leigh T, Steele M, et al: The relation of attachment status, psychiatric classification and response to psychotherapy. J Consult Clin Psychol 64:22–31, 1996

Fonagy P, Redfern S, Charman A: The relationship between belief-desire reasoning and a projective measure of attachment security (SAT). B J Dev Psychol 15:51–61, 1997a

Fonagy P, Steele H, Steele M, et al: Attachment and theory of mind: overlapping constructs? Association of Child Psychology and Psychiatry Occasional Papers 14:31–40, 1997b

Fonagy P, Steele M, Steele H, et al: Reflective-Functioning Manual for Application to Adult Attachment Interviews, Version 4.1. London, Psychoanalysis Unit, Sub-Department of Clinical Health Psychology, University College London, 1997c

Fonagy P, Target M, Gergely G: Attachment and borderline personality disorder: a theory and some evidence. Psychiatr Clin North Am 23:103–122, 2000

Fonagy P, Gergely G, Jurist EL, et al: Affect Regulation, Mentalization and the Development of the Self. New York, Other Press, 2002a

Fonagy P, Target M, Cottrell D, et al: What Works for Whom? A Critical Review of Treatments for Children and Adolescents. New York, Guilford, 2002b

Fonagy P, Twemlow SW, Vernberg E, et al: Creating a peaceful school learning environment: the impact of an antibullying program on educational attainment in elementary schools. Med Sci Monit 11:317–325, 2005

Fonagy P, Gergely G, Target M: The parent-infant dyad and the construction of the subjective self. J Child Psychol Psychiatry 48:288–328, 2007

Foxman P: Tolerance for ambiguity and self-actualization. J Pers Assess 40:67–72, 1976

Fraiberg S, Adelson E, Shapiro V: Ghosts in the nursery: a psychoanalytic approach to the problems of impaired infant-mother relationships. J Am Acad Child Psychiatry 14:387–421, 1975

Franco F: Infant pointing: Harlequin, servant of two masters, in Joint Attention: Communication and Other Minds. Edited by Eilan N, Hoerl C, McCormack T, et al. New York, Oxford University Press, 2005, pp 129–164

Frank JD: Persuasion and Healing. New York, Schocken Books, 1961

Frankfurt HG: On Bullshit. Princeton, NJ, Princeton University Press, 2005

Freud S: Project for a scientific psychology (1895), in The Origins of Psycho-Analysis: Letters to Wilhelm Fleiss, Drafts and Notes: 1887–1902. Edited by Bonaparte M, Freud A, Kris E. New York, Basic Books, 1954, pp 347–445

Freud S: The Interpretation of Dreams (1900). New York, Avon, 1965

Freud S: Remembering, repeating and working-through (1914), in The Standard Edition of the Complete Psychological Works of Sigmund Freud, Vol 12. Edited and translated by Strachey J. London, Hogarth Press, 1958, pp 147–156

Freud S: Civilization and Its Discontents (1929). New York, Norton, 1961

Freyd JJ: Betrayal Trauma: The Logic of Forgetting Childhood Abuse. Cambridge, MA, Harvard University Press, 1996

Frith CD, Corcoran R: Exploring "theory of mind" in people with schizophrenia. Psychol Med 26:521–530, 1996

Frith U, Frith CD: Development and neurophysiology of mentalizing. Philos Trans R Soc Lond B Biol Sci 358:459–473, 2003

Frith U, Morton J, Leslie AM: The cognitive basis of a biological disorder: autism. Trends Neurosci 14:433–438, 1991

Fruzzetti AE, Shenk C, Lowry K, et al: Emotion regulation, in Cognitive-Behavior Therapy: Applying Empirically Supported Techniques in Your Practice. Edited by O'Donohue JE, Fisher SC. New York, Wiley, 2003, pp 152–159

Fruzzetti AE, Shenk C, Hoffman PD: Family interaction and the development of borderline personality disorder: a transactional model. Dev Psychopathol 17:1007–1030, 2005

Gabbard GO: When is transference work useful in dynamic psychotherapy? Am J Psychiatry 163:1667–1669, 2006

Gabbard GO, Wilkinson SM: Management of Countertransference With Borderline Patients. Washington, DC, American Psychiatric Press, 1994

Gabbard GO, Miller LA, Martinez M: A neurobiological perspective on mentalizing and internal object relations in traumatized patients with borderline personality disorder, in Handbook of Mentalization-Based Treatment. Edited by Allen JG, Fonagy P. Chichester, UK, Wiley, 2006, pp 123–140

Gallagher HL, Frith CD: Functional imaging "theory of mind." Trends Cogn Sci 7:77–83, 2003

Gallagher HL, Jack AI, Roepstorff A, et al: Imaging the intentional stance in a competitive game. Neuroimage 16:814–821, 2002

Gallese V: The "shared manifold" hypothesis: from mirror neurons to empathy. Journal of Consciousness Studies 8:33–50, 2001

Gallese V, Keysers C, Rizzolatti G: A unifying view of the basis of social cognition. Trends Cogn Sci 9:396–403, 2004

Garland AF, Landsverk JL, Hough RL, et al: Type of maltreatment as a predictor of mental health service use for children in foster care. Child Abuse Negl 20:675–688, 1996

Gergely G: The obscure object of desire—"nearly, but clearly not, like me": contingency preference in normal children versus children with autism. Bull Menninger Clin 65:411–426, 2001

Gergely G: The social construction of the subjective self: the role of affect mirroring, markedness and ostensive communication in self development, in Developmental Science and Psychoanalysis. Edited by Mayes LC, Fonagy P, Target M. London, Karnac, 2007

Gergely G, Csibra G: Teleological reasoning in infancy: the naive theory of rational action. Trends Cogn Sci 7:287–292, 2003

Gergely G, Csibra G: The social construction of the cultural mind: imitative learning as a mechanism of human pedagogy. Interaction Studies 6:463–481, 2005

Gergely G, Watson JS: The social biofeedback theory of parental affect-mirroring: the development of emotional self-awareness and self-control in infancy. Int J Psychoanal 77:1181–1212, 1996

Gergely G, Watson JS: Early social-emotional development: contingency perception and the social biofeedback model, in Early Social Cognition: Understanding Others in the First Months of Life. Edited by Rochat P. Hillsdale, NJ, Erlbaum, 1999, pp 101–137

Gergely G, Nadasdy Z, Csibra G, et al: Taking the intentional stance at 12 months of age. Cognition 56:165–193, 1995

Gergely G, Egyed K, Király I: On pedagogy. Dev Sci 10:139–146, 2007

Giedd JN: The anatomy of mentalization: a view from neuroimaging. Bull Menninger Clin 67:132–142, 2003

Gilbert DT, Driver-Linn E, Wilson TD: The trouble with Vronsky: impact bias in the forecasting of future affective states, in The Wisdom in Feeling: Psychological Processes in Emotional Intelligence. Edited by Feldman Barrett L, Salovey P. New York, Guilford, 2002, pp 114–143

Glodich A: Psychoeducational groups for adolescents exposed to violence and abuse: assessing the effectiveness of increasing knowledge of trauma to avert reenactment and risk-taking behaviors. Doctoral dissertation, Smith College, Northampton, MA, 1999

Glodich A, Allen JG, Arnold L: Protocol for a trauma-based psychoeducational group intervention to decrease risk-taking, reenactment and further violence exposure: Application to the public high school setting. Journal of Child and Adolescent Group Psychotherapy 11:87–107, 2001

Glodich A, Allen JG, Fultz J, et al: School-based psychoeducational groups on trauma designed to decrease reenactment, in Community-Based Clinical Practice. Edited by Lightburn A, Sessions P. New York, Oxford University Press, 2006, pp 349–363

Godfrey-Smith P: On folk psychology and mental representation, in Representation in Mind: New Approaches to Mental Representation. Edited by Clapin H, Staines P, Slezak P. Amsterdam, Elsevier, 2004, pp 147–162

Goldberg E: The Executive Brain: Frontal Lobes and the Civilized Mind. New York, Oxford University Press, 2001

Goldberg S, Benoit D, Blokland K, et al: Atypical maternal behavior, maternal representations and infant disorganized attachment. Dev Psychopathol 15:239–257, 2003

Goldie P: Emotion, feelings and knowledge of the world, in Thinking about Feeling: Contemporary Philosophers on Emotions. Edited by Solomon RC. New York, Oxford University Press, 2004a, pp 91–106

Goldie P: Emotion, reason and virtue, in Emotion, Evolution and Rationality. Edited by Evans D, Cruse P. New York, Oxford University Press, 2004b, pp 249–267

Goldman AI: Simulating Minds: The Philosophy, Psychology and Neuroscience of Mindreading. New York, Oxford University Press, 2006

Golomb A, Ludolph P, Westen D, et al: Maternal empathy, family chaos and the etiology of borderline personality disorder. J Am Psychoanal Assoc 42:525–548, 1994

Gómez JC: Apes, Monkeys, Children and the Growth of Mind. Cambridge, MA, Harvard University Press, 2004

Gómez JC: Joint attention and the notion of subject: insights from apes, normal children and children with autism, in Joint Attention: Communication and Other Minds. Edited by Eilan N, Hoerl C, McCormack T, et al. New York, Oxford University Press, 2005, pp 65–84

Goodwin FK, Jamison KR: Manic-Depressive Illness: Bipolar Disorders and Recurrent Depression, 2nd Edition. New York, Oxford University Press, 2007

Gopnik A, Meltzoff AN: Words, Thoughts and Theories. Cambridge, MA, MIT Press, 1997

Gottman JM, Katz LF, Hooven C: Parental meta-emotion philosophy and the emotional life of families: theoretical models and preliminary data. J Fam Psychol 10:243–268, 1996

Grayling AC: The Reason of Things: Living With Philosophy. London, Weidenfeld Nicolson, 2002

Grayling AC: Among the Dead Cities: The History of Moral Legacy of the WWII Bombing of Civilians in Germany and Japan. New York, Walker, 2006

Green J, Goldwyn R: Annotation: Attachment disorganisation and psychopathology: new findings in attachment research and their potential implications for developmental psychopathology in childhood. J Child Psychol Psychiatry 43:835–846, 2002

Greenwald R: The power of suggestion—comment on EMDR and Mesmerism: a comparative historical analysis. J Anxiety Disord 13:611–615, 1999

Grienenberger J, Kelly K, Slade A: Maternal reflective functioning, mother-infant affective communication and infant attachment: exploring the link between mental states and observed caregiving behavior in the intergenerational transmission of attachment. Attach Hum Dev 7:299–311, 2005

Grossmann KE, Grossmann K, Zimmermann P: A wider view of attachment and exploration: stability and change during the years of immaturity, in Handbook of Attachment: Theory, Research and Clinical Applications. Edited by Cassidy J, Shaver PR. New York, Guilford, 1999, pp 760–786

Gunderson JG: Borderline Personality Disorder: A Clinical Guide. Washington, DC, American Psychiatric Publishing, 2001

Gunderson JG, Sabo AN: The phenomenological and conceptual interface between borderline personality disorder and PTSD. Am J Psychiatry 150:19–27, 1993

Gunderson JG, Bender D, Sanislow C, et al: Plausibility and possible determinants of sudden "remissions" in borderline patients. Psychiatry 66:111–119, 2003

Gunderson JG, Daversa MT, Grilo CM, et al: Predictors of 2-year outcome for patients with borderline personality disorder. Am J Psychiatry 163:822–826, 2006a

Gunderson JG, Weinberg I, Daversa MT, et al: Descriptive and longitudinal observations on the relationship of borderline personality disorder and bipolar disorder. Am J Psychiatry 163:1173–1178, 2006b

Guttman HA, Laporte L: Empathy in families of women with borderline personality disorder, anorexia nervosa and a control group. Fam Process 39:345–358, 2000

Hahn TN: The Miracle of Mindfulness: A Manual on Meditation. Boston, MA, Beacon Press, 1975

Hamilton CE: Continuity and discontinuity of attachment from infancy through adolescence. Child Dev 71:690–694, 2000

Hare RD: A research scale for the assessment of psychopathy in criminal populations. Pers Individ Dif 1:111–119, 1980

Hare RD, Hart SD, Harpur TJ: Psychopathy and the DSM-IV criteria for antisocial personality disorder. J Abnorm Psychol 100:391–398, 1991

Hariri AR, Mattay VS, Tessitore A, et al: Neocortical modulation of the amygdala response to fearful stimuli. Biol Psychiatry 53:494–501, 2003

Harris PL: Individual differences in understanding emotion: the role of attachment status and psychological discourse. Attach Hum Dev 1:307–324, 1999

Harvey AG, Bryant RA: The effect of attempted thought suppression in acute stress disorder. Behav Res Ther 36:583–590, 1998

Haslam-Hopwood GTG, Allen JG, Stein A, et al: Enhancing mentalizing through psychoeducation, in Handbook of Mentalization-Based Treatment. Edited by Allen JG, Fonagy P. Chichester, UK, Wiley, 2006, pp 249–267

Hatfield E, Cacioppo JT, Rapson RL: Emotional Contagion. Paris, Cambridge University Press, 1994

Heal J: Mind, Reason and Imagination. New York, Cambridge University Press, 2003

Henderson AJZ, Bartholomew K, Dutton DG: He loves me; he loves me not: attachment and separation resolution of abused women. J Fam Violence 12:169–191, 1997

Herman JL: Complex PTSD: a syndrome in survivors of prolonged and repeated trauma. J Trauma Stress 5:377–391, 1992a

Herman JL: Trauma and Recovery. New York, Basic Books, 1992b

Herman JL, Perry C, van der Kolk BA: Childhood trauma in borderline personality disorder. Am J Psychiatry 146:490–495, 1989

Herpertz SC: Emotional processing in personality disorder. Curr Psychiatry Rep 5:23–27, 2003

Herpertz SC, Dietrich TM, Wenning B, et al: Evidence of abnormal amygdala functioning in borderline personality disorder: a functional MRI study. Biol Psychiatry 50:292–298, 2001a

Herpertz SC, Werth U, Lukas G, et al: Emotion in criminal offenders with psychopathy and borderline personality disorder. Arch Gen Psychiatry 58:737–745, 2001b

Hobson RP: The Cradle of Thought: Exploring the Origins of Thinking. New York, Oxford University Press, 2002

Hobson RP: What puts the jointness into joint attention? in Joint Attention: Communication and Other Minds. Edited by Eilan N, Hoerl C, McCormack T, et al. New York, Oxford University Press, 2005, pp 185–204

Hobson RP, Patrick MPH, Crandell LE, et al: Personal relatedness and attachment in infants of mothers with borderline personality disorder. Dev Psychopathol 17:329–347, 2005

Hoermann S, Clarkin JF, Hull JW, et al: The construct of effortful control: an approach to borderline personality disorder heterogeneity. Psychopathology 38:82–86, 2005

Hofer MA: The emerging neurobiology of attachment and separation: how parents shape their infant's brain and behavior, in September 11: Trauma and Human Bonds. Edited by Coates SW, Rosenthal JL, Schechter DS. New York, Guilford, 2003, pp 191–209

Holmes J: Defensive and creative uses of narrative in psychotherapy: an attachment perspective, in Healing Stories: Narrative in Psychiatry and Psychotherapy. Edited by Roberts G, Holmes J. London, Oxford University Press, 1999, pp 49–66

Holmes J: Mentalizing from a psychoanalytic perspective: what's new? in Handbook of Mentalization-Based Treatment. Edited by Allen JG, Fonagy P. Chichester, UK, Wiley, 2006, pp 31–49

Horwitz AV, Widom CS, McLaughlin J, et al: The impact of childhood abuse and neglect on adult mental health: a prospective study. J Health Soc Behav 42:184–201, 2001

Horwitz L, Gabbard GO, Allen JG, et al: Borderline Personality Disorder: Tailoring the Therapy to the Patient. Washington, DC, American Psychiatric Press, 1996

Hoven CW, Mandell DJ, Duarte CS: Mental health of New York City public school children after 9/11, in September 11: Trauma and Human Bonds. Edited by Coates SW, Rosenthal JL, Schechter DS. Hillsdale, NJ, Analytic Press, 2003, pp 51–74

Hughes C, Cutting A: Nature, nurture and individual differences in early understanding of mind. Psychol Sci 10:429–432, 1999

Hughes C, Dunn J: Understanding mind and emotion: longitudinal associations with mental-state talk between young friends. Dev Psychol 34:1026–1037, 1998

Hughes C, Dunn J: "When I say a naughty word"—children's accounts of anger and sadness in self, mother and friend: longitudinal findings from ages four to seven. Br J Dev Psychol 20:515–535, 2002

Hughes C, Ensor R: Social cognition and disruptive behavior disorders in young children: families matter, in Social Cognition and Developmental Psychopathology. Edited by Sharp C, Fonagy P, Goodyer IM. New York, Oxford University Press (in press)

Hughes C, Jaffee SR, Happe F, et al: Origins of individual differences in theory of mind: from nature to nurture? Child Dev 76:356–370, 2005

Humphrey NK: The social function of intellect, in Machiavellian Intelligence: Social Expertise and the Evolution of Intellect in Monkeys, Apes and Humans. Edited by Byrne RW, Whiten A. New York, Oxford University Press, 1988, pp 13–26

Hurry A: Psychoanalysis and developmental therapy, in Psychoanalysis and Developmental Therapy. Edited by Hurry A. Madison, CT, International Universities Press, 1998, pp 32–73

Iacoboni M, Koski LM, Brass M, et al: Reafferent copies of imitated actions in the right superior temporal cortex. Proc Natl Acad Sci USA 98:13995–13999, 2001

Ickes W, Simpson JA, Orina M: Empathic accuracy and inaccuracy in close relationships, in Other Minds: How Humans Bridge the Divide between Self and Others. Edited by Malle BF, Hodges SD. New York, Guilford, 2005, pp 310–322

Ingram RE, Miranda J, Segal ZV: Cognitive Vulnerability to Depression. New York, Guilford, 1998

Inoue Y, Tonooka Y, Yamada K, et al: Deficiency of theory of mind in patients with remitted mood disorder. J Affect Disord 82:403–409, 2004

Jackson PL, Meltzoff AN, Decety J: How do we perceive the pain of others? A window into the neural processes involved in empathy. Neuroimage 24:771–779, 2005

Janis IB, Veague HB, Driver-Linn E: Possible selves and borderline personality disorder. J Clin Psychol 62:387–394, 2006

Janoff-Bulman R. Shattered Assumptions: Towards a New Psychology of Trauma. New York, Free Press, 1992

Jeannerod M: The Cognitive Neuroscience of Action. Oxford, UK, Blackwell, 1997

Johnson JG, Cohen P, Smailes E, et al: Childhood verbal abuse and risk for personality disorders during adolescence and early adulthood. Compr Psychiatry 42:16–23, 2001

Johnson JG, Cohen P, Gould MS, et al: Childhood adversities, interpersonal difficulties and risk for suicide attempts during late adolescence and early
adulthood. Arch Gen Psychiatry 59:741–749, 2002

Johnson JG, Cohen P, Chen H, et al: Parenting behaviors associated with risk for
offspring personality disorder during adulthood. Arch Gen Psychiatry
63:579–587, 2006

Jost JT, Kruglanski AW, Nelson TO: Social metacognition: an expansionist review. Pers Soc Psychol Rev 2:137–154, 1998

Judd LL, Akiskal HS, Schettler PJ, et al: The long-term natural history of the
weekly symptomatic status of bipolar I disorder. Arch Gen Psychiatry
59:530–537, 2002

Jurist EL: Mentalized affectivity. Psychoanal Psychol 22:426–444, 2005

Karmiloff-Smith A: Beyond Modularity: A Developmental Perspective on Cognitive Science. Cambridge, MA, MIT Press, 1992

Katz LF, Gottman JM: Buffering children from marital conflict and dissolution.
J Clin Child Psychol 26:157–171, 1997

Kekes J: The Roots of Evil. Ithaca, NY, Cornell University Press, 2005

Keltner D, Ekman P, Gonzaga GC, et al: Facial expression of emotion, in Handbook of Affective Science. Edited by Davidson RJ, Scherer KR, Goldsmith
HH. New York, Oxford University Press, 2003, pp 415–432

Kernberg OF: Borderline Conditions and Pathological Narcissism. New York,
Aronson, 1975

Kernberg OF: Object relations theory and character analysis. J Am Psychoanal
Assoc 31:247–271, 1983

Kerr N, Dunbar RIM, Bentall RP: Theory of mind deficits in bipolar affective
disorder. J Affect Disord 73:253–259, 2003

Keysers C, Wicker B, Gazzola V, et al: A touching sight: SII/PV activation during the observation and experience of touch. Neuron 42:335–346, 2004

Kim-Cohen J, Caspi A, Moffitt TE, et al: Prior juvenile diagnoses in adults with
mental disorder. Arch Gen Psychiatry 60:709–717, 2003

Klerman GL, Weissman MM, Rounsaville BJ, et al: Interpersonal Psychotherapy
of Depression. New York, Basic Books, 1984

Klin A, Schultz R, Cohen DJ: Theory of mind in action: developmental perspectives on social neuroscience, in Understanding Other Minds: Perspectives
from Developmental Cognitive Neuroscience, 2nd Edition. Edited by
Baron-Cohen S, Tager-Flusberg H, Cohen DJ. New York, Oxford University
Press, 2000, pp 357–388

Kobak R, Cassidy J, Lyons-Ruth K, et al: Attachment stress and psychopathology: a developmental pathways model, in Developmental Psychopathology, 2nd Edition, Vol 1: Theory and Method. Edited by Cicchetti D, Cohen
DJ. New York, Wiley, 2006, pp 334–369

Kochanska G: Emotional development in children with different attachment
histories: the first three years. Child Dev 72:474–490, 2001

Kochanska G, Murray KT: Mother-child mutually responsive orientation and
conscience development: from toddler to early school age. Child Dev
71:417–431, 2000

Kochanska G, Murray KT, Jacques TY, et al: Inhibitory control in young children
and its role in emerging internalization. Child Dev 67:490–507, 1996

Kochanska G, Murray KT, Coy KC: Inhibitory control as a contributor to conscience in childhood: from toddler to early school age. Child Dev 68:263–277, 1997

Kochanska G, Murray KT, Harlan E: Effortful control in early childhood: continuity and change, antecedents and implications for social development. Dev Psychol 36:220–232, 2000

Kochanska G, Coy KC, Murray KT: The development of self-regulation in the first four years of life. Child Dev 72:1091–1111, 2001

Koós O, Gergely G: A contingency-based approach to the etiology of "disorganized" attachment: the "flickering switch" hypothesis. Bull Menninger Clin 65:397–410, 2001

Koren-Karie N, Oppenheim D, Dolev S, et al: Mothers' insightfulness regarding their infants' internal experience: relations with maternal sensitivity and infant attachment. Dev Psychol 38:534–542, 2002

Korfine L, Hooley JM: Directed forgetting of emotional stimuli in borderline personality disorder. J Abnorm Psychol 109:214–221, 2000

Koriat A: The feeling of knowing: some metatheoretical implications for consciousness and control. Conscious Cogn 9:149–171, 2000

Koriat A, Ma'ayan H, Niussinson R: The intricate relationships between monitoring and control in metacognition: lessons for the cause-and-effect relation between subjective experience and behavior. J Exp Psychol Gen 135:36–69, 2006

Korsgaard CM: Morality and the distinctiveness of human action, in Primates and Philosophers: How Morality Evolved. Edited by Macedo S, Ober J. Princeton, NJ, Princeton University Press, 2006, pp 98–119

Kreppner JM, O'Connor TG, Rutter M: Can inattention/overactivity be an institutional deprivation syndrome? J Abnorm Child Psychol 29:513–528, 2001

Kringelbach ML: The human orbitofrontal cortex: linking reward to hedonic experience Nat Rev Neurosci 6:691–702, 2005

Krystal H: Integration and Self-Healing: Affect, Trauma, Alexithymia. Hillsdale, NJ, Analytic Press, 1988

Lakatos K, Toth I, Nemoda Z, et al: Dopamine D4 receptor (DRD4) gene polymorphism is associated with attachment disorganization in infants. Mol Psychiatry 5:633–637, 2000

Lalonde C, Chandler MJ: False belief understanding goes to school: on the social-emotional consequences of coming early or late to a first theory of mind. Cogn Emot 9:167–185, 1995

Lambert M, Bergin AE, Garfield S: Introduction and historical overview, in Bergin and Garfield's Handbook of Psychotherapy and Behavior Change. Edited by Lambert M. New York, Wiley, 2004, pp 3–15

Lane RD: Neural correlates of conscious emotional experience, in Cognitive Neuroscience of Emotion. Edited by Lane RD, Nadel L. New York, Oxford University Press, 2000, pp 345–370

Lawrence EJ, Shaw P, Giampietro VP, et al: The role of "shared representations" in social perception and empathy: an fMRI study. Neuroimage 29:1173–1184, 2006

Lebell S: Epictetus: The Art of Living. New York, HarperCollins, 1995

Lecours S, Bouchard MA: Dimensions of mentalisation: outlining levels of psychic transformation. Int J Psychoanal 78:855–875, 1997

LeDoux J: The Emotional Brain. New York, Simon and Schuster, 1996

Lee CW, Taylor G, Drummond PD: The active ingredient in EMDR: is it traditional exposure or dual focus of attention? Clin Psychol Psychother 13:97–107, 2006

Lee L, Harkness KL, Sabbagh MA, et al: Mental state decoding abilities in clinical depression. J Affect Disord 86:247–258, 2005

LeGris J, van Reekum R: The neuropsychological correlates of borderline personality disorder and suicidal behavior. Can J Psychiatry 51:131–142, 2006

Leichsenring F, Sachsse U: Emotions as wishes and beliefs. J Pers Assess 79:257–273, 2002

Lenzenweger MF, Clarkin JF, Fertuck EA, et al: Executive neurocognitive functioning and neurobehavioral systems indicators in borderline personality disorder: a preliminary study. J Pers Disord 18:421–438, 2004

Leslie AM: Pretense and representation: the origins of "theory of mind." Psychol Rev 94:412–426, 1987

Levinson A, Fonagy P: Offending and attachment: the relationship between interpersonal awareness and offending in a prison population with psychiatric disorder. Can J Psychoanal 12:225–251, 2004

Levy KN: The implications of attachment theory and research for understanding borderline personality disorder: a preliminary study. Dev Psychopathol 17:959–986, 2005

Lewis L: Enhancing mentalizing capacity through Dialectical Behavior Therapy skills training and Positive Psychology, in Handbook of Mentalization-Based Treatment. Edited by Allen JG, Fonagy P. Chichester, UK, Wiley, 2006, pp 171–182

Lewis L, Kelly KA, Allen JG: Restoring Hope and Trust: An Illustrated Guide to Mastering Trauma. Baltimore, MD, Sidran Press, 2004

Lieb K, Zanarini MC, Schmahl C, et al: Borderline personality disorder. Lancet 364:453–461, 2004

Liebenluft E, Gobbini MI, Harrison T: Mothers' neural activation in response to pictures of their children and other children. Biol Psychiatry 56:225–232, 2004

Lieberman AF: Toddlers' internalization of maternal attributions as a factor in quality of attachment, in Attachment and Psychopathology. Edited by Atkinson L, Zucker K. New York, Guilford, 1997, pp 277–299

Lieberman AF: Child-parent psychotherapy: a relationship-based approach to the treatment of mental health disorders in infancy and early childhood, in Treating Parent-Infant Relationship Problems: Strategies for Intervention. Edited by Sameroff AJ, McDonough SC, Rosenblum KL. New York, Guilford, 2004, pp 97–122

Lieberman AF, Padron E, Van Horn P, et al: Angels in the nursery: the intergenerational transmission of benevolent parental influences. Infant Ment Health J 26:504–520, 2005

Lieberman MD: Intuition: a social cognitive neuroscience approach. Psychol Bull 126:109–137, 2000

Lieberman MD: Social cognitive neuroscience: a review of core processes. Annu Rev Psychol 58:18.1–18.31, 2007

Lieberman MD, Eisenberger NI, Crockett MJ, et al: Putting feelings into words: affect labeling disrupts amygdala activity to affective stimuli. Psychol Sci 18:421–428, 2007

Lightburn A, Sessions P (eds): Handbook of Community-Based Clinical Practice. New York, Oxford University Press, 2006

Linehan MM: Cognitive-Behavioral Treatment of Borderline Personality Disorder. New York, Guilford, 1993a

Linehan MM: Skills Training Manual for Treating Borderline Personality Disorder. New York, Guilford, 1993b

Liszkowski U, Carpenter M, Henning A, et al: Twelve-month-olds point to share attention and interest. Dev Sci 7:297–307, 2004

Livesley WJ, Jackson DN: Guidelines for developing, evaluating and revising the classification of personality disorders. J Nerv Ment Dis 180:609–618, 1992

Loewald HW: On the therapeutic action of psycho-analysis. Int J Psychoanal 41:16–33, 1960

Loewald HW: Psychoanalytic theory and the psychoanalytic process. Psychoanal Study Child 25:45–68, 1970

Long AA: Epictetus: A Stoic and Socratic Guide to Life. New York, Oxford University Press, 2002

Ludolph PS, Westen D, Misle B, et al: The borderline diagnosis in adolescents: symptoms and developmental history. Am J Psychiatry 147:470–476, 1990

Lukens EP, McFarlane WR: Psychoeducation as evidence based practice: considerations for practice, research and policy. Brief Treat Crisis Interv 4:205–225, 2004

Lundy BL: Father- and mother-infant face-to-face interactions: differences in mind-related comments and infant attachment? Infant Behav Dev 26:200–212, 2003

Lyons-Ruth K: Dissociation and the parent-infant dialogue: a longitudinal perspective from attachment research. J Am Psychoanal Assoc 51:883–911, 2003

Lyons-Ruth K, Jacobvitz D: Attachment disorganization: unresolved loss, relational violence and lapses in behavioral and attentional strategies, in Handbook of Attachment: Theory, Research and Clinical Applications. Edited by Cassidy J, Shaver PR. New York, Guilford, 1999, pp 520–554

Lyons-Ruth K, Yellin C, Melnick S, et al: Expanding the concept of unresolved mental states: hostile/helpless states of mind on the Adult Attachment Interview are associated with disrupted mother-infant communication and infant disorganization. Dev Psychopathol 17:1–23, 2005

Macedo S, Ober J (eds): Primates and Philosophers: How Morality Evolved. Princeton, NJ, Princeton University Press, 2006

Macfie J, Cicchetti D, Toth SL: The development of dissociation in maltreated preschool-aged children. Dev Psychopathol 13:233–254, 2001

Macfie J, McElwain NL, Houts RM, et al: Intergenerational transmission of role reversal between parent and child: dyadic and family systems internal working models. Attach Hum Dev 7:51–65, 2005

MacLean PD: The Triune Brain in Evolution: Role in Paleocerebral Functions. New York, Plenum, 1990

Main M: Metacognitive knowledge, metacognitive monitoring and singular (coherent) vs. multiple (incoherent) models of attachment, in Attachment Across the Life Cycle. Edited by Parkes CM, Stevenson-Hinde J, Marris P. London, Routledge, 1991, pp 127–159

Main M: Recent studies in attachment: overview with selected implications for clinical work, in Attachment Theory: Social, Developmental and Clinical Perspectives. Edited by Goldberg S, Muir R, Kerr J. Hillsdale, NJ, Analytic Press, 1995, pp 407–474

Main M: Attachment theory: eighteen points with suggestions for future studies, in Handbook of Attachment: Theory, Research and Clinical Applications. Edited by Cassidy J, Shaver PR. New York, Guilford, 1999, pp 845–887

Main M, Goldwyn R: Adult Attachment Scoring and Classification Systems. Berkeley, Department of Psychology, University of California Berkeley, 1994

Main M, Hesse E: Parents' unresolved traumatic experiences are related to infant disorganized attachment status: is frightened and/or frightening parental behavior the linking mechanism? in Attachment in the Preschool Years: Theory, Research and Intervention. Edited by Greenberg MT, Cicchetti D, Cummings EM. Chicago, IL, University of Chicago Press, 1990, pp 161–182

Main M, Solomon J: Procedures for identifying infants as disorganized/disoriented during the Ainsworth Strange Situation, in Attachment in the Preschool Years: Theory, Research and Intervention. Edited by Greenberg MT, Cicchetti D, Cummings EM. Chicago, IL, University of Chicago Press, 1990, pp 121–160

Main M, Kaplan N, Cassidy J: Security in infancy, childhood and adulthood: a move to the level of representation, in Growing Points of Attachment Theory and Research. Edited by Bretherton I, Waters E. Chicago, University of Chicago Press, 1985, pp 66–104

Maldonado-Duran JM (ed): Infant and Toddler Mental Health: Models of Clinical Intervention With Infants and Their Families. Washington, DC, American Psychiatric Publishing, 2002

Malle BF: How the Mind Explains Behavior: Folk Explanations, Meaning, and Social Interaction. Cambridge, MA, MIT Press, 2004

Malle BF: Three puzzles of mindreading, in Other Minds: How Humans Bridge the Divide between Self and Others. Edited by Malle BF, Hodges SD. New York, Guilford, 2005, pp 26–43

Malle BF, Hodges SD (eds): Other Minds: How Humans Bridge the Divide between Self and Others. New York, Guilford, 2005

Marks I, Lovell K, Noshirvani H, et al: Treatment of posttraumatic stress disorder by exposure and/or cognitive restructuring. Arch Gen Psychiatry 55:317–325, 1998

Mayer JD: A field guide to emotional intelligence, in Emotional Intelligence in Everyday Life. Edited by Ciarrochi J, Forgas JP, Mayer JD. Philadelphia, PA, Psychology Press, 2001, pp 3–24

Mayer JD, Salovey P, Caruso DR: Models of emotional intelligence, in Handbook of Intelligence. Edited by Sternberg R. Cambridge, UK, Cambridge University Press, 2000, pp 396–420

Mayes LC: A developmental perspective on the regulation of arousal states. Semin Perinatol 24:267–279, 2000

Mayr E: Toward a New Philosophy of Biology: Observations of an Evolutionist. Cambridge, MA, Harvard University Press, 1988

McCabe K, Houser D, Ryan L, et al: A functional imaging study of cooperation in two-person reciprocal exchange. Proc Natl Acad Sci USA 98:11832–11835, 2001

McCallum M, Piper WE: Psychological mindedness. Psychiatry 59:48–63, 1996

McEwen BS: The End of Stress as We Know It. Washington, DC, Joseph Henry Press, 2002

McGlashan TH, Grilo CM, Sanislow CA, et al: Two-year prevalence and stability of individual DSM-IV criteria for schizotypal, borderline, avoidant, and obsessive-compulsive personality disorders: toward a hybrid model of Axis II disorders. Am J Psychiatry, 162:883–889, 2005

McKinnon DF, Pies R: Affective instability as rapid cycling: theoretical and clinical implications for borderline personality and bipolar spectrum disorders. Bipolar Disord 8:1–14, 2006

McLean LM, Gallop R: Implications of childhood sexual abuse for adult borderline personality disorder and complex posttraumatic stress disorder. Am J Psychiatry 160:369–371, 2003

McNally RJ: EMDR and Mesmerism: a comparative historical analysis. J Anxiety Disord 13:225–236, 1999a

McNally RJ: On eye movements and animal magnetism: a reply to Greenwald's defense of EMDR. J Anxiety Disord 13:617–620, 1999b

Meins E: Security of Attachment and the Social Development of Cognition. East Sussex, UK, Psychology Press, 1997

Meins E, Fernyhough C, Russell J, et al: Security of attachment as a predictor of symbolic and mentalising abilities: a longitudinal study. Soc Dev 7:1–24, 1998

Meins E, Fernyhough C, Fradley E, et al: Rethinking maternal sensitivity: mothers' comments on infants' mental processes predict security of attachment at 12 months. J Child Psychol Psychiatry 42:637–648, 2001

Meins E, Fernyhough C, Wainwright R, et al: Maternal mind-mindedness and attachment security as predictors of theory of mind understanding. Child Dev 73:1715–1726, 2002

Meins E, Fernyhough C, Wainwright R, et al: Pathways to understanding mind: construct validity and predictive validity of maternal mind-mindedness. Child Dev 74:1194–1211, 2003

Meins E, Fernyhough C, Johnson F, et al: Mind-mindedness in children: individual differences in internal-state talk in middle childhood. Br J Dev Psychol 24:181–196, 2006

Meloy JR: Antisocial personality disorder, in Treatment of Psychiatric Disorders, 3rd Edition, Vol 2. Edited by Gabbard GO. Washington DC, American Psychiatric Publishing, 2001, pp 2251–2271

Meltzoff AN, Moore MK: Explaining facial imitation: theoretical model. Early Development and Parenting 6:179–192, 1997

Menninger KA: The Human Mind. New York, Knopf, 1930

Menninger WC: A Psychiatrist for a Troubled World (1947). New York, Viking, 1967

Michels R: Epilogue: Thinking about mentalization, in Handbook of Mentalization-Based Treatment. Edited by Allen JG, Fonagy P. Chichester, UK, Wiley, 2006, pp 327–333

Minzenberg MJ, Grossman R, New AS, et al: Blunted hormone responses to ip-
    sapirone are associated with trait impulsivity in personality disorder pa-
    tients. Neuropsychopharmacology 31:197–203, 2006a
Minzenberg MJ, Poole JH, Vinogradov S: Adult social attachment disturbance
    is related to childhood maltreatment and current symptoms in borderline
    personality disorder. J Nerv Ment Dis 194:341–348, 2006b
Mithen S: The Prehistory of the Mind: The Cognitive Origins of Art and Science.
    London, Thames and Hudson, 1996
Monk R: How to Read Wittgenstein. New York, Norton, 2005
Moran PM, Bifulco A, Ball C, et al: Exploring psychological abuse in childhood,
    I: developing a new interview scale. Bull Menninger Clin 66:213–240, 2002
Moran R: Authority and Estrangement: An Essay on Self-Knowledge. Prince-
    ton, NJ, Princeton University Press, 2001
Morey LC, Zanarini MC: Borderline personality: traits and disorder. J Abnorm
    Psychol 109:733–737, 2000
Morris JS, Frith CD, Perrett DI, et al: A differential neural response in the human
    amygdala to fearful and happy facial expressions. Nature 383:812–815,
    1996
Morris JS, Ohman A, Dolan RJ: Conscious and unconscious emotional learning
    in the human amygdala. Nature 393:467–470, 1998
Morton J: The origins of autism. New Sci 1694:44–47, 1989
Moses LJ: Executive functioning and children's theories of mind, in Other
    Minds: How Humans Bridge the Divide between Self and Others. Edited
    by Malle BF, Hodges SD. New York, Guilford, 2005, pp 11–25
Moses LJ, Baldwin DA, Rosicky JG, et al: Evidence for referential understanding
    in the emotions domain at twelve and eighteen months. Child Dev 72:718–
    735, 2001
Moskowitz GB: Social Cognition: Understanding Self and Others. New York,
    Guilford, 2005
Moss E, Bureau JF, Cyr C, et al: Correlates of attachment at age 3: construct va-
    lidity of the preschool attachment classification system. Dev Psychol
    40:323–334, 2004
Mundy P: Annotation: The neural basis of social impairments in autism: the role
    of the dorsal medial-frontal cortex and the anterior cingulate system.
    J Child Psychol Psychiatry 44:793–809, 2003
Mundy P, Neal R: Neural plasticity, joint attention and a transactional social-
    orienting model of autism, in International Review of Mental Retardation:
    Autism, Vol 23. Edited by Glidden LM. San Diego, CA, Academic Press,
    2001, pp 139–168
Munich RL: Integrating mentalization-based treatment and traditional psycho-
    therapy to cultivate common ground and promote agency, in Handbook of
    Mentalization-Based Treatment. Edited by Allen JG, Fonagy P. Chichester,
    UK, Wiley, 2006, pp 143–156
Murdoch I: The Sovereignty of Good. London, Routledge, 1971
Murdoch I: Metaphysics as a Guide to Morals. London, Penguin, 1992
Murdoch I: Existentialists and Mystics: Writings on Philosophy and Literature.
    New York, Penguin, 1999
Neiman S: Evil in Modern Thought: An Alternative History of Philosophy. Prin-
    ceton, NJ, Princeton University Press, 2002

Nelson TO: Consciousness and metacognition. Am Psychol 51:102–116, 1996

New AS, Buchsbaum MS, Hazlett EA, et al: Fluoxetine increases relative metabolic rate in prefrontal cortex in impulsive aggression. Psychopharmacology 176:451–458, 2004

Nishitani N, Avikainen S, Hari R: Abnormal imitation-related cortical activation sequences in Asperger's syndrome. Ann Neurol 55:558–562, 2004

Nolen-Hoeksema S: The role of rumination in depressive disorders and mixed anxiety/depressive symptoms. J Abnorm Psychol 109:504–511, 2000

Nussbaum MC: Upheavals of Thought: The Intelligence of the Emotions. Cambridge, UK, Cambridge University Press, 2001

Ogrodniczuk JS, Piper WE, Joyce AS, et al: Different perspectives of the therapeutic alliance and therapist technique in two forms of dynamically oriented psychotherapy. Can J Psychiatry 45:452–458, 2000

O'Hagan KP: Emotional and psychological abuse: problems of definition. Child Abuse Negl 19:449–461, 1995

Oliver JE: Intergenerational transmission of child abuse: rates research and clinical implications. Am J Psychiatry 150:1315–1324, 1993

Onishi KH, Baillargeon R: Do 15-month-old infants understand false beliefs? Science 308:255–258, 2005

Oppenheim D, Koren-Karie N: Mothers' insightfulness regarding their children's internal worlds: the capacity underlying secure child-mother attachment. Infant Ment Health J 23:593–605, 2002

Osofsky JD (ed): Young Children and Trauma: Intervention and Treatment. New York, Guilford, 2004

Pagano ME, Skodol AE, Stout RL, et al: Stressful life events as predictors of functioning: findings from the Collaborative Longitudinal Personality Disorders Study. Acta Psychiatr Scand 110:421–429, 2004

Paris J: Personality Disorders over Time: Precursors, Course and Outcome. Washington, DC, American Psychiatric Publishing, 2003

Paris J: Sociocultural factors in the treatment of personality disorders, in Handbook of Personality Disorders: Theory and Practice. Edited by Livesley WJ. New York, Wiley, 2004, pp 135–147

Parker AG, Boldero JM, Bell RC: Borderline personality disorder features: the role of self-discrepancies and self-complexity. Psychol Psychother 79:309–321, 2006

Parker G, Barrett E: Personality and personality disorder: current issues and directions. Psychol Med 30:1–9, 2000

Parrott WG: The functional utility of negative emotions, in The Wisdom in Feeling: Psychological Processes in Emotional Intelligence. Edited by Feldman Barrett L, Salovey P. New York, Guilford, 2002, pp 341–359

Pearlman LA, Courtois CA: Clinical applications of the attachment framework: relational treatment of complex trauma. J Trauma Stress 18:449–459, 2005

Pearlman LA, Saakvitne KW: Trauma and the Therapist: Countertransference and Vicarious Traumatization in Psychotherapy With Incest Survivors. New York, WW Norton, 1995

Pears KC, Fishler PH: Emotion understanding and theory of mind among maltreated children in foster care. Dev Psychopathol 17:47–65, 2005

Perner J: Understanding the Representational Mind. Cambridge, MA, MIT Press, 1991

Perner J, Lang B: Theory of mind and executive function: is there a developmental relationship? in Understanding Other Minds: Perspectives from Developmental Cognitive Neuroscience, 2nd Edition. Edited by Baron-Cohen S, Tager-Flusberg H, Cohen DJ. New York, Oxford University Press, 2000, pp 150–181

Perry JC, Banon E, Ianni F: Effectiveness of psychotherapy for personality disorders. Am J Psychiatry 156:1312–1321, 1999

Phillips ML, Young AW, Senior C, et al: A specific neural substrate for perceiving facial expressions. Nature 389:495–498, 1997

Phillipson H: The Object Relations Technique. London, Tavistock Press, 1955

Pine F: The interpretive moment: variations on classical themes. Bull Menninger Clin 48:54–71, 1984

Piper WE, Joyce AS, McCallum M, et al: Concentration and correspondence of transference interpretations in short-term psychotherapy. J Consult Clin Psychol 61:586–595, 1993

Pitman RK, Altman B, Greenwald E, et al: Psychiatric complications during flooding therapy for posttraumatic stress disorder. J Clin Psychiatry 52:17–20, 1991

Pliszka SR: Neuroscience for the Mental Health Clinician. New York, Guilford, 2003

Poa E: Trapped in transition: the complex young adult patient. Bull Menninger Clin 70:29–52, 2006

Posner MI, Rothbart MK: Attention, self-regulation and consciousness. Philos Trans R Soc Lond B Biol Sci 353:1915–1927, 1998

Posner MI, Rothbart MK: Developing mechanisms of self-regulation. Dev Psychopathol 12:427–441, 2000

Posner MI, Rothbart MK, Vizueta N, et al: Attentional mechanisms of borderline personality disorder. Proc Natl Acad Sci USA 99:16366–16370, 2002

Post RM, Weiss SRB, Smith M, et al: Kindling versus quenching: implications for the evolution and treatment of posttraumatic stress disorder, in Psychobiology of Posttraumatic Stress Disorder. Edited by Yehuda R, McFarlane AC. New York, New York Academy of Sciences, Volume 823, 1997, pp 285–295

Premack D, Woodruff G: Does the chimpanzee have a theory of mind? Behav Brain Sci 1:515–526, 1978

Preston SD, de Waal F: Empathy: its ultimate and proximate bases. Behav Brain Sci 25:1–20, 2002

Preston SD, Bechara A, Damasio H, et al: The neural substrates of cognitive empathy. Soc Neurosci 2:254–275, 2007

Pribram KH, Gill MM: Freud's "Project" Re-assessed: Preface to Contemporary Cognitive Theory and Neuroscience. New York, Basic Books, 1976

Putnam KM, Silk KR: Emotion dysregulation and the development of borderline personality disorder. Dev Psychopathol 17:899–925, 2005

Rachman S: Emotional processing. Behav Res Ther 18:51–60, 1980

Raine A: Features of borderline personality and violence. J Clin Psychol 49:277–281, 1993

Rapaport D: On the psychoanalytic theory of affects, in The Collected Papers of David Rapaport. Edited by Gill MM. New York, Basic Books, 1967, pp 476–512

Reddy V: Before the "third element": understanding attention to the self, in Joint Attention: Communication and Other Minds. Edited by Eilan N, Hoerl C, McCormack T, et al: New York, Oxford University Press, 2005, pp 85–109

Repacholi BM, Gopnik A: Early reasoning about desires: evidence from 14- and 18-month-olds. Dev Psychol 33:12–21, 1997

Resick PA, Schnicke MK: Cognitive processing therapy for sexual assault victims. J Consult Clin Psychol 60:748–756, 1992

Richardson RD: William James: In the Maelstrom of American Modernism. Boston, MA, Houghton Mifflin, 2006

Rizzolatti G, Craighero L: The mirror-neuron system. Annu Rev Neurosci 27:169–192, 2004

Rizzolatti G, Luppino G: The cortical motor system. Neuron 31:899–901, 2001

Rizzolatti G, Fogassi L, Gallese V: Neurophysiological mechanisms underlying the understanding and imitation of action. Nat Rev Neurosci 2:661–670, 2001

Robbins TW: Arousal systems and attentional processes. Biol Psychiatry 45:57–71, 1997

Rogers CR: Client-Centered Therapy: Its Current Practice, Implications and Theory. Boston, MA, Houghton Mifflin, 1951

Rogosch FA, Cicchetti D, Aber JL: The role of child maltreatment in early deviations in cognitive and affective processing abilities and later peer relationship problems. Dev Psychopathol 7:591–609, 1995

Rolls ET: The Brain and Emotion. New York, Oxford University Press, 1999

Rosenthal MZ, Cukrowicz KC, Cheavens JS, et al: Self-punishment as a regulation strategy in borderline personality disorder. J Pers Disord 20:232–246, 2006

Ross SM: Risk of physical abuse to children of spouse abusing parents. Child Abuse Negl 20:589–598, 1996

Roth A, Fonagy P: What Works for Whom? A Critical Review of Psychotherapy Research, 2nd Edition. New York, Guilford, 2005

Rothbaum BO: A controlled study of Eye Movement Desensitization and Reprocessing in the treatment of posttraumatic stress disorder. Bull Menninger Clin 61:317–334, 1997

Rothbaum BO, Astin MC, Marsteller F: Prolonged exposure versus Eye Movement Desensitization and Reprocessing (EMDR) for PTSD rape victims. J Trauma Stress 18:607–616, 2005

Ruffman T, Perner J, Parkin L: How parenting style affects false belief understanding. Soc Dev 8:395–411, 1999

Russ E, Heim A, Westen D: Parental bonding and personality pathology assessed by clinician report. J Pers Disord 17:522–536, 2003

Rutter M: Temperament, personality and personality disorder. Br J Psychiatry 150:443–458, 1987

Rutter M, Giller H, Hagell A: Antisocial Behaviour by Young People. Cambridge, UK, Cambridge University Press, 1998

Ryan RM: The developmental line of autonomy in the etiology, dynamics and treatment of borderline personality disorders. Dev Psychopathol 17:987–1006, 2005

Ryan RM, Deci EL: On assimilating identities to the self: a self-determination theory perspective on internalization and integrity within cultures, in Handbook of Self and Identity. Edited by Leary MR, Tangney JP. New York, Guilford, 2003, pp 253–272

Ryan RM, Kuczkowski R: The imaginary audience, self-consciousness and public individuation in adolescence. J Pers 62:219–238, 1994

Sabbagh MA, Callanan MA: Metarepresentation in action: 3-, 4-, and 5-year-old's developing theories of mind in parent-child conversations. Dev Psychol 34:491–502, 1998

Sadler LS, Slade A, Mayes LC: Minding the Baby: a mentalization-based parenting program, in Handbook of Mentalization-Based Treatment. Edited by Allen JG, Fonagy P. Chichester, UK, Wiley, 2006, pp 271–288

Sameroff AJ, McDonough SC, Rosenblum KL (eds): Treating Parent-Infant Relationship Problems: Strategies for Intervention. New York, Guilford, 2004

Samson D, Apperly IA, Kathirgamanathan U, et al: Seeing it my way: a case of selective deficit in inhibiting self-perspective. Brain 128:1102–1111, 2005

Sanislow CA, Grilo CM, Morey LC, et al: Confirmatory factor analysis of DSM-IV criteria for borderline personality disorder: findings from the Collaborative Longitudinal Personality Disorders Study. Am J Psychiatry 159:284–290, 2002

Sartre JP: The Emotions: Outline of a Theory. New York, Philosophical Library, 1948

Satpute AB, Lieberman MD: Integrating automatic and controlled processes into neurocognitive models of social cognition. Brain Res 1079:86–97, 2006

Saxe R, Kanwisher N: People thinking about people: the role of the temporo-parietal junction in "theory of mind." Neuroimage 19:1835–1842, 2003

Saxe R, Carey S, Kanwisher N: Understanding other minds: linking developmental psychology and functional neuroimaging. Annu Rev Psychol 55:87–124, 2004

Scanlon TM: What We Owe to Each Other. Cambridge, MA, Harvard University Press, 1998

Schacter DL: The seven sins of memory: insights from psychology and cognitive neuroscience. Am Psychol 54:182–203, 1999

Schlomerich A, Lamb ME, Leyendecker B, et al: Mother-infant teaching interactions and attachment security in Euro-American and Central-American immigrant families. Infant Behav Dev 20:165–174, 1997

Schmahl CG, Vermetten E, Elzinga BM, et al: Magnetic resonance imaging of hippocampal and amygdala volume in women with childhood abuse and borderline personality disorder. Psychiatr Res 122:193–198, 2003

Schmideberg M: The treatment of psychopathic and borderline patients. Am J Psychother 1:45–71, 1947

Schnell K, Dietrich T, Schnitker R, et al: Processing of autobiographical memory retrieval cues in borderline personality disorder. J Affect Disord 97:253–259, 2006

Schore AN: Effects of a secure attachment relationship on right brain development, affect regulation and infant mental health. Infant Ment Health J 22:7–66, 2001

Scott JP: The emotional basis of attachment and separation, in Attachment and the Therapeutic Processes: Essays in Honor of Otto Allen Will, Jr, MD. Edited by Sacksteder JL, Schwartz DP, Akabane Y. Madison, CT, International Universities Press, 1987, pp 43–62

Segal ZV, Gemar M, Williams S: Differential cognitive response to a mood challenge following successful cognitive therapy or pharmacotherapy for depression. J Abnorm Psychol 108:3–10, 1999

Segal ZV, Williams JMG, Teasdale JD: Mindfulness-Based Cognitive Therapy for Depression: A New Approach to Preventing Relapse. New York, Guilford, 2002

Seidler GH, Wagner FE: Comparing the efficacy of EMDR and trauma-focused cognitive-behavioral therapy in the treatment of PTSD: a meta-analytic study. Psychol Med 36:1515–1522, 2006

Semerari A, Carcione A, Dimaggio G, et al: How to evaluate metacognitive functioning in psychotherapy? The Metacognition Assessment Scale and its applications. Clin Psychol Psychother 10:238–261, 2003

Shapiro F: Efficacy of Eye Movement Desensitization procedure in the treatment of traumatic memories. J Trauma Stress 2:199–223, 1989

Shapiro F: Eye Movement Desensitization and Reprocessing: Basic Principles, Protocols and Procedures. New York, Guilford, 1995

Sharp C: Mentalizing problems in childhood disorders, in Handbook of Mentalization-Based Treatment. Edited by Allen JG, Fonagy P. Chichester, UK, Wiley, 2006, pp 101–121

Sharp C, Fonagy P, Goodyer IM: Imagining your child's mind: psychosocial adjustment and mothers' ability to predict their children's attributional states. Br J Dev Psychol 24:197–214, 2006

Sharp C, Croudace TJ, Goodyer IM: Biased mentalizing in children aged 7–11: latent class confirmation of response styles to social scenarios and associations with psychopathology. Soc Dev 16:181–202, 2007

Shaw M: The Object Relations Technique: Assessing the Individual. Manhasset, NY, ORT Institute, 2002

Shea MT, Stout RL, Yen S, et al: Associations in the course of personality disorders and Axis I disorders over time. J Abnorm Psychol 113:499–508, 2004

Siegel DJ: The Developing Mind: Toward a Neurobiology of Interpersonal Experience. New York, Guilford, 1999

Siever LJ, Torgersen S, Gunderson JG, et al: The borderline diagnosis III: identifying endophenotypes for genetic studies. Biol Psychiatry 51:964–968, 2002

Silk KR, Lee S, Hill EM, et al: Borderline personality disorder symptoms and severity of sexual abuse. Am J Psychiatry 152:1059–1064, 1995

Silverman RC, Lieberman AF: Negative maternal attributions, projective identification and the intergenerational transmission of violent relational patterns. Psychoanalytic Dialogues 9:161–186, 1999

Singer T, Seymour B, O'Doherty J, et al: Empathy for pain involves the affective but not sensory components of pain. Science 303:1157–1162, 2004

Singer T, Seymour B, O'Doherty J, et al: Empathic neural responses are modulated by the perceived fairness of others. Nature 439:466–469, 2006

Skodol AE, Siever LJ, Livesley WJ, et al: The borderline diagnosis, II: biology, genetics and clinical course. Biol Psychiatry 51:951–963, 2002

Skodol AE, Gunderson JG, Shea MT, et al: The Collaborative Longitudinal Personality Disorders Study (CLPS): overview and implications. J Pers Disord 19:487–504, 2006

Slade A: Keeping the baby in mind: a critical factor in perinatal mental health. Zero to Three, June/July, 10–16, 2002

Slade A: Parental reflective functioning: an introduction. Attach Hum Dev 7:269–281, 2005

Slade A: Reflective parenting program: theory and development. Psychoanalytic Inquiry 26:640–657, 2006

Slade A: Working with parents in child psychotherapy: engaging the reflective function, in Reflecting on the History of Psychoanalysis: Mentalization, Internalization, and Representation. Edited by Jurist E, Slade A, Bergner S. New York, Other Press (in press)

Slade A, Sadler LS, Currier J, et al: Minding the Baby: A Manual. New Haven, CT, Yale Child Study Center, 2004

Slade A, Grienenberger J, Bernbach E, et al: Maternal reflective functioning, attachment and the transmission gap: a preliminary study. Attach Hum Dev 7:283–298, 2005

Slomkowski C, Dunn J: Young children's understanding of other people's beliefs and feelings and their connected communication with friends. Dev Psychol 32:442–447, 1996

Smith JD, Shields WE, Washburn DA: The comparative psychology of uncertainty monitoring and metacognition. Behav Brain Sci 26:317–373, 2003

Smith M, Walden T: Understanding feelings and coping with emotional situations: a comparison of maltreated and nonmaltreated preschoolers. Soc Dev 8:93–116, 1999

Sodian B, Taylor C, Harris PL, et al: Early deception and the child's theory of mind: false trails and genuine markers. Child Dev 62:468–483, 1992

Soloff PH, Kelly TM, Strotmeyer SJ, et al: Impulsivity, gender and response to fenfluramine challenge in borderline personality disorder. Psychiatr Res 119:11–24, 2003a

Soloff PH, Meltzer CC, Becker C, et al: Impulsivity and prefrontal hypometabolism in borderline personality disorder. Psychiatr Res 123:153–163, 2003b

Solomon J, George C, Dejong A: Children classified as controlling at age six: evidence of disorganized representational strategies and aggression at home and at school. Dev Psychopathol 7:447–463, 1995

Solomon RC: Emotions, thoughts and feelings: emotions as engagements with the world, in Thinking about Feeling: Contemporary Philosophers on Emotions. Edited by Solomon RC. New York, Oxford University Press, 2004, pp 76–88

Solomon RC: True to Our Feelings: What Our Emotions are Really Telling Us. New York, Oxford University Press, 2007

Sperber D, Wilson D: Pragmatics, modularity and mind-reading. Mind and Language 17:3–23, 2002

Sroufe A: Emotional Development: The Organization of Emotional Life in the Early Years. New York, Cambridge University Press, 1996

Sroufe A, Egeland B, Carlson EB, et al: The Development of the Person: The Minnesota Study of Risk and Adaptation from Birth to Adulthood. New York, Guilford, 2005

Steele H, Steele M, Fonagy P: Associations among attachment classifications of mothers, fathers and their infants. Child Dev 67:541–555, 1996

Stein H: Does mentalizing promote resilience? in Handbook of Mentalization-Based Treatment. Edited by Allen JG, Fonagy P. Chichester, UK, Wiley, 2006, pp 305–326

Stein H, Allen D, Allen JG, et al: Supplementary Manual for Scoring Bifulco's Childhood Experiences of Care and Abuse Interview (M-CECA): Version 2.0. Technical Report No 00–0024. Topeka, KS, The Menninger Clinic Research Department, 2000

Stern DN: The Interpersonal World of the Infant: A View From Psychoanalysis and Developmental Psychology. New York, Basic Books, 1985

Stern DN: The Present Moment in Psychotherapy and Everyday Life. New York, WW Norton, 2004

Stern DN, Sander LW, Nahum JP, et al: Non-interpretive mechanisms in psychoanalytic therapy: the "something more" than interpretation. Int J Psychoanal 79:903–921, 1998

Stone MH: The Fate of Borderline Patients: Successful Outcome and Psychiatric Practice. New York, Guilford, 1990

Stone VE: The role of the frontal lobes and the amygdala in theory of mind, in Understanding Other Minds: Perspectives from Developmental Cognitive Neuroscience, 2nd Edition. Edited by Baron-Cohen S, Tager-Flusberg H, Cohen DJ. New York, Oxford University Press, 2000, pp 253–273

Strenger C: Between Hermeneutics and Science: An Essay on the Epistemology of Psychoanalysis. Madison, CT, International Universities Press, 1991

Strentz T: The Stockholm Syndrome: Law enforcement policy and hostage behavior, in Victims of Terrorism. Edited by Ochberg FM, Soskis DA. Boulder, CO, Westview Press, 1982, pp 149–163

Stuart J, Westen D, Lohr NE, et al: Object relations in borderlines, depressives and normals: an examination of human responses on the Rorschach. J Pers Assess 55:296–318, 1990

Stueber KR: Rediscovering Empathy: Agency, Folk Psychology, and the Human Sciences. Cambridge, MA, MIT Press, 2006

Tager-Flusberg H: Language and understanding minds: connections in autism, in Understanding Other Minds: Perspectives from Developmental Cognitive Neuroscience, 2nd Edition. Edited by Baron-Cohen S, Tager-Flusberg H, Cohen DJ. New York, Oxford University Press, 2000, pp 124–149

Taliaferro C: Evidence and Faith: Philosophy and Religion Since the Seventeenth Century. Cambridge, UK, Cambridge University Press, 2005

Target M: Outcome research on the psychosocial treatment of personality disorders. Bull Menninger Clin 62:215–230, 1998

Target M, Fonagy P: Playing with reality, II: the development of psychic reality from a theoretical perspective. Int J Psychoanal 77:459–479, 1996

Tarrier N, Pilgrim H, Sommerfield C, et al: A randomized trial of cognitive therapy and imaginal exposure in treatment of chronic posttraumatic stress disorder. J Consult Clin Psychol 67:13–18, 1999

Taylor GJ, Bagby RM: New trends in alexithymia research. Psychother Psychosom 73:68–77, 2004

Taylor M, Carlson SM: The relation between individual differences in fantasy and theory of mind. Child Dev 68:436–455, 1997

Taylor S, Thordarson DS, Maxfield L, et al: Comparative efficacy, speed and adverse effects of three PTSD treatments: exposure therapy, EMDR and relaxation training. J Consult Clin Psychol 71:330–338, 2003

Tomasello M: The Cultural Origins of Human Cognition. Cambridge, MA, Harvard University Press, 1999

Tomasello M, Call J: Primate Cognition. New York, Oxford University Press, 1997

Tomlin D, Kayali MA, King-Casas B, et al: Agent-specific responses in the cingulate cortex during economic exchanges. Science 312:1047–1050, 2006

Torgersen S, Lygren S, Oien PA, et al: A twin study of personality disorders. Compr Psychiatry 41:416–425, 2000

Toth SL, Cicchetti D, Macfie J, et al: Narrative representations of caregivers and self in maltreated pre-schoolers. Attach Hum Dev 2:271–305, 2000

Twemlow SW, Fonagy P: The prevalence of teachers who bully students in schools with differing levels of behavioral problems. Am J Psychiatry 162:2387–2389, 2005

Twemlow SW, Fonagy P: Transforming violent social systems into non-violent mentalizing systems: an experiment in schools, in Handbook of Mentalization-Based Treatment. Edited by Allen JG, Fonagy P. Chichester, UK, Wiley, 2006, pp 289–306

Twemlow SW, Sacco FC, Williams P: A clinical and interactionist perspective on the bully-victim-bystander relationship. Bull Menninger Clin 60:296–313, 1996

Twemlow SW, Fonagy P, Sacco FC: The role of the bystander in the social architecture of bullying and violence in schools and communities. Ann NY Acad Sci 1036:215–232, 2004

Twemlow SW, Fonagy P, Sacco FC: A developmental approach to mentalizing communities, I: a model for social change. Bull Menninger Clin 69:265–281, 2005a

Twemlow SW, Fonagy P, Sacco FC: A developmental approach to mentalizing communities, II: the Peaceful Schools experiment. Bull Menninger Clin 69:282–304, 2005b

Twemlow SW, Fonagy P, Sacco FC, et al: Teachers who bully students: a hidden trauma. Int J Soc Psychiatry 52:187–198, 2006

Tyrer P, Bateman AW: Drug treatments for personality disorders. Adv Psychiatr Treat 10:389–398, 2004

Umilta MA, Kohler E, Gallese V, et al: I know what you are doing: a neurophysiological study. Neuron 31:155–165, 2001

Ursano RJ, Grieger TA, McCarroll JE: Prevention of posttraumatic stress: consultation training and early treatment, in Traumatic Stress: The Effects of Overwhelming Experience on Mind, Body and Society. Edited by van der Kolk BA, McFarlane AC, Weisaeth L. New York, Guilford, 1996, pp 441–462

Van Boven L, Loewenstein G: Empathy gaps in emotional perspective taking, in Other Minds: How Humans Bridge the Divide between Self and Others. Edited by Malle BF, Hodges SD. New York, Guilford, 2005, pp 284–297

van der Kolk BA: The compulsion to repeat the trauma: reenactment, revictimization and masochism. Psychiatr Clin North Am 12:389–411, 1989

van der Kolk BA: The body keeps the score: memory and the evolving psychobiology of posttraumatic stress. Harv Rev Psychiatry 1:253–265, 1994 van der Kolk BA, Perry JC, Herman JL: Childhood origins of self-destructive behavior. Am J Psychiatry 148:1666–1671, 1991

van der Kolk BA, McFarlane AC, van der Hart O: A general approach to treatment of posttraumatic stress disorder, in Traumatic Stress: The Effects of Overwhelming Experience on Mind, Body and Society. Edited by van der Kolk BA, McFarlane AC, Weisaeth L. New York, Guilford, 1996, pp 417–440

van IJzendoorn MH: Adult attachment representations, parental responsiveness and infant attachment: a meta-analysis of the predictive validity of the Adult Attachment Interview. Psychol Bull 117:387–403, 1995

van IJzendoorn MH, Bakermans-Kranenburg MJ: Intergenerational transmission of attachment: a move to the contextual level, in Attachment and Psychopathology. Edited by Atkinson L, Zucker KJ. New York, Guilford, 1997, pp 135–170

van IJzendoorn MH, van Vliet-Visser S: The relationship between quality of attachment in infancy and IQ in kindergarten. J Genet Psychol 149:23–28, 1988

van IJzendoorn MH, Schuengel C, Bakermans-Kranenburg MJ: Disorganized attachment in early childhood: meta-analysis of precursors, concomitants and sequelae. Dev Psychopathol 11:225–249, 1999

Vinden PG: Parenting attitudes and children's understanding of mind: a comparison of Korean American and Anglo-American families. Cogn Dev 16:793–809, 2001

Volkmar FR, Lord C, Bailey A, et al: Autism and pervasive developmental disorders. J Child Psychol Psychiatry 45:135–170, 2004

Vollm BA, Taylor ANW, Richardson P, et al: Neuronal correlates of theory of mind and empathy: a functional magnetic resonance imaging study in a nonverbal task. Neuroimage 29:90–98, 2006

Vygotsky LS: Mind in Society: The Development of Higher Psychological Processes. Cambridge, MA, Harvard University Press, 1978

Walker LE: The Battered Woman. New York, Harper and Row, 1979

Ward MJ, Carlson EA: Associations among adult attachment representations, maternal sensitivity and infant-mother attachment in a sample of adolescent mothers. Child Dev 66:69–79, 1995

Waters E, Merrick SK, Trebous D, et al: Attachment security from infancy to early adulthood. Child Dev 71:684–689, 2000

Wegner DM: Ironic processes of mental control. Psychol Rev 101:34–52, 1994

Weil S: Human personality (1943), in Simone Weil: An Anthology. Edited by Miles S. New York, Grove Press, 1986, pp 49–78

Weinfield NS, Sroufe A, Egeland B: Attachment from infancy to early adulthood in a high risk sample: continuity, discontinuity, and their correlates. Child Dev 71:695–702, 2000

Weinfield NS, Whaley GJ, Egeland B: Continuity, discontinuity and coherence in attachment from infancy to late adolescence: sequelae of organization and disorganization. Attach Hum Dev 6:73–97, 2004

Weiss M, Zelkowitz P, Feldman RB, et al: Psychopathology in offspring of mothers with borderline personality disorder: a pilot study. Can J Psychiatry 41:285–290, 1996

Weissman MM, Markowitz JC, Klerman GL: Comprehensive Guide to Interpersonal Psychotherapy. New York, Basic Books, 2000

Wellman HM, Lagattuta KH: Developing understandings of mind, in Understanding Other Minds: Perspectives from Developmental Cognitive Neuroscience, 2nd Edition. Edited by Baron-Cohen S, Tager-Flusberg H, Cohen DJ. New York, Oxford University Press, 2000, pp 21–49

Wells A: Emotional Disorders and Metacognition: Innovative Cognitive Therapy. Chichester, UK, Wiley, 2000

Wells A, King P: Metacognitive therapy for generalized anxiety disorder: an open trial. J Behav Ther Exp Psychiatry 37:206–212, 2006

Wertsch JV: Mind as Action. New York, Oxford University Press, 1998

Westen D, Lohr NE, Silk KR, et al: Object relations and social cognition in borderlines, major depressives and normals: a TAT analysis. Psychol Assess 2:355–364, 1990a

Westen D, Ludolph P, Lerner H, et al: Object relations in borderline adolescents. J Am Acad Child Adolesc Psychiatry 29:338–348, 1990b

Whalen PJ, Rauch SL, Etcoff NL, et al: Masked presentations of emotional facial expressions modulate amygdala activity without explicit knowledge. J Neurosci 18:411–418, 1998

White HR, Bates ME, Buyske S: Adolescence-limited versus persistent delinquency: extending Moffitt's hypothesis into adulthood. J Abnorm Psychol 110:600–609, 2001

Wicker B, Keysers C, Plailly J, et al: Both of us disgusted in my insula: the common neural basis of seeing and feeling disgust. Neuron 40:655–664, 2003

Widom CS: Posttraumatic stress disorder in abused and neglected children grown up. Am J Psychiatry 156:1223–1229, 1999

Widom CS, Morris S: Accuracy of adult recollections of childhood victimization, part 2: childhood sexual abuse. Psychol Assess 9:34–46, 1997

Widom CS, Shepard RL: Accuracy of adult recollections of childhood victimization, part 1: childhood physical abuse. Psychol Assess 8:412–421, 1996

Wilkinson-Ryan T, Westen D: Identity disturbance in borderline personality disorder: an empirical investigation. Am J Psychiatry 157:528–541, 2000

Williams JHG, Whiten A, Suddendorf T, et al: Imitation, mirror neurons and autism. Neurosci Biobehav Rev 25:287–295, 2001

Williams L, Fonagy P, Target M, et al: Training psychiatry residents in mentalization-based therapy, in Handbook of Mentalization-Based Treatment. Edited by Allen JG, Fonagy P. Chichester, UK, Wiley, 2006, pp 223–231

Williams LM: Recovered memories of abuse in women with documented child sexual victimization. J Trauma Stress 8:649–673, 1995

Wilson SA, Becker LA, Tinker RH: Eye Movement Desensitization and Reprocessing (EMDR) treatment for psychologically traumatized individuals. J Consult Clin Psychol 63:928–937, 1995

Wilson SA, Becker LA, Tinker RH: Fifteen-month follow-up of Eye Movement Desensitization and Reprocessing (EMDR) treatment for posttraumatic stress disorder and psychological trauma. J Consult Clin Psychol 65:1047–1056, 1997

Wilson SM, Saygun AP, Sereno MI, et al: Listening to speech activates motor areas involved in speech production. Nat Neurosci 7:701–702, 2004

Wimmer H, Perner J: Beliefs about beliefs: representation and constraining function of wrong beliefs in young children's understanding of deception. Cognition 13:103–128, 1983

Winnicott DW: Playing and Reality. London, Routledge, 1971

Wittgenstein L: Philosophical Investigations (1953). Malden, MA, Blackwell, 2001

Wolock I, Horowitz B: Child maltreatment as a social problem: the neglect of neglect. Am J Orthopsychiatry 54:530–542, 1984

Yen S, Shea MT, Battle CL, et al: Traumatic exposure and posttraumatic stress disorder in borderline, schizotypal, avoidant and obsessive-compulsive personality disorders: findings from the Collaborative Longitudinal Personality Disorders Study. J Nerv Ment Dis 190:510–518, 2002

Yen S, Shea MT, Pagano ME, et al: Axis I and Axis II disorders as predictors of prospective suicide attempts: findings from the Collaborative Longitudinal Personality Disorders Study. J Abnorm Psychol 112:375–381, 2003

Young JE, Klosko JS, Weishaar ME: Schema Therapy: A Practitioner's Guide. New York, Guilford, 2003

Yudofsky SC: Fatal Flaws: Navigating Destructive Relationships With People With Disorders of Personality and Character. Washington DC, American Psychiatric Publishing, 2005

Zahn-Waxler C, Radke-Yarrow M, Wagner E, et al: Development of concern for others. Dev Psychol 28:126–136, 1992

Zanarini MC (ed): Role of Sexual Abuse in the Etiology of Borderline Personality Disorder. Washington DC, American Psychiatric Press, 1997

Zanarini MC, Gunderson JG, Frankenberg FR: Discriminating borderline personality disorder from other Axis II disorders. Am J Psychiatry 147:161–167, 1990

Zanarini MC, Williams AA, Lewis RE, et al: Reported pathological childhood experiences associated with the development of borderline personality disorder. Am J Psychiatry 154:1101–1106, 1997

Zanarini MC, Frankenburg FR, DeLuca CJ: The pain of being borderline: dysphoric states specific to borderline personality disorder. Harv Rev Psychiatry 6:201–207, 1998

Zanarini MC, Frankenberg FR, Hennen J, et al: The longitudinal course of borderline psychopathology: 6-year prospective follow-up of the phenomenology of borderline personality disorder. Am J Psychiatry 160:274–283, 2003

Zanarini MC, Frankenberg FR, Hennen J, et al: Axis I comorbidity in patients with borderline personality disorder: 6-year follow-up and prediction of time to remission. Am J Psychiatry 161:2108–2114, 2004

Zanarini MC, Frankenberg FR, Hennen J, et al: The McLean Study of Adult Development (MSAD): overview and implications of the first six years of prospective follow-up. J Pers Disord 19:505–523, 2006

Zittel-Conklin C, Westen D: Borderline personality disorder in clinical practice. Am J Psychiatry 162:867–875, 2005

Zweig-Frank H, Paris J: Parents' emotional neglect and overprotection according to the recollections of patients with borderline personality disorder. Am J Psychiatry 148:648–651, 1991

Recommended Reading

Allen JG: Traumatic Relationships and Serious Mental Disorders. Chichester, UK, Wiley, 2001

Allen JG: Coping With Trauma: Hope Through Understanding. Washington, DC, American Psychiatric Publishing, 2005

Allen JG, Fonagy P (eds): Handbook of Mentalization-Based Treatment. Chichester, UK, Wiley, 2006

Allen JG, Gergely G (eds): Special Issue: Cognitive and Interactional Foundations of Attachment. Bull Menninger Clin 65(3), 2001

Allen JG, Munich RL (eds): Special Issue: Clinical Implications of Attachment and Mentalization: Efforts to Preserve the Mind in Contemporary Treatment, Parts I and II. Bull Menninger Clin 67(3, 4), 2003

Baron-Cohen S: Mindblindness: An Essay on Autism and Theory of Mind. Cambridge, MA, MIT Press, 1995

Baron-Cohen S, Tager-Flusberg H, Cohen DJ (eds): Understanding Other Minds: Perspectives on Developmental Cognitive Neuroscience, 2nd Edition. New York, Oxford University Press, 2000

Bateman A, Fonagy P: Psychotherapy for Borderline Personality Disorder: Mentalization-Based Treatment. New York, Oxford University Press, 2004

Bateman A, Fonagy P: Mentalization-Based Treatment for Borderline Personality Disorder: A Practical Guide. New York, Oxford University Press, 2006

Dimaggio G, Semerari A, Carcione A, et al: Psychotherapy of Personality Disorders: Metacognition, States of Mind and Interpersonal Cycles. New York, Routledge, 2007

Elan N, Hoerl C, McCormack T, Roessler J (eds): Joint Attention: Communication and Other Minds. New York, Oxford University Press, 2005

Fonagy P: Attachment Theory and Psychoanalysis. New York, Other Press, 2001

Fonagy P, Gergely G, Jurist EL, Target M: Affect Regulation, Mentalization, and the Development of the Self. New York, Other Press, 2002

Goldman AI: Simulating Minds: The Philosophy, Psychology, and Neuroscience of Mindreading. New York, Oxford University Press, 2006

Hobson P: The Cradle of Thought: Exploring the Origins of Thinking. New York, Oxford University Press, 2002

Malle BF: How the Mind Explains Behavior: Folk Explanations, Meaning, and Social Interaction. Cambridge, MA, MIT Press, 2004

Malle BF, Hodges SD (eds): Other Minds: How Humans Bridge the Divide Between Self and Others. New York, Guilford, 2005

Perner J: Understanding the Representational Mind. Cambridge, MA, MIT Press, 1991

Stueber KR: Rediscovering Empathy: Agency, Folk Psychology, and the Human Sciences. Cambridge, MA, MIT Press, 2006

Tomasello M: The Cultural Origins of Human Cognition. Cambridge, MA, Harvard University Press, 1999

Index

*Page numbers printed in **boldface** type refer to tables or figures.*